D0153221

# DIAGNOSIS
# AND EVALUATION
# IN SPEECH PATHOLOGY

## Third Edition

**Lon L. Emerick**
*Northern Michigan University—Marquette*

**William O. Haynes**
*Auburn University—Alabama*

PRENTICE-HALL, INC., Englewood Cliffs, New Jersey 07632

*Library of Congress Cataloging-in-Publication Data*

Emerick, Lon L.
  Diagnosis and evaluation in speech pathology.

  Includes bibliographies and index.
  1. Speech, Disorders of—Diagnosis.  2. Speech,
Disorders of—Case Studies.  I. Haynes, William O.
II. Title.  [DNLM: 1. Speech Disorders—diagnosis.
WM 475 E52d]
RC423.E58  1986      616.85′5′075      85-12390
ISBN 0-13-208646-8

RC423
.H3826
1986x

© 1973, 1979, 1986 by Prentice-Hall, Inc., Englewood Cliffs, New Jersey 07632

All rights reserved. No part of this book may be
reproduced, in any form or by any means,
without permission in writing from the publisher.

Printed in the United States of America

10  9  8  7  6  5  4  3  2  1

ISBN 0-13-208646-8 01

Prentice-Hall International (UK) Limited, *London*
Prentice-Hall of Australia Pty. Limited, *Sydney*
Prentice-Hall Canada, Inc., *Toronto*
Prentice-Hall Hispanoamericana, S.A., *Mexico*
Prentice-Hall of India Private Limited, *New Delhi*
Prentice-Hall of Japan, Inc., *Tokyo*
Prentice Hall of Southeast Asia Pte. Ltd., *Singapore*
Editora Prentice-Hall do Brasil, Ltda., *Rio de Janeiro*
Whitehall Books Limited, *Wellington, New Zealand*

# CONTENTS

OCT 2 2 1999

**CHAPTER SIX**
## STUTTERING                                                                    189

**CHAPTER SEVEN**
## THE ASSESSMENT OF APHASIA IN ADULTS                                           245

**CHAPTER EIGHT**
## VOICE DISORDERS                                                               287

**CHAPTER NINE**
**THE DIAGNOSTIC REPORT**                                                318

**APPENDIX A**
**CHILD LANGUAGE ASSESSMENT INTERVIEW PROTOCOL**                          334

**APPENDIX B**
**CODING SHEET FOR EARLY MULTIWORD ANALYSIS**                             338

**APPENDIX C**
**SUMMARY SHEET FOR EARLY MULTIWORD ANALYSIS**                            339

**APPENDIX D**
**DATA CONSOLIDATION FOR CHILD LANGUAGE EVALUATION**                      340

**NAME INDEX**                                                           344

**SUBJECT INDEX**                                                        347

# PREFACE

With this third edition we invite a new group of students to look over the shoulders of speech clinicians as they go about their appointed diagnostic rounds. We were pleased that so many readers of the prior editions found in them the imprint of clinical relevance, that they too shared our primary concern with *people,* not speech defects or complex analytical models of communication.

We regret that we could not find a better way to use gender pronouns than alternating "he" and "she." The form s/he was tried, but it interfered with the flow of the message. Perhaps the time has come for the creation of a new pronoun.

As working clinicians and teachers, we have gained much from the novel insights, open enthusiasm, and challenging questions of our clients and students—and it is to them that this book is dedicated.

L.L.E.
W.O.H.

# CHAPTER ONE
# INTRODUCTION

Speech pathology is a wonderfully diverse profession that requires a practitioner to possess a wide range of skills, knowledge, and personal characteristics. A speech clinician[1] works as a case selector, case evaluator, diagnostician, interviewer, parent counselor, teacher, coordinator, record keeper, researcher, and student. Because the boundaries between these various duties are not clearly defined, and because the clinician must move continuously from one area to another, it is inevitable that no one person can expect to be equally competent in all areas. The ultimate goal is to maximize one's strengths in all aspects to provide the best possible service to the communicatively handicapped.

Diagnosis is one of the most comprehensive and difficult tasks of the speech clinician. An evaluation of a client requires a synthesis of the entire field: knowledge of norms and testing techniques, skills in observation, an ability to relate effectively and empathically, and a great deal of creative intuition. Furthermore, because speech is a function of the entire person, the diagnostician must try to scrutinize all aspects of behavior. She must remember that she is not simply working with speech sounds or the sounds of speech but rather with changing people in a changing environment. The experienced diagnostician does not look at objective scores of articulatory skill, point scales of vocal quality disorders, or language age as ends in themselves but rather as aspects of an individual's communication ability—

---

[1] While recognizing that it is currently popular to use the designation speech-language clinician, we shall refer to the practitioner as speech clinician or speech pathologist in this text.

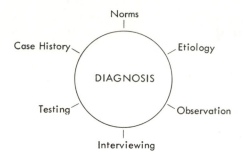

**FIGURE 1.1**
Diagnosis synthesizes knowledge and skills.

*we diagnose communicators, not communication.* That revelation is a major factor in the transition from technician to professional.

Because our diagnostic tools are crude, being largely in the experimental stages, and because communication disorders are by nature complex and perplexing, many of our diagnostic undertakings are incomplete and ambiguous. The lack of absolute and definitive answers to the various questions of diagnosis is often frustrating and demoralizing to the clinician. The ambiguous findings that sometimes culminate a diagnostic evaluation must be dealt with in a fashion that perpetuates the evaluative undertaking rather than closes the door on further probing. Diagnosis is a continuous and open-ended venture that results in answers or partial answers that themselves are open to revision with added information.

## DIAGNOSIS DEFINED

The term *diagnosis* in the original Greek means to understand thoroughly.[2] The process of understanding—observing, measuring, describing, distinguishing—we shall refer to as *evaluation*. There are essentially three interrelated and overlapping aspects to diagnosis:

1.  Determining the reality of the problem
2.  Determining the etiology of the problem
3.  Providing clinical focus

### Diagnosis to Determine the Reality of the Problem

The first task of diagnosis is to determine whether the presenting speech pattern does indeed constitute a handicap.[3] Before this is possible, however, it is necessary to have a clear idea of what constitutes a speech disorder. Van Riper's definition of a speech disorder is widely quoted: "Speech is abnormal when it deviates so far from the speech of other people that it calls attention to itself, inter-

---

[2] The prefix *dia-* means "through" or "between"; *gnosis* translates as "to know."

[3] Schultz (1972) has developed a model of clinical decision making. Compare Schultz's "decision axis" concept with the present discussion.

feres with communication, or causes the speaker or his listeners to be distressed" (Van Riper and Emerick, 1984: 34). We propose further that there are three essential aspects of the communicative act that are important in defining speech: the acoustic characteristics of the individual's speech signal; the influence of the acoustic signal on the intelligibility of the message; and, finally, the handicapping condition that results from the first two aspects. A communication *difference* involves signal alterations, a communication *disturbance* involves a breakdown of message transmission, and a communication *disorder* involves a handicapping condition. The first relates to speech signals, the second to information transmission, and the third to people.

*The speech signal.* We can quantify the physical characteristics of the speech signal through recording, measurement, and observation. Speech spectographs, pitch meters, and other instruments are available to help the diagnostician obtain an objective measure of the acoustic nature of the individual's speech. But these data are of limited value unless it can be determined what *difference* a particular speech difference makes. In other words, we must scrutinize the physical characteristics of the speech signal and judge its *quality*.

The state of the art has not progressed to where we can simply take the quantified data, compare them with established numerical norms, and determine the correctness of the speech sample. Unfortunately, there is no registered standard /s/ phone; thus, each diagnostician must develop his own frame of reference. The physician is able to scrutinize data from a laboratory test and make an immediate diagnosis regarding the normalcy of an individual's blood count, but this kind of reference information is not yet available to the speech clinician. The question of whether the presenting speech difference is different enough to be of concern thus becomes a matter of human judgment. This judgment involves filtering incoming data through many synaptic junctions whose thresholds may have been worn thin by bias and experience. An inordinately critical or uncritical acoustic system is a hazard with far-reaching implications.

Each clinician must find some way to realistically judge adequate speech production. Pronovost (1966:179) asks, "Do we consider ourselves self-appointed enforcers of society's standards of speech?" Even more perplexing is the question of

**FIGURE 1.2  Components of a definition of a speech disorder.**

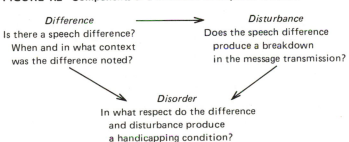

whether we should appoint ourselves *determiners* of that standard. Should we protect some absolute standard of speech production? Is that the function of our profession or the function of society? If the speech difference we hear appears to have no impact on the speaker or his environment, should the speech clinician consider it a problem and set out to correct it?

Many speech clinicians in the schools have recently begun to abandon the traditional screening process for case detection in favor of parent and teacher referral. This trend reflects an awareness that the determination of how much a difference is important in speech production is primarily made by society rather than professionals. Some states have been even more restrictive in their definition of speech handicap by mandating that clinical speech services only be provided to those children whose communicative differences have a proven detrimental effect on their educational growth. By this criterion many or all of the traditional articulation disorders and voice disorders would not qualify for clinical speech services.

Studies of the incidence of speech disorders provide a great deal of information about the researchers as well as the subjects. One has only to compare the often-quoted figure (7 to 10 percent) of the incidence of speech disorders as provided in speech pathology literature with the 0.65 percent figure that was obtained in a Public Health Service report cited by Newman (1961). Although the Public Health Service data no doubt are open to some criticism, they were obtained from a house-to-house interview study and may more accurately reflect the general population's concept of defective speech. Incidence figures are notoriously self-fulfilling prophecies; they are also reports about someone *by someone*. If you *expect* that 10 percent of all grade-school children will have speech disorders, the probability that you will find just that percentage is greatly enhanced.

Johnson (1946) has emphasized the concept of the "participants of a problem," implying that in the final analysis the diagnostician becomes a part of the defect by identifying and labeling it. The widely varying estimates of the percentage of children in the schools with speech defects underscore the point that speech disorders are sometimes born in the ear of the listener as well as in the mouth of the speaker. In his admonishing and thought-provoking article, Van Riper (1966) emphasizes the importance of the client's self-image in rehabilitative efforts. If our diagnosis fixates a self-image and perpetuates the error rather than helping to eradicate it, then our selection criteria must be broadened to include more than simply the acoustic nature of the speech. We are charged with the responsibility to prevent or reduce abnormality, not to cause it.

What constitutes normal behavior? There are several definitions available, but we will discuss only two, representing the diverging philosophies with which each clinician must contend in establishing her own concept. The first theory we shall call the concept of *cultural norms*. The assumption is that there are behaviors that society considers aberrant in terms of *group* characteristics. According to this model, each bit of behavior can be judged against a real or theoretical standard, the nature of which is independent of the individual's personal idiosyncrasies. The second theory we shall call the concept of *individual norms*. Advocates of this model assume that each individual has made his unique adjustment to life based on his own previous experiences, his physical limitations, and his environment's reactions to him. Any judgment as to the normalcy of a bit of behavior must be contingent upon individual characteristics such as age, intelligence, and experience.

Taken to the extreme, of course, the latter model would assert that each person is normal no matter what he does, since his behavior is the end product of all that plays upon his being; and to this extent the concept of individual norms loses meaning. But a case example may help to clarify and give perspective. The audiologist who examines the hearing of a seventy-five-year-old individual and obtains the "typical" presbycusic audiometric curve could make a case for the judgment that this person has "normal" hearing. According to personal norms, this is average or normal behavior for a person of seventy-five; but according to cultural norms, the individual's hearing level is below the average for the total population. Follow-up procedures would be based, then, on the practical matter of getting a more efficient communication system for the individual and also on providing counseling so that the person will understand the nature of his hearing. Therefore, both cultural and personal norms play a part in diagnostic judgments and rehabilitative programs.

A severely retarded ten-year-old with a frontal lisp may not be judged to have defective speech, whereas an eight-year-old presenting a similar speech pattern, but a different intellectual potential, may be enrolled. Such judgments have implications for case selection, and the clinician must reconcile the variances between the physical differences in the sounds involved and individual variables in conjunction with what is normal for the population as a whole. Each clinician must continually use both concepts of normalcy in his diagnostic work. Every five-year-old "lisper" who leaves the kindergarten classroom for his semiweekly speech therapy session is most probably a victim of a one-dimensional definition of normal.

Far too many clinicians view diagnosis simply as a labeling process, but the actual labeling, or categorizing, is only a small part of the total assessment process. Classification systems within our profession are poor at best, and high-level abstractions (for example, lisping) tend to emphasize the similarities within a population rather than the individual differences. The keen diagnostician looks upon classifications as communication conveniences to be viewed with suspicion; he is continually alert for "hardening of the categories." Of course, the convenience factor is important, and each clinician making a determination of the reality of the problem must be willing to label it. This must of necessity, however, follow an orderly description of the characteristics of the disorder so that it can be clear what route the diagnostician took in arriving at the final classification. A diagnosis that only describes the characteristics of the problem, without judging its type or class, is a dead end. The opposite path is also dangerous; the diagnostician who is willing to begin an evaluation by labeling the problem has reversed the orderly sequence of acquiring knowledge and often effectively closes her mind to factors that may later point away from her premature "diagnosis" (see Chapter 1 Highlight on page 18).

*Intelligibility of the message.*    The intelligibility of a speech signal relates to the degree of agreement between what the speaker intends and what the listener perceives. Many factors play a part in both the encoding and decoding processes, and the diagnostician must be capable of representing the standard for his society when listening and making judgments. The essential judgment to be made is, how well did the intentions of the speaker match the perceptions of the listener, and what are the factors that affect this? Are there attributes of the signal that distract the listener, thus altering the message? Is the signal indistinct, thus allowing only partial transmission of information? Is the signal distinct but conveying a message other than that intended by the speaker? Is the signal distinct but conveying a message (albeit the one selected by the speaker) that is inappropriate for the context?

We have, in the main, been content with clinical insight and intuitive estimates when we have judged the impact of speech differences upon intelligibility. Only a few research investigations have been concerned with this important problem (Yorkston and Beukelman, 1981). No research has clearly quantified the effect of a lateral lisp, for example, and yet each working day practicing clinicians must decide on the importance of such acoustic characteristics. What is needed is a massive study of how each type of speech disorder influences the transmission of information to the listener. The speech clinician is able to count the phoneme errors, quantify the number of repetitions per sentence, and establish a type-token ratio, but as yet he is unable to assess the intelligibility of the transmitted message with any degree of reliability.[4]

*Handicapping condition.*    The most important variable in the determination of the reality of a communication problem is the determination of whether anyone is handicapped by the signal or intelligibility differences. The diagnostician does not simply identify the error and assess its influence on the intelligibility of the message; she must also prepare a description of the person and the ways in which the symptoms shape that person's adjusting characteristics. What impact does the speech pattern have on the person's life (Emerick, 1984)?

> In the final analysis this third aspect justifies the existence of our profession. If the speech difference has no discernible impact on the child's behavior, and ultimately on his adjusting abilities and learning potential, there is little justification for concern on the part of the speech clinician. Although it is not feasible to compile a listing of all of the possible conditions under which a communication difference would become handicapping, it is generally agreed that communicative differences are considered handicapping when
>
> — the transmission and/or perception of messages is faulty
> — the person is placed at an economic disadvantage

[4]Several clinicians have attempted to devise objective measures of intelligibility. Most of the tests rely exclusively on the impact of speech sound errors on the accurate transmission of a message. A recent contribution, the *Weiss Intelligibility Test* (1983), employs the utterance of twenty-five isolated words and a contextual speech sample to assess intelligibility of children and adolescents. The work of Yorkston and Beukelman (1981) describes a technique for quantifying dysarthric speech based on single-word intelligibility.

 —the person is placed at a learning disadvantage
 —the person is placed at a social disadvantage
 —there is a negative impact upon the emotional growth of the person
 —the problem causes physical damage or endangers the health of the person

Among the three factors taken into account in determining the reality of a disorder, a variety of relationships are possible (see Figure 1.3): Condition *A* of Figure 1.3 represents a condition in which the speech signal is significantly aberrant, although intelligibility and impact on the communication are minimal; this may be the case with certain voice disorders. In condition *B* there is little signal variation and similarly negligible impact on the intelligibility, but the communicants are significantly affected by the difference.

Mrs. Norton brought her four-year-old son into our office ostensibly for evaluation of his speech. Initial testing revealed an inconsistent frontal lisp which was easily stimulable to correction. Our first inclination was to simply

**FIGURE 1.3** Possible relationships of signal distortion, intelligibility, and impact upon communicants.

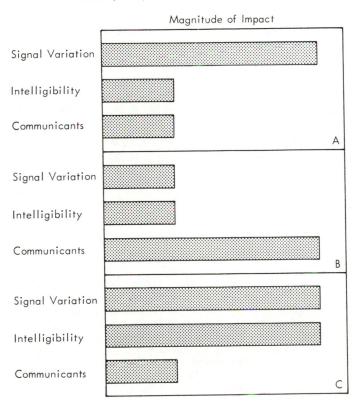

inform Mrs. Norton that her child's speech was within normal limits and conclude the session, but better judgment prevailed. It was noted earlier in the interview that Mrs. Norton was firmly convinced of the existence of the problem and considered it quite severe.

The last condition in Figure 1.3 reflects a situation that may be a bit more controversial. Some would argue that the severely retarded individual who lacks effective communication is not handicapped by this condition since the impairment is not central to her disability. The addition of communication skill, it is postulated, would not effectively alter her condition. Taking this line of thinking to its logical conclusion, it would then be possible to have an individual with significant signal differences that have a marked impact on intelligibility but that do not handicap the speaker.

Predisposing factors are generally thought to be important because of their potential link with a third agent. A classic example of predisposing factors is the higher than normal incidence of left-handedness among stutterers. The left-handedness itself is of little consequence, but the implication of basic underlying neurological differences has perplexed researchers for decades. The wary diagnostician must watch for factors that occur with high regularity in association with certain communication disorders. Such data could ultimately be instrumental in uncovering some basic information regarding the nature of the disorder.

Precipitating factors are generally no longer operating and as such may or may not be identifiable. There is a philosophical question of whether we need to search for precipitating factors if they are not still operating, and the point is well taken. Each moment, however, there is created a new set of precipitating factors that, acting as characteristics of the past, perpetuate behaviors of the present. Speech disorders generally are not static entities developed at a given point and perpetuated without modification through time; rather they are ever-changing characteristics that are constantly influenced by intrinsic and extrinsic factors. Precipitating factors are best considered as the agents that brought the disorder to its present state.

The perpetuating factors are those variables currently at work on the individual. Almost without exception, habit strength is a prime perpetuating factor in developmental speech disorders. Other factors are also crucial, however, and it is the diagnostician's task to uncover the environmental and physical factors that are reinforcing and thus perpetuating the disorder.

Mrs. Mudge was an alert, intense person with an extremely high energy level. The referring physician's report described her as "hyper," and the description was apt indeed. Although such people do not always develop vocal nodules, they certainly seem predisposed to them. Mrs. Mudge's vocal nodules had been surgically removed but were beginning to show signs of recurrence when we first saw her. In the initial interview several facts became apparent. First, it was evident that Mrs. Mudge was overwhelmed by the pressures of motherhood (five children under seven years of age) and the routine and often unfulfilling chores of the daily household. She had, over the past five years, developed a method of control over the children which could best be described as the "holler and hit" technique. Unfortunately for Mrs. Mudge's vocal folds, she resorted to too much hollering and too little hitting.

Mrs. Mudge's case illustrates the importance of all three types of etiological factors. The personality characteristics clearly predisposed her to the resulting disorder; the intrusion of children into her life precipitated the vocal disorder by raising her anxiety and greatly increasing her vocal output; and the perpetuating influence of habit strength and the continuation of the original "irritants" were currently evident.

### Diagnosis to Determine the Etiology of the Problem

"Cause" has different meanings depending on its distance from the problem. As you look at a client in a diagnostic session, you search for reasons for his presenting behaviors. In fact, many of these reasons may be buried in the past and can only be revealed by painstaking effort. In many cases, cause and effect may be layered in complex patterns. Swift's pithy quatrain describes it best:

So, naturalists observe, a flea
Hath smaller fleas that on him prey;
And these have smaller still to bite 'em;
And so proceed *ad infinitum.*

Not only must we search through the client's past experience in order to uncover events that may help us alter current behaviors but we must also guard against looking for causes in only one dimension of behavior. Johnny's brain damage, once identified, is probably not the only etiological factor, because speech is a complicated human function. Social, learning, motivational, and many other factors enter into the total process.

Classically, etiology has been defined in terms of *predisposing, precipitating,* and *perpetuating* factors. Agents that dispose or incline an individual toward communication impairment are designated as predisposing causes. Precipitating factors actually bring about the onset of the problem, whereas perpetuating variables are responsible for the persistence of the abnormality.

### Diagnosis to Provide Clinical Focus

Although it is important to know the causes of the disorder, it is substantially more important to know the *causes of the correction of the condition.* It is at this point that diagnosis and clinical management overlap. Finding the cause of the cure is an ongoing process that incorporates sound testing and evaluative procedures along with clinical management. Determining what will bring about change raises many questions, both diagnostic and clinical in nature:

What do I know about this condition?
   What are the usual etiologies?
   What are the usual effective procedures for correction?

What is the typical prognosis?
etc.
What do I know about this person?
What is the level of impact upon the person?
What are the person's strengths and weaknesses?
What do I know about other important personal variables—age, sex, environment, etc.?
How is this person like others I have worked with?
How is this person different from others I have worked with?
etc.
What do I know about my own skills in management of this person and this disorder type?
How do I effectively approach similar problems?
How do I effectively approach similar people?
What do I know about the services of other professionals available for this person?
What referrals need to be made?
What factors need to be removed, altered, or added to improve the possibility of correction?
What inhibiting environmental factors exist?
What organic factors need alteration?
What new motivating procedures could be effective?
etc.

If diagnosis is to be of utmost benefit it must be goal-oriented. Every classroom teacher has experienced the frustration of receiving a report from a school psychometrist stating that the child she referred because of behavioral problems does indeed have behavioral problems. Such a diagnosis fails to provide the crucial final link: recommendations for remedial procedures. Diagnosis is an empty exercise in test administration, data collection, and client evaluation if it fails to provide logical suggestions for treatment.

There are several major diagnostic philosophies that the speech clinician must be aware of in order to formulate her own logical and professionally comfortable personal model.

The *medical,* or *disease, model* of diagnosis appears to be based on a few solidly entrenched tenets. First, diagnosis must be completed *before* treatment. The assumption is that curative procedures are much more efficient if the etiological factors are known. Symptomatic medicine is considered tantamount to quackery. This model holds that diagnosis and treatment are two discernibly different tasks. Seldom is it possible for a physician to engage in a procedure that serves both diagnostic and therapeutic functions.

Another assumption of the medical model is that physical disturbances are generally related to organic causes. If the temperature is high, there is a structural explanation to be pursued within the soma. Identification of the site of the lesion is thus paramount in determining the cause-effect relationship. Classifications generally pertain to the site of the lesion, and it is generally assumed that the lesion is within the client. The application of this model to speech and language has been criticized because it restricts the scope of the investigation.

Medical diagnosis is generally concluded in an *absolute* manner. Hypotheses regarding etiology, nature of the problem, and prognosis are generally presented to other professionals and to the client as facts. This most useful technique serves to build confidence and may actually hasten the recovery process. Few of us would return to a physician who vacillated regarding the diagnosis of our ailment. The therapeutic value of an omniscient clinical demeanor is a lesson well learned by most physicians. Absolutism is indeed a luxury, but at times a very useful one.

There is no single *educational model* of diagnosis, but recent discussions by Ysseldyke and Salvia (1974), Bateman (1967), and others have described a variety of philosophies. Ysseldyke and Salvia describe the *ability training model* in which the teacher attempts to identify strengths and weaknesses in order to prescribe remedial approaches. Teaching is carried out using careful diagnosis and prescription with the assumption that knowledge of the cause and work on underlying skills will have a positive impact on target behaviors. Since we have not determined what particular abilities are necessary for each educational skill, much of what is currently being done in this area is experimental in nature. Englemann (1967) criticizes such approaches because they end up teaching splinter tasks that may be irrelevant to the actual educational goal. Most speech clinicians would identify the ITPA, Frostig, or perceptual motor programs with this model.

The *task analysis model* of diagnosis could logically be included as a behavioral model, but it is often presented as a separate concept. Advocates of the task analysis viewpoint stress the need to know where the child is along the ladder of skills necessary for achievement of a particular terminal behavior. The child's performance is not judged relative to norms but relative to the sequence of tasks assumed to be a part of the final product. Crucial counterparts of task analysis training are clearly presented behavioral objectives and the development of *behavioral philosophies. Task analysis teaching* and *behavioral objectives* written in clearly defined terms have enjoyed a mutually supporting growth.

Another closely related model of educational diagnosis and teaching is *data-based instruction.* The basic tenets of this contribution are that intervention procedures should be based on continuous and systematic measurement of child performance on relevant behaviors. Instructional goals are directly related to the level of performance, and the criteria for moving from one performance level to another are determined by reference to a task ladder and to child performance. Obviously, this model is directly related to the task analysis model.

The *operant,* or *behavioral, paradigm* offers several applicable concepts that speech clinicians are beginning to incorporate into their working philosophies (Sloane and MacAulay, 1968; Starkweather, 1984). Typically, the operant model disavows interest in the factors that intervene between stimulus and response, as such factors are at best only hypothetical. Probably the primary characteristic of the model is the belief that discriminative stimuli and resultant behaviors are observable, measurable, and quantifiable, and the establishment of "baseline," or presenting, behaviors is paramount to further therapeutic measures. The second major undertaking is to determine what reinforcers exist for the person. In other words, the diagnostician must determine what systematic relationship exists between behaviors and the variables that control those behaviors. Detailed examination of the subject, his environment, and his current behavioral repertoire should lead the diagnostician to some conclusion regarding the terminal behaviors desired. This task is of vital importance in operant theory but strangely has been neglected in much of the speech therapy literature. Once goal behavior has been described, it will be necessary to delineate the exact progression of steps necessary to achieve the goal. Precision recording is necessary in order for the diagnostician to guide the clinician's work toward the proper level of difficulty and appropriateness.

Although there is no single *clinical speech model* of diagnosis, elements of many of the previously mentioned models are frequently found in the literature of speech pathology. Our profession has historically had a keen interest in etiology and has based much of its remedial programs on the assumptions of the ability training model. As an example, many articulation approaches are based on diagnostic findings of poor auditory discrimination skills, on the assumption that auditory discrimination is an underlying skill that has an impact on articulation. In fact, elements of every diagnostic model are found in the working skills of most speech clinicians. Each concept makes a contribution to the diagnostic venture and each presents major pitfalls that must be avoided. For further information on models of communication as they apply to diagnosis, refer to the works of Nation and Aram (1977) and Schultz (1972).

The philosophy of diagnosis dictates the uses of diagnostic information; however, there are several widely accepted ways in which diagnosis helps direct the clinical effort. The diagnosis should identify the problem, indicate the logical entry level for clinical work, identify the etiological factors that affect the problem, identify the avenues of input and output that will best serve the individual, determine the most appropriate methods to approach the problem, establish a most logical setting and timetable for clinical work, determine the appropriate stimuli and reinforcers, and determine the level of motivation and desire for change.

## DIAGNOSIS—SCIENCE AND ART

Diagnosis demands a unique blend of science and art (Silverman, 1984). The scientific method is applicable to our work as diagnosticians, both in guiding our procedures and in focusing our attitude of operation. The scientific method directs the diagnostician to observe "all" of the available factors, formulate testable hypotheses using clearly stated and answerable questions, test those hypotheses to determine their validity, and formulate conclusions based on the tested hypotheses. The method demands rigorous adherence to standardized procedures and has as its favorable characteristics objectivity, quantifiability, and structure. The "scientific" diagnostician tends to rely on tests, test data, and other procedures that lend themselves to quantification.

As an attitude of operation the scientific method implies that the diagnostician has not predetermined his test findings and that he is not biased in seeking the proof or disproof of his hypotheses. The diagnostician sees his hypotheses as something to be tested rather than something to be defended. Many things are implied in this attitude. We have all experienced the biased clinician who finds what he expects to find in each diagnosis. The self-fulfilling prophecy is a lethal but almost universal human characteristic; it must be counterbalanced by a scientific approach to testing. The writers are familiar with one youngster who had traveled all over the country in search of a diagnostic explanation for his delay in language development that would be compatible with his parents' precepts. When we saw the child, his father brought with him a case file thick with reports from various noted authorities (the "fat folder" syndrome). Each report revealed more about the examiner than the child as it cited facts in support of a theory of etiology congruent with the diagnostician's particular specialty. Such youngsters—or diagnostic vagabonds, as we might call them—are victims of misguided but persistent parents and nonscientific diagnosticians.

The beginning student must also guard against the "recent article" syndrome to which we all fall prey upon occasion. Typically, the behavioral pattern goes something like this: You read an article that depicts a particular syndrome and explains the distinctive characteristics of a disorder; for a few weeks thereafter every child you see appears to fall into the pattern described in the publication.

Speech pathology witnessed a significant increase in the incidence of "apraxia" in children following the publication of a series of articles on the topic. The way to overcome the "recent article" syndrome, of course, is to be aware that it exists and, incidentally, to have a thorough understanding of the nature of human perception.

> In nearly all matters the human mind has a strong tendency to judge in the light of its own experience, knowledge, and prejudices rather than on the evidence presented. Thus new ideas are judged in the light of prevailing beliefs. (Beveridge, 1951: 103)

The strict adherence to fact that is demanded by the pure scientific method is often a bit confining. That, in part, may explain why we all practice the "art" of diagnosis at times. The artistic approach has several specific characteristics. The "artist" is less dependent on specific observations for the formation of hypotheses than on her casual and nonstructured scrutiny. This type of clinician is perfectly willing to disregard formal test results or standard testing procedures in favor of what appears obvious to her on the basis of her clinical expertise. The hunch, or clinical intuition, plays a significant part in such evaluations. The diagnostician will contend that facts can be approached from several directions and that she is capable of assessing the same kinds of behaviors that are measured by formal tests. Such contentions are disconcerting to the test-bound person who has come to expect that the only valid way to gain information is through standardized procedures.

It is obvious that, in the extreme, there are weaknesses in both approaches. The scientist may tend to become so dependent on his objective methods of measurement that he fails to see the client through the maze of percentile scores and age norms. The whole is greater than the sum of its parts, and every diagnostician must guard against simply measuring the isolated characteristics without getting a full picture of the individual. The client is often made to fit the test results even when circumstances clearly contraindicate such a conclusion. We recently received a report from a clinician who claimed great frustration with a particular child because "his ITPA results are not consonant with his classroom performance. He is not as low in psycholinguistic abilities as his test performance would indicate." This person believed that the child had poorer abilities than his classroom performance indicated and that there must have been something invalid about his daily behavior. Could it not be that the test results do not tell us as much as the child's everyday performance? Test data become an artifact of the child's total behavior and should be so judged, while the daily behavior may hold much more meaning for the future remedial program. Don't build altars to any testing device; every objective instrument was once only a hunch in someone's mind.

The other end of the science-art continuum is just as precarious, if not more so. The possibility of a diagnostician projecting more than a modest amount of himself into his evaluation is greater when he is less scientific in his approach. Clinical intuitions are often simply clinical biases, and it is very easy to make new evidence fit old categories. The diagnostician must find the proper admixture of each philosophy in establishing his own diagnostic procedures (Deutscher, 1983; Ringel and Trachtman and Prutting, 1984).

### The Diagnostician as a Factor

Ultimately, however, the most important diagnostic tool is the diagnostician himself. The children we assess have seldom read the test manual, and the rigid structures of the testing situation may not be compatible with the child's fluid and nonstructured style of behavior. Tests are abstractions of behavior, and as such they represent only a fraction of the child's total repertoire of responses to his environment. What better measure of an individual's behavior than that behavior itself? Thus, the diagnostician becomes an important aspect of the evaluating situation as he selects, interacts, responds, and assembles information.

What skills are necessary to develop in order to become an effective, nontest-bound diagnostician? How do you develop them? There are no easy answers to these questions. Experience in the diagnostic process is an absolute necessity, but experience in terms of number of children seen is not enough; there is little value in one diagnostic experience reduplicated 1,000 times. The diagnostician must be able to gain from new experiences, and this demands *flexibility*. The stereotyped and stagnant diagnostician learns little from increased exposure to people and new situations, but those who use their experience as a pattern to be compared against, rather than as a mold into which all new experiences must fit, will continue to grow and learn.

The diagnostician must be flexible enough within the testing situation to shift from predetermined plans to new modes of evaluation as the client presents unpredicted behaviors. The examiner who steadfastly plods through a series of tests even though a child has not interacted in any significant degree may well have lost the opportunity to gain information by other means. It is not atypical for beginning speech clinicians to panic in the face of an unexpected performance and become intransigent in their application of a series of formal tests. In this regard, continued experience in diagnosis may provide the flexibility needed to move freely to other avenues of information.

> A graduate student was recently observed attempting to administer a comprehensive language inventory to Mr. Dodds, a sixty-three-year-old aphasic. Despite the student's determined attempts to complete the formal testing, Mr. Dodds continued commenting on the test room, the diagnostician, and other subjects irrelevant to the test. His most persistent topic was his altered life circumstances and his frustrations. The diagnostic session ended with two unfulfilled participants. The student could not understand why Mr. Dodds would not cooperate and came away with none of the data he desired regarding the client's language ability. Indeed, upon later discussion it became evident that the student even failed to gain much insight into the patient's current concerns because he worried only about completing predetermined procedures. Mr. Dodds, on the other hand, left the session feeling that the diagnostician lacked any understanding of his problem, thereby adding to his feelings of futility.

Practicing clinicians often eagerly accept new and novel techniques as they become available. We have noted a generation gap within the field of speech pathology in the past few years. As the profession moves into new, uncharted areas of concern, many new materials, tests, and techniques have become available. The old guard tends to scoff at something new, and the young clinicians bristle with frustration at the inflexibility of the veteran therapists. New techniques must not be accepted or rejected carte blanche but rather must be scrutinized for their merit. Techniques grossly foreign to experience tend to threaten and bewilder the inflexible diagnostician because she perceives them as attacks on her trusted and time-proven methods. Is it possible that training programs that emphasize testing and therapy techniques and materials are more likely to produce an inflexible therapist than those programs that emphasize theory, problem-solving ability, and creativity?

A clinician must possess many important personal attributes. Rogers (1942) speaks of empathy, congruency, and unconditional positive regard as necessary characteristics of the clinician, and they most certainly apply to the diagnostic process as well. Generally these qualities must be nurtured through consistent effort and proper guidance. Video- and audiotape equipment now allows the developing clinician to observe her own behaviors in the testing situation in order to understand more fully her own performance. Equally important in developing these characteristics is skillful guidance from a master diagnostician.

If the term *sensitivity* may be defined as a keenness of sense or a heightened awareness of incoming sensory data, then this much-maligned term has meaning for the diagnostician. She must be able to detect subtle physical, psychological, or interactional changes in a client's behavior, as these small changes have the most significant meaning in the diagnostic process. For further reading in enhancing awareness skills, see the works of Johnson (1972) and others (Emerick and Hood, 1975; Buscaglia, 1982).

*Insight* into the meaning of behaviors must be developed from a thorough grounding in the basic processes requisite for the speech act. Each diagnostician must become so familiar with the normal process of language acquisition and normal speech functioning that he has a built-in set of standards on which to base judgment. The insightful clinician is the knowledgeable professional who is capable of quickly comparing the client's behavior with the norm.

The development of an *evaluative attitude* is often a rather difficult task for the beginning clinician. We are, to a large extent, slaves to our experience; each clinician tends to bring the "social attitude" into the testing setting. Rather than looking upon the client's performance as having meaning for the evaluative process, we consult our own responses and formulate our own points of view in the give-and-take of the conversation. The critical, questioning attitude must be developed so that the clinician looks upon the behaviors in terms of their meaning rather than in terms of the response expected of him. Social interaction lends itself to superficiality, whereas the flow of the diagnostic interaction must, by design, lend itself to uncovering the meaning of the incorporated behavior. Effective diagnosticians tend to question the surface validity of behaviors and search for motivations, explanations, and interpretations that are not readily apparent.

Closely allied with the concept of the evaluative attitude is the idea of *persistent curiosity*. The diagnostician must develop an inquisitiveness that will make him persistent in his search for explanations. Answers are seldom apparent at first, and continuous effort is imperative. The directors of training institutions foster weakness in this area when they assign clients to students and expect therapy to get underway in a "reasonable" period of time. They are so bound to the rigid university timetables that therapy is often discontinuous. In an attempt to give each student a variety of clinical experiences, they often tend to sever clinical undertakings with a client at each semester's end, knowing full well that the diagnostic or therapeutic process is not best served in this way. The student may not always understand that these have been decisions based on program convenience rather than client need and may develop the notion that diagnosis is a temporary therapy-initiating exercise to be completed in an hour or two. The curious and persistent clinician, however, continues to place the client in situations that will permit additional scrutiny.

*Objectivity* comes from practicing the art of controlled involvement. The diagnostician must cultivate objectivity because she is subject to human errors. She must be warm, understanding, and accepting on the one hand and objective, evaluative, and detached on the other. Without some degree of balance between the two extremes, the diagnostician may so severely distort the interaction between herself and the client that she obtains little of value. Objectivity demands more than simply guarding against undue emotional involvement. The examiner must be objective about *herself*, her skills, knowledge, and personal characteristics. In other words, she must know herself to a sufficient degree that she can judge her own successes and failures and continue to grow in professional skill.

*Rapport* may be defined as the establishment of a working relationship, based on mutual respect, trust, and confidence, that encourages optimum performance on the part of both client and clinician. Rapport is developed over a period of time and is not easily established in a single session or during a few minutes at the initiation of one therapeutic encounter. Rapport must not only be developed, it must be maintained, and this calls for continued effort. The list of characteristics that enhance rapport is endless, but the factor we have found to be universally important is the *ability to maintain a nonthreatened posture throughout the testing session.* The student or clinician who is easily threatened in interpersonal interaction tends to have greater difficulty establishing rapport than one who can work with people and experience little threat from unpredictable or hostile reactions. The link between this characteristic and ego strength is probably quite strong and should be seriously contemplated by the beginning diagnostician.

Although much standardization is possible through strict adherence to test routines, the lowest common denominator in diagnostic evaluations is the examiner himself. Test results are the product of the subject, examiner, test, and test circumstance, each of which has certain influence. Examinations are clearly selected as a result of the experiences and biases of the examiner. Just as the answers we receive to questions are in part a function of the questions we ask and how we ask them, the diagnostic findings we obtain are in part a function of the tests we administer and the way they are administered. A "defective speech pattern" may be partially due to a defective testing pattern or a defective tester.

## PUTTING THE DIAGNOSIS TO WORK

As mentioned previously, the most important variable in the success of a diagnosis is the diagnostician. The available body of knowledge and set of skills set the stage for success or failure. The diagnostician brings knowledge of individual behavior, normal human behavior, normal speech and language development, concepts of testing and evaluation, test selection, communicative disorders, and a variety of other information, all of which culminates in skillful application of test administration, interviewing, and observation. The most knowledgeable and skillful diagnostician, however, may fail to achieve adequate results if he lacks the inquisitiveness necessary to encourage continuous effort and if he does not have the professional integrity to serve each individual to the maximum of his potential. Each of us is subject to individual variations in daily behavior that can have a direct effect on performance; however, it is incumbent upon every professional to control those variations so as to provide each individual with the best professional service available.

Perhaps the most demanding of all diagnostic ventures is the ultimate synthesis of findings into a coherent statement of the nature of the problem. The skilled clinician draws the findings together using the data available, past experience,

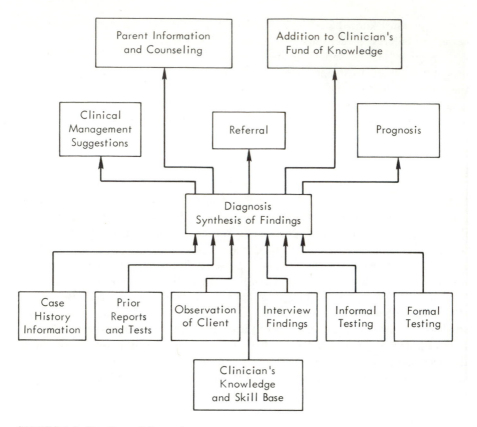

**FIGURE 1.4  Paradigm of diagnosis.**

knowledge, and intuition to formulate a total picture of the condition. At this point textbooks, research findings, and academic lectures fail to provide all of what is needed to succeed. Maturation of skills will only develop in an extensive practicum under the close supervision of a knowledgeable diagnostician.

The essence of the synthesis process is comparison of what is observed with what we expect to observe from our knowledge of the normal process. The incongruities between the observed and the normal provide the building blocks for completion of the picture. Figure 1.4 identifies diagnosis as a synthesis of findings and shows a number of outcomes to which this synthesis might lead.

HIGHLIGHT  *Diagnostic Observation*

A diagnostic session begins with observation and must ultimately return to observation for validation of the measures obtained. The ability to observe carefully, then, is a crucial clinical skill. Looking, listening, even touching are common yet powerful ways of obtaining information about an individual.

But clinical observation involves more than simply watching a person—it requires skills acquired by many hours of hard work.

One of the very real problems in acquiring observational skills is the tendency all of us have to bring our perceptual biases into a clinical setting. For each of us, the way in which we see the world seems to be the normal, the right, the proper way to see it. We call this the *illusion of centrality*. Someone once wrote:

> In matters controversial
> My perception's rather fine;
> I always see both points of view—
> The one that's right and mine.

In order to foster the orderly acquisition of information—and to minimize perceptual bias—we advocate a sequence of five steps in diagnostic observation: *focus, depth, description, interpretation,* and *implications* (Johnson, 1946: 127).

*Focus.* Probably the most difficult aspect of observation for the beginning student is focusing on the pertinent aspects of behavior. It is important for the student to remind himself that *no behavior has meaning unto itself,* and thus not only must he look at the presenting conduct of the client but he ·must also determine what aspects of the environment serve as stimuli or antecedent events to that behavior and what aspects serve as perpetuators. Quantification of behaviors forces the observer to become objective and he should carefully analyze the effect of the action on the environment. If the behavior is of high incidence, the events that succeed it must be suspect as maintainers and as such are of prime importance. The casual and untrained observer usually cannot focus on the descriptive level. He tends to categorize behavior as good or bad, normal or abnormal, cooperative or uncooperative, shy or outgoing, and so forth. The first step in observation, then, is to focus on a very descriptive level so that the examiner can present the actual behaviors the client exhibited rather than generalizations regarding the meaning of those actions. In order to underscore the importance of focusing attention in the observational task, we often ask students to observe some single aspect of behavior in a therapy session and report on that one characteristic. Recently five students were assigned to observe one of the following aspects of a given therapy session: (1) how much of the session was consumed by the clinician talking; (2) the amount of eye contact between child and clinician; (3) the percentage of the total therapy session in which goal-directed behaviors were exhibited by both the clinician and the child; (4) the mother's facial expressions and remarks as the session progressed; and (5) the entire therapy process. The interesting result of this experiment was that each of the first four students came up with suggestions that were pertinent to the therapy process, while the last student could only add general suggestions. These microscopic observations must eventually enable the student to make general conclusions from the total situation; our experience has led us to believe that it is best to start with such a finite focal point.

*Depth.* The depth of the observation is determined to a large degree by circumstance, but the diagnostician must find ways to observe the client interacting with many different people and stimuli. The diagnostician cannot expect to gain a great deal of information from fleeting observations; she must be willing to spend the time and energy necessary to observe a significant amount of behavior.

Observation of the child in many and varied settings must have a reference point, and that point must be normal behavior. Never let an exception to a general state go unnoticed! The unexpected may take any one of several forms. It may be bizarre and out of place with no observable precipitant, it may be the lack of response where one is naturally expected, or it may be expected in terms of the stimuli presented but bizarre in some other aspect such as intensity, frequency, or length of response.

*Description.* Simply selecting the proper focus and observing ample and varied behavior is not going to lead to a productive session; the diagnostician must attempt to put those observations into words. The translation from observation to description is often a much more difficult step than the novice suspects. In the early stages the diagnostician must train herself to describe behavior in writing as objectively, explicitly, and completely as possible. During these first attempts to communicate the findings of the observation, the clinician must withstand the temptation to jump to conclusions. She must stick to what she observes and what she can describe. The authors recently assigned several students to the same diagnostic session and asked them to record their observations; here are two samples of their reports:

*Student A.* Timmy entered the testing room and was very shy and unhappy. He was afraid of the examiner and wanted his mother. He continued to act in this spoiled manner until his mother was brought into the room. Once Mrs. Hopper was in the room, Timmy began to behave himself, and the testing could be undertaken.

*Student B.* Timmy stood in the doorway, held his head down, and refused to move into the room for three or four minutes until the clinician physically picked him up and closed the door. Timmy stood by the door and cried, while the clinician attempted to engage him in such play activities as card games, lotto, and ball. Timmy continued to cry for approximately fifteen minutes throughout all of these attempts until the clinician went out and brought Mrs. Hopper into the room. Timmy immediately crawled up on his mother's lap, and the clinician gave the articulation testing cards to the mother to show Timmy. After five minutes of encouragement by the mother, Timmy began to name the pictures.

Careful examination of these two accounts shows that one student was willing to make judgments, classify behavior, and generally draw conclusions without clearly specifying just what behavior was observed; the other student made a valiant effort to report the observables. Either approach can be taken to an extreme and thus interfere with the orderly transmission of information, but we strongly recommend that the beginning clinician make every attempt to keep the early accounts of her observations descriptive.

*Interpretation.*   Once all pertinent behaviors have been described, it is incumbent upon the observer to make *interpretations.* Without moving to this level, the observations are of little value (unless the worker is willing to allow someone else to make an interpretation based on his descriptive data). At this point the observer makes inferences regarding the meaning of behaviors; he attempts to generalize and classify behaviors and draw conclusions as to the meaning of what he observed. All of this can only be done, however, after sufficient purely descriptive information has been compiled. Interpretations drawn from objective quantified data are much more easily checked against reality than are interpretations made from desultory observations.

While making interpretative statements it is generally best to provide the reader with specific examples of the types of observational information that lead to such conclusions. For example, the examiner concludes that Mrs. King is having some difficulty with behavior management, which may have an influence on Jason's language disorder:

> During the interview session Jason emptied his mother's purse on the floor, pulled the testing materials off the table, took his shoes and socks off, and pinched his mother's leg until large red marks appeared. Following each of these episodes Mrs. King twice asked Jason to stop, with no result.

*Implications.*   Finally, the observer is expected to explain the *implications* of the observed behavior. Implications may be found by evaluating the consistency of the disorder in various settings, the degree of intelligibility in contextual speech, and so on. Information on the etiology of the problem may also be available through observation, and such interpretations as are warranted must be ventured. Similarly, the observed behavior can be assigned a meaning in order to direct the therapeutic effort.

Notice the definite sequence in the five steps of observation: The diagnostician moves from the nonverbal level of sensing and observing to the verbal levels of describing, labeling, and interpreting and finally draws conclusions and states some implications. Leaving out the steps of focus, depth, and description would allow too much distorting subjectivity and projection on the part of the observer. Adherence to the logical order of observation leads to accurate and more defensible conclusions.

## BIBLIOGRAPHY

BATEMAN, B. (1967). "Three Approaches to Diagnosis and Educational Planning for Children with Learning Disabilities." *Academic Therapy Quarterly,* 3: 11–16.

BEVERIDGE, W. (1951). *The Art of Scientific Investigation.* New York: W. W. Norton & Co.

BUSCAGLIA, L. (1982). *Living, Loving and Learning.* New York: Ballantine.

DEUTSCHER, M. (1983). *Subjecting and Objecting.* Oxford, Eng.: Basil Blackwell Publishers, Ltd.

EMERICK, L. (1984). *Speaking for Ourselves: Self-Portraits of the Speech or Hearing Handicapped.* Danville, Ill.: Interstate Printers and Publishers.

EMERICK, L., and S. HOOD (1975). *The Client-Clinician Relationship.* Springfield, Ill.: Chas.
C Thomas.

ENGLEMANN, S. (1967). *The Basic Concept Inventory.* Chicago: Follett.

JOHNSON, D. (1972). *Reaching Out.* Englewood Cliffs, N.J.: Prentice-Hall, Inc.

JOHNSON, W. (1946). *People in Quandaries.* New York: Harper & Row.

NATION, J., and D. ARAM (1977). *Diagnosis of Speech and Language Disorders.* St. Louis:
C. V. Mosby.

NEWMAN, P. (1961). "Speech Impaired?" *ASHA,* 3: 9–10.

PRONOVOST, W. (1966). "Case Selection in the Schools: Articulatory Disorders." *ASHA,* 8:
179–181.

RINGEL, R., L. TRACHTMAN, and C. PRUTTING (1984). "The Science in Human Communication Sciences." *Journal of American Speech and Hearing Association,* 26: 33–36.

ROGERS, C. (1942). *Counseling and Psychotherapy.* Boston: Houghton Mifflin.

SCHULTZ, M. (1972). *An Analysis of Clinical Behavior in Speech and Hearing.* Englewood
Cliffs, N.J.: Prentice-Hall, Inc.

SILVERMAN, F. (1984). *Speech: Language Pathology and Audiology.* Columbus, Ohio: Chas.
E. Merrill.

SLOAN, H., and B. MacAULEY, eds. (1968). *Operant Procedures in Remedial Speech and
Language Training.* Boston: Houghton Mifflin.

STARKWEATHER, C. W. (1984). *Speech and Language: Principles and Processes of Behavioral
Change.* Englewood Cliffs, N.J.: Prentice-Hall, Inc.

VAN RIPER, C. (1966). "Guilty?" *WMU Journal of Speech Therapy,* 2: 2–3.

VAN RIPER, C., and L. EMERICK (1984). *Speech Correction: An Introduction to Speech
Pathology.* Englewood Cliffs, N.J.: Prentice-Hall, Inc.

WEISS, C. (1983). *Weiss Intelligibility Test.* Tigard, Ore.: C. C. Publications.

YORKSTON, K., and D. BEUKELMAN (1981). *Assessment of Intelligibility of Dysarthric
Speech.* Tigard, Oreg.: C. C. Publications.

YSSELDYKE, J., and J. SALVIA (1974). "Diagnostic-Prescriptive Teaching: Two Models."
*Exceptional Children,* 41: 181–185.

# CHAPTER TWO
# INTERVIEWING

The clinician sets in motion the process of recovery at the very first contact with a client. This is accomplished through the vehicle of the spoken word, in short, by means of the initial interview. Because the intake interview ushers the client into treatment, it is *the* key link in the evaluation process. In order to assess and treat persons with disorders of oral language, it is essential that we know how to talk with them in a manner that reflects our expertise and inspires confidence and trust.

## THE IMPORTANCE OF INTERVIEWING

Although clinical evaluation obviously involves more than proficiency at conducting interviews, it is central to the role of the diagnostician. By means of verbal exchange we gather data about the individual, transmit information, and establish and sustain a working relationship. The interview is also the means by which treatment is carried out and, as such, serves both as a tool and as a relationship (Figure 2.1). For the clinical speech pathologist, interviewing is an extremely important activity.

Although widely used, interviewing is one of the least understood aspects of the worker's role. Prospective speech clinicians are expected to acquire an impressive array of knowledge, but often it is merely presumed that they know how to communicate effectively with clients. The mastery of interviewing is either taken for granted or expected to accrue somehow as an incidental artifact of required course work and practicum experiences.

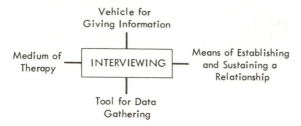

FIGURE 2.1   **Interviewing is central in speech pathology.**

Some clinicians consider interviewing to be secondary; they use paper to re-place personal interaction. An elaborate case history form containing a plethora of questions is mailed to the parents, and they are requested to fill it out and return it before the diagnostic appointment. The rationale for this procedure is that it saves the clinician time and alerts her to problem areas she can then explore in the personal interview. Although the clinician certainly should get some idea of the problem before the diagnostic examination, she seldom needs a twelve-page ques-tionnaire. There are several reasons for disenchantment with the paper approach: (a) The questions are generic—they cover *all* possible respondents—and thus are ambiguous or not applicable to many *particular* clients; a parent may not under-stand the relationship between the questions posed and the child's speech problem. Face-to-face interviews permit greater flexibility in formulating precise and germane inquiries. (b) The queries may be threatening or engender guilt, and the clinician is not present to observe these reactions or to support and assist the respondent as he searches for an answer. Does the mailed questionnaire allow time for the respon-dent to plan a defense? Is it more likely that we end up with a view of what the respondent wants us to see? More complete information can be obtained in an interview, where primary questions may be followed up with pertinent secondary inquiries. (c) The questions, if answered by the respondent in one particular way, may prevent her from developing any other possible answers. Spoken language does tend to create a reality for the individual, but writing lends an air of permanence. During an interview, however, the clinician can determine not only *what* a client says but also *how* she says it—for example, how does she assign priority to items, how does she associate items with one another, how does she reveal attitudes by vocal quality or body language? (d) Mailed case history forms also tend to bias the diagnostician toward a set of expectancies that are difficult to change. The main objection, however, is the impersonal, routine nature of the procedure. It denies the uniqueness of each client and implies that the agency simply wants to compile a fund of information for its files.

## THE NATURE OF INTERVIEWING

An interview is essentially a *process,* not an entity—a process of verbal and non-verbal intercourse between a trained professional worker and a client seeking his services. More specifically, an interview, in a clinical diagnostic sense, is a *purpose-*

*ful* exchange of meanings between two persons, a directed conversation that pro-
ceeds in an orderly fashion to obtain data, to convey certain information, and to
provide release and support. The professional worker, by reason of his position and
clinical expertise, is expected to (and usually does) provide the direction for the
verbal exchange. Thus, an interview is not just an ordinary conversation in terms of
a desultory exchange of opinions and ideas but rather a specialized pattern of verbal
interaction directed toward a specific purpose and focused on specific content. The
roles of interviewer and respondent are more highly specified in a professional interview than in a conversation. An interview differs from a social conversation in a
number of other important respects: (a) the time and location of an interview is
specified formally; (b) the inquiries are generally unilateral—the clinician may ask
about the parents' relationship with their child, for example, but it is not expected
that the client will reciprocate with questions about the worker's children; and
(c) the clinician does not necessarily avoid unpleasant topics in the interest of social
propriety.

In a good diagnostic interview, the clinician and client must become coworkers, multiplying their efforts by creating a mutual feeling of cooperation. It is
futile to expect straightforward answers to simple questions. A good diagnostic
interview always involves more than making queries and recording answers.

Interviewing is a unique kind of conversation. Perhaps for the first time the
respondent can talk freely without fear of criticism or admonishment. The *clinician*
knows that an interview is a unique and distinct mode of verbal exchange, but does
the *client* need to know? Probably not. Indeed, we typically advise students to refer
to an interview as a "chat" or "a chance to share information" when they contact
clients or parents to request an appointment time. An "interview" sounds rather
ominous and frightening, perhaps even like a summons to account for one's failings.

In summary, a diagnostic interview is a directed conversation, carried out for
specific purposes such as fact finding, informing, or altering attitudes and opinions.
The clinician's efforts are directed toward the creation of mutual respect and team
effort in the understanding and solution of the communication problem.


## COMMON INTERVIEWING PROBLEMS

Several factors can prevent the establishment of effective communicative bonds between a speech clinician and those he interviews. Although the list could obviously
be expanded, we have picked several aspects which in our experience are the most
common interviewing barriers.

### Fears of the Clinician

There are two points in a student clinician's career when her anxiety rises to
very high levels: the confrontation with her first therapy case and her first diagnostic interview. It is—and should be—an awesome responsibility to undertake the professional treatment of another human being. There is always an element of risk in
offering help. As a matter of fact, if a student does not get somewhat tense in this

situation, we suspect her suitability for the profession, since either she is so dumb she knows no fear or she doesn't care enough to be afraid. We certainly are not applauding anxiety, but we should accept and recognize our fears, specify their nature, and develop effective ways to channel the nervous energy into improving our performance. The client's needs, not the clinician's feelings of adequacy, are salient.

Perhaps the most common fear expressed by beginning interviewers is that clients will not accept them in a professional role because of their youth. They doubt they can bridge the age gap, especially when they deal with parents: "Who am I to be asking questions and giving suggestions to them when they are older and more experienced?" They sigh, "Won't parents consider me a pipsqueak? Won't they look down on me if I don't have children?" Most of this is pure projection on the student's part. If the interviewer indicates his deep concern for the welfare of the child, then nearly every parent will respond in a positive manner, without scrutinizing the clinician for wrinkles, grey hairs, or diaper-pail hands. The clinician, of course, should not communicate the uncertainty he may feel in the interview situation, or he will never establish his competence or inspire confidence. The worker must abandon all thoughts of himself, his doubts and fears, how well he is doing, and channel all his energy into making the client feel that he is a co-worker.

Another common fear among incipient interviewers—and one that is also largely projected—is that the interviewee will become defensive or resentful during questioning. We have seen students omit a whole series of important questions when a client, especially a parent, responded curtly or showed mild annoyance. While it is not uncommon for parents to feel ashamed because they think of their child's speech disorder as an outward and visible sign of their own failure, few in our experience are resentful or defensive about the clinician's sincere efforts to determine the nature of the child's problem. The important point is, again, to make the interviewees feel that they have done the best they could do, and now, with some assistance from the clinician, they can do better. As we suggested in Chapter 1, the clinician should *always maintain a nonthreatened posture in the clinical transaction.*

Many beginning interviewers are leery of questions directed at them. "What do you do when the client starts asking *you* questions?" the student interviewer frequently despairs. "Will I be able to explain to them adequately what they need to know? How will I know if I have gotten it across if they just sit there and nod?" We shall return to this important topic of clients' questions in a later section of this chapter.

*Memory failure.* A common deterrent to communication in an interview is loss of memory. Clients simply will not remember things that the clinician needs to know in order to plan best a program of therapy.

*Emotional barriers.* Sometimes an interviewee cannot or will not give information because emotional blocks prevent free communication. Self-disclosure is often difficult, and the respondent may not be able to identify a payoff for revealing personal information.

*The language gap.*   The clinician must remember that laypeople often have a markedly different way of talking about a speech or hearing problem. If there is a language gap and the clinician does not take steps to close it, the interview will be unsuccessful: the greatest barrier to communication is the assumption of it.

*The lack of specific purpose.*   Many beginning interviewers either have purposes that are too broad and general or interviewing goals that are too nebulous. It is important to write out carefully and rather explicitly the purposes for the interview before meeting with the client. We must know *why* we want the answers to the questions we ask. Specifying the purposes of an interview is also an effective way to reduce the interviewer's uncertainty and anxiety. Kadushin (1972: 2) summarizes the importance of planning in this way:

> To know is to be prepared; to be prepared is to experience reduced anxiety; to reduce anxiety is to increase the interviewer's freedom to be fully responsive to the interviewee.

The clinician should keep in mind, however, that thorough planning does not mean the application of an inflexible routine.


## AN APPROACH TO INTERVIEWING

We now present an interviewing approach, an eclectic product of our experience in social work, speech pathology, and clinical audiology, together with an intensive study of relevant bibliographic materials. No doubt the reader will want to modify it to suit his individual setting. It is desirable that he do so, for only through critical self-evaluation and modification can any clinician acquire an interviewing procedure that is uniquely his own.

There are three basic goals in diagnostic interviews: to obtain information, to give information, and to provide release and support. For the purpose of discussion each goal will be considered separately, a procedure rarely possible to do in an actual interview.

### Goal One: Obtain Information

Although it may seem obvious, it is worth restating that as clinicians we must listen before we speak. There are essentially three reasons for this: (1) it gives clients an opportunity to talk out problems, to ventilate fears and feelings, thus enabling them to profit better from the direction and advice that the speech clinician will offer; (2) it gives the clinician an idea of the nature and scope of the information the client will need; and (3) it allows the clinician to formulate hypotheses concerning the individual's communication disorder.

*Setting the tone.*   The first important task of the clinician is to set the right tone for the interview, to get a structured conversation initiated and channeled in the proper direction. How does one go about that? Research by McQuire and Lorch

(1968) has underscored the importance of proper structuring. Their findings indicate that the initial style of interaction may well determine the style of interaction for the entire interview (see the work of Matarazzo and Wiens, 1972). We find that defining the roles is an effective procedure for setting the tone:

> Mrs. Seelos, I'm Miss Sullivan, Terry's speech clinician. I really appreciate the opportunity to chat with you about Terry and the things we are doing in speech. First, though, you can be of great help to me since you know Terry so much better than I do. There are several things about his early development and how his speech seems to be at home that I need to understand before planning a long-range therapy program. Before you came in today, I made some notes for myself so that we could best use this half hour before my next session.

It is helpful to think of the interview as a kind of role-playing situation. The clinician defines the roles for the client and indicates the rules and responsibilities that accrue to these roles. She tells who she is, what she intends to do, and what she expects of the client. In other words, the interviewer structures the situation by explaining the purposes of the interview—why the information is wanted and what will be done with it. Initially, of course, the client accepts the respondent role because of the nature of the situation and the official sanction of the interviewer's position. Then it is up to the worker to demonstrate her empathy and clinical expertise in order to solicit further cooperation. Two problems sometimes arise here. First, some clients may be inhibited by such explicit role definitions; respondents from lower middle or lower social classes have had little experience in holding directed conversations. In this case, a clinician can prolong the small-talk phase, emphasize the nature of the interview as a chat, and gently ease into the more structured situation as the relationship develops.[1]

The second, more difficult, problem concerns the site of the interview. Although it is generally best to conduct interviews in a clinical setting, sometimes this is not possible and one has to seek out the client or parents at home. This is rarely satisfactory, not only because of the distractions inherent in the situation (children, pets, and neighbors) but also because the interview frequently becomes a social visit.

It is vital that the interviewer convey his sincere interest in the situation as the client sees it. He must demonstrate to the client that he is genuinely trying to comprehend what the problem is and what it means to the client personally. The clinician can show his interest by carefully attending to the respondent: Assume a relaxed, natural posture; maintain eye contact; and offer minimal verbal encouragements that reveal that he is listening ("Yes," "I see," etc.).

Rapport, of course, is not a separate substance that one pours into a session; it is mutual respect and trust, a feeling of confidence in the clinician, and a large

---

[1]When two or more people meet together, even for serious purposes, a certain amount of social and idle talk seems to foster positive attitudes toward continued interaction. Czikszentmihalyi (1975) describes this feature of group interaction as "flow."

measure of understanding. Empathy, warmth, and acceptance are crucial aspects; the worker must strive for the ability to understand sensitively and accurately the interviewee's situation. He should also try to be genuine, not contrived, with a professional character armor that signals "clinician on duty." As a matter of fact, it is helpful to avoid interposing a desk—a symbol of authority—between the respondent and the interviewer. The interview is more effective without such a barrier. In addition to the words spoken, a number of forces shape the interview. Some things are conveyed by the setting and by the dress, manners, and expressions of the participants. If our office is located in a boiler room or a storage area, we have already conveyed something of our attitude toward the client and his problem by the very physical space that we use. In professional interviewing, the goal is to provide an atmosphere that fosters communication between client and clinician (Staples and Sloane, 1976).

*Asking the questions.*    Preferably, the clinician should use an interview guide rather than one of the more elaborate questionnaires—that is, instead of a formal set of questions written out to be read and answered, she should use a form that indicates areas to explore. The interview is much more spontaneous and meaningful if the speech clinician words her questions in keeping with her understanding of the individual's situation rather than reading prepared ones. In most cases, formal questionnaires operate as another type of barrier or crutch for the insecure interviewer.

The specific content of the queries addressed to a respondent depend on, among other things, the age of the client, the nature of the problem, and the purposes of the interview.[2] Because we intend to focus on style of interviewing in this chapter, we will not include lists of questions that pertain to particular disorders of communication. There are, however, seven general topics or areas of inquiry that are useful in any diagnostic session:

1. *What is the respondent's perception of the problem?* We seek here a global description of the communication disorder. In a parent interview, for example, we frequently open the session with an open-ended question, "Tell me why you brought Jamie to the speech clinic."

2. *When and under what conditions did the communication disorder arise?* The purpose of this question is to determine the history of a child's development and the onset of the problem. This line of inquiry is particularly important in evaluating a child with delayed language—we want to know as much as possible about the youngster's motor, social, and cognitive development.

3. *In what ways has the communication disorder changed since its onset?* When interviewing parents of a child exhibiting early signs of stuttering, for example, we are interested in how the speech disfluency has changed since first noticed.

---

[2] Most clinicians find that the younger the client being evaluated, the more important is the parent interview. Hodges et al. (1982) devised a *Child Assessment Schedule* that elicits a school-aged youngster's responses to items pertaining to school, friends, and family. Sigelman (1982) offers a multiple-choice technique (using pictures) that we have found useful in diagnostic interviews with mentally retarded persons.

4. *What are the consequences (the handicapping conditions) of the problem?* In what manner—socially, educationally, occupationally—does the communication disorder affect the person's life? In what ways has she adapted to the disorder?

5. *How has the client and her family attempted to cope with the problem?* What lay remedies have been tried by the client and her family? How has she responded to them?

6. *What impact has the client's communication disorder had on the rest of the family?* When a child has a handicapping condition, it creates fertile ground for familial confict (see Featherstone, 1980). In order to obtain a description of the child's ongoing behavior, and how he fits into the family regimen, ask the parents to describe a "typical" day, from the time the youngster gets up until he goes to bed.

7. *What are the client's (or parents') expectations regarding the diagnostic session?*

Students frequently ask what type of interviewers they should strive to be: directive, nondirective, behavioristic, psychoanalytic, neo-Freudian, and so forth. The best answer that we have been able to give—although it sounds facetious—is that they must use whatever techniques seem to be best for the job that they need to do. Often we feel that a beginning clinician concentrates too hard on being behavioristic or Rogerian rather than focusing on what he must do to meet the needs of a particular client. Some writers feel that the direct interview is unpleasant, although there is no evidence to support this assumption. As a matter of fact, one research team (Richardson, Dohrenwend, and Klein, 1965) discovered that the lack of structure inherent in the pure nondirective interview produced anxiety in some respondents, especially the less educated ones. Actually, the whole matter is an academic question, because a good diagnostic interview is characterized by a shifting of styles: objective questions that ask for specifics, subjective queries that deal with feelings and attitudes, and finally the indeterminate questions like: "Tell me more" that keep the respondent going.

A far better question for the clinician to direct to himself is, "Why am I asking these questions?" He should have his purposes clearly in mind. Classically, the interviewer should start with the least anxiety-provoking queries, mostly objective questions that have high specificity (Woolf, 1971), and then proceed to more subjective questions as the relationship develops.

Quite often, however, we find it useful to employ a "funnel" sequence of inquiry during the course of a diagnostic interview—starting with broad, open-ended questions and then progressing to more specific or closed questions (Stewart and Cash, 1974). Here is an example of a funnel sequence from a recent parent interview:

—How does Jimmy function in the family setting?
—How does he get along with his siblings?
—How does his older sister "help" him to communicate?
—Can you describe an instance in which she talked for him?

The "inverted funnel" approach, proceeding from specific to general, is also useful. It is best to avoid the checklist or long series of "tunnel" questions that call for information on one level of specificity and all of which are asked in a similar style (for example, "Did your child have earaches, fevers, head injury, etc.?").

*The presenting story.*    Most persons who anticipate visiting a clinic or discussing a speech problem with a public school speech clinician will have mentally rehearsed what they intend to say.[3] In some cases they may even have a pseudo-conversation with the worker. We must allow this story to be unraveled, or the respondent will be left with a sense of frustration and lack of closure. A question such as, "What seems to be the problem?" will permit the flow of conversation to begin. The clinician should remember that this is how the *client* perceives the problem—it is her unique way of looking at the situation. It may be grossly inaccurate, but the interviewer should hear her out; nothing turns a respondent off more quickly than for the interviewer to suggest by word or action that his views are silly or misguided. Sometimes the presenting story will become a motif that recurs again and again during the course of the interview.

This is generally a crucial point in an interview. The interviewee may cautiously extend a portion of himself verbally, carefully scan the interviewer's response, and then decide whether or not to tell the whole story. Sometimes a respondent may even set up a straw man to see how the interviewer deals with it:

Mrs. Dimitri, mother of Ivan, a fifth-grader who possessed a serious lateral lisp, appeared to see herself as a modern, informed parent. At our initial interview, she launched into a lengthy diatribe about the school reading program, explaining in great detail why Ivan couldn't read. We listened intently for a time and when she paused to recycle her complaints, we praised her for her concern and suggested that she bring this up at the next PTA meeting and with Ivan's teacher. Apparently Mrs. Dimitri expected a debate, and she was much mollified that we had heard her out. We then proceeded to an excellent review of her insights into the child's speech problem.

This is not the proper time for the clinician to debate an issue with the client. His story can be accepted initially on the level of feeling, and later in the interview—when rapport is stronger—the point can be discussed more fully. We feel very strongly that these initial stories, these primitive theories, should be respected as the best possible answer clients have been able to come up with. This does not mean agreeing with their conclusions; it just means we accept their judgment with understanding so that we can form a basis for further communication.

Actually, the presenting information can be a very rich source of clinical hypotheses to be explored during the course of the interview. How do the client

---

[3] Often the interviewer will have to contend with events that occurred prior to the session—the family car failing to start, a burned breakfast, absence of a convenient parking place. A few words to reveal the worker's understanding of the distracting antecedents will generally assist the respondent in shifting to the topic of the interview.

and parent present themselves (Goffman, 1959)—as long-suffering, anxious, diffident? How do they associate ideas or items of information sequentially? What priorities do they assign to issues they raise? Do they seem to be realistic in their expectations regarding the diagnostic session and treatment?

*Nonverbal messages.*    Respondents do not communicate by words alone, and the discerning clinician attends to body as well as oral language during an interview. As a matter of fact, some observers (Bosmajian, 1971; Hinde, 1972; Mehrabian, 1972; Harrison, 1974) suggest that a large portion of the total message—particularly messages involving strong feelings—is carried by nonverbal cues. However, the diagnostician should resist the urge to interpret a client's every twitch; each instance of nonverbal behavior should be related to the *content* of the oral message and the *context* in which it occurs (Birdwhistle, 1970; Knapp, 1972; Feldman, 1973):

> If a parent leaves her coat on during an interview it may mean she feels vulnerable and the garment provides a bit of protective armor. It may also mean that she has a spot on her dress, or that all the hangers in the waiting room were taken again by forgetful students, or that the room is chilly. However, if she shifts her chair away from the clinician, sits with her arms and legs tightly crossed, avoids eye contact, and responds to questions with one-word answers, then it may be concluded that she is defensive and guarded in the clinical setting.

The issue here is to avoid making one item of nonverbal behavior the sole basis for interpretation; the interviewer should be on the lookout for patterns (Weitz, 1974).

Although research into the nonverbal facets of dyadic interviewing is still in its early stages, there are several useful questions that can assist the examiner's scrutiny of body language (Egolf and Chester, 1973):

1. What clues are evident during the initial contact with the client? Does he enter the room hesitantly and wait to be seated? What can be discerned from his clothing or personal grooming? Does he avoid eye contact and shake hands limply?
2. Is the respondent's facial expression congruent with the content of his oral message? Does his face flush or show other emotions when discussing different aspects of his speech problem? Does he reveal tension by constant bunching of his jaw muscles?
3. How does the respondent use eye gaze during the course of the interview? As a general rule, persons maintain less eye contact when talking than listening, particularly when responding to questions that provoke reflection and recall. The amount of mutual gaze between two individuals is increased markedly when they like each other and are involved in a joint concern. Keep in mind, however, that unwavering eye contact by the clinician, particularly when asking questions, may be interpreted as a threat signal or an attempt to dominate (Argyle and Cook, 1976).
4. Attend to the client's body movements and postural shifts: What is the rate and extent of movement, and the degree of tension shown? Does the respondent's postural shifting congruently mirror that of the interviewer?

5. How does the client speak with his hands? Does he use mainly pronated or supinated gestures? Are his hands tightly clasped? Does he wring them, or play continually with his ring? Does he use a number of "adaptors" (Knapp, 1972), such as adjusting his clothing, scratching, or inspecting his fingernails?

6. How does the respondent communicate by use of the available space? In which chair does a client choose to sit with respect to proximity with the interviewer?

7. What can be discerned by attending to nuances of the client's use of pitch, loudness, or vocal quality? Does his rate reflect apprehension, excitement, or depression? Is the respondent's recital of the presenting story punctuated by heavy sighs?

8. In what respect do the stigmata associated with various communication disorders (for example, stuttering, cerebral palsy) interfere with or confound nonverbal messages (Goffman, 1963; Eisenberg and Smith, 1971)? How does body language vary with respect to the factors of sex, age, and culture (Morsbach, 1973)?

The most important thing to look for may be lack of congruence between the respondent's verbal and nonverbal messages; in cases where the two conflict, body language is a more accurate indicator of how a person feels about an issue:

> During a recent diagnostic session we opened the parent interview by asking the parent to describe the nature of his child's speech problem (the child was multiply handicapped). Before the parent responded verbally, he made a short, chopping gesture with his right hand, stamped his right foot, and wrinkled his face in a fleeting expression of disgust. However, he then proceeded to tell us calmly what a wonderful relationship he had with his son. The nonverbal message occurred so swiftly that later we were uncertain if we had really seen it; when we played back the videotape, however, the graphic body language was evident even to the father. This vivid self-confrontation seemed to release some long-repressed feelings, and the father then talked at length about how disappointed he was in his son, how much attention his wife devoted to the child—often, he felt, at his expense, and what a financial drain the various treatment programs had been. The consequence of the interview was a referral to a family service agency where both parents received the type of counseling they needed.

Although persons vary in terms of their skill at "reading" nonverbal cues, it is possible to improve with training (Rosenthal et al., 1974). Since body language is continuous—there is no way to turn it off, not even for the clinician—the interviewer will want to investigate the topic of nonverbal communication more fully (Scheflen, 1972; Spiegel and Machotka, 1974; Leathers, 1976; Duncan and Fiske, 1977; Ekman, 1980).

*Things to avoid in the interview.*   Beginning interviewers commit several common errors. The list that follows is not meant to be exhaustive, but it does cover the most glaring mistakes.

1. It is usually best to avoid questions that may be answered by a simple yes or no. Although open-ended questions do produce longer responses in general, it is

interesting to note that respondents from lower socioeconomic groups, who have less education, become more anxious as the questions become less structured. We have interviewed several clients who are confirmed yes-men. No matter what the clinician asks, no matter what comments he makes, these respondents simply nod in passive agreement. Perhaps they are fearful of exposing their ignorance and feel that it is better to remain silent and be thought a fool than to say something and make it obvious.

We find that requesting the client to rate himself on some simple scale is more effective than either-or questions. We frequently ask the client to tell us not whether something is difficult or easy but to what degree. A simple rating procedure, with low values (1 or 2) indicating relative ease and higher values (4 or 5) indicating relative difficulty, may be used.

2. Avoid phrasing questions in such a way that they inhibit freedom of response. Do not say: "You don't have any difficulty with ringing in your ears, do you?" or "You don't tell Billy to stop and start over again, do you?" Such leading questions are not effective interviewing. The beginning interviewer tends to be anxious about asking open-ended questions. He is afraid that silence will result and that this will damage his relationship with the client. So he will ask an open-ended question and then close it. For example, "How do you feel about David's stuttering; does it bother you?" Leave it open! Although open-end questions consume more time and may produce some rambling and irrelevant responses, there are many advantages to recommend their use:

> They let the respondent do the talking while the interviewer plays his role as listener and observer. The freedom to determine the nature and amount of information the respondent will give may communicate to him that you are interested in him, as well as his answers, and that you respect his ability to give accurate and relevant data. (Stewart and Cash, 1974: 28)

Try also to avoid abrupt shifts in your line of questioning. For example, if you are exploring the client's feelings or attitudes on a particular issue (subjective questions), don't suddenly ask an objective question. Inexperienced interviewers, fearful that they are too deep in an area, tend to jump around; often they persist with objective queries and, once a pattern of response is established, the client finds it difficult to shift to more elaborate answers.

3. Avoid talking too much. This is perhaps the most common mistake of the beginning interviewer. He feels he must fill up every pause with his own verbiage. It is much better to rephrase what the respondent has said or make some comment like, "I see," "Tell me more," or "Anything else?" Sometimes a smile and an understanding nod are effective when it is felt that the client has more to say but needs some silent time to conjure it up. If there is a positive attitude—a good rapport—and the person feels comfortable in the situation, then these encouragements increase the length of the response; if the topic or situation is neutral, these comments tend to expand the message. However, if the topic is negative or the individual feels uncomfortable, the "hmm, hmm" may be taken as a criticism—that is, if she *cannot*

respond at length, she will feel that she is being pressured to do so.[4] Parents with little education are perhaps the most vulnerable to this kind of pressure.

Be careful not to fall into stereotyped verbal habits. One of our students used "very good" as reinforcement so frequently with a severely aphasic patient that one day, after making a particularly effective response to a problem, the patient—who had said very little since his stroke—finished the clinician's "very" with a resounding "good," surprising them both.

4. Avoid concentrating on the physical symptoms and the etiological factors to the exclusion of the client's feelings and attitudes. There is a little bit of Dr. Kildare in all of us; we yearn to play the role of omniscient healer. This is further compounded by instructors who dwell interminably on causation in their courses dealing with speech disorders. But it is possible to track each suspicious symptom with such zeal that we fail to obtain a basis for understanding the emotional and environmental complications of a speech or hearing disability. The interviewer should remind herself to distinguish between items of information that are simply interesting and background information that she really needs to know.

5. Avoid providing information too soon. There will be plenty of time to clear up misconceptions later in the interview. The surest way to cut off the flow of information is to stop a parent, for instance, after he says, "I just tell Michael to stop, take a deep breath, and start all over again," and counsel him on the proper responses to nonfluency.

6. Avoid qualifying and hemming and hawing when asking questions. Ask them in a straightforward fashion and maintain eye contact. Rather than asking, "Did you find that, well, you know, when you were, ah, shall we say . . . with child—did you experience any untoward conditions?" say, "Did anything unusual happen during your pregnancy?" Instead of inquiring, "Did you discover, hmm, I mean, well, after your father, ah, passed away, did your stuttering problem increase?" say, "What impact did your father's death have on your speech?"

7. Avoid negativistic or moralistic responses, verbal or nonverbal, to the client's statements (avoid even the response "good," as it implies a value judgment). The flow of information will stop rapidly and the relationship will be impaired severely if the individual senses that we find him or his behavior distasteful. We do not have to subscribe to a person's values or code of behavior for us to show compassion and understanding for his situation. Use inquiries that begin with "why" very sparingly, since the word is often perceived as a challenge or a threat; it is too reminiscent of disciplinary sessions (Why were you late for class? Why can't you behave properly?). In a clinical setting we must not let our values obscure our perception of the client's frame of reference (Benjamin, 1974).

8. When the client causes the interview to wander, avoid abrupt transitions to bring it back to the point. Most of those whom you will interview have had little

---

[4] The "activity" level of the clinician appears to be a critical factor in his perceived effectiveness: interviewers who talked more (and interrupted respondents more often) were rated at higher levels of accurate empathy (Matarazzo and Wiens, 1972).

experience in directed, orderly conversation. They tend to follow chance associations and wander far afield. The experienced interviewer has the ability to make smooth transitions. How does one go about getting the interview back on track? The best way is by building a bridge to the respondent's previous statements. For example: "That's interesting, Mrs. Davis, maybe we can come back to that in a little while; now earlier you were mentioning that your child's loss of hearing occurred suddenly . . . ." The key here is to use respondent antecedents—things that the person has said earlier in the interview. If we use only the interviewer's antecedents—questions that the interviewer has asked before—the client will not feel understood and will sense that what he has said was of little consequence. The inexperienced interviewer asks lots of questions either with no antecedents or with her own antecedents. She is afraid of losing control of the interview and thus becomes preoccupied with formulating the next question.

9. Avoid allowing the interview to produce only superficial answers. We need ways to get deeper, more significant responses from our clients. There are several interviewing devices, termed *probes,* that the clinician will find helpful:

*Crosshatch,* or *interlocking,* questions are useful when we need to elicit more detail about a topic that has been glossed over. Often there are discrepancies that must be resolved. Essentially, the way to go about this is to ask the same thing in different ways and at different points during the interview. For instance, the father of a young stutterer responded in a superficial manner to our query about his relationship with the child. He assured us that he had a "loving relationship" with his son and then complained at length about his working conditions. Later in the interview when we asked him to describe the sorts of things he did with the child, he was unable to mention a single one. We don't mean to imply that the clinician should attempt to catch the client lying and then demand an explanation. The clinician must check out discrepancies, however, in order to enhance her understanding of the problem, since they could have a significant effect on the mode of treatment.

*Pauses* can be very helpful. When there is a lull in the interview, it may mean simply that the client has exhausted his store of information, that a memory barrier has prevented further recall, or that he senses he is not being understood. It can also mean, however, that a sensitive area has been touched upon. Do not feel that pauses harm the interview. Much significant information can be forthcoming if we keep quiet and indicate with a smile or a nod that we expect more.

Another aid is to encourage *time regression* and *association.* Memories are weak. In order to pinpoint some significant data, we may have to take the person back in time to find a memory peg such as a wedding, a natural calamity, or the like, that may call forth more information. One father, a long-time air force sergeant, cataloged everything in terms of the make and model of car he was driving. Another client, an inveterate bird-watcher, remembered incidents by the times he had seen the marbled godwit or the prothonotary warbler.

The *summary probe* is one of the best ways to keep the interview moving smoothly. The clinician summarizes periodically what the client has said, ending perhaps with a request for clarification or further information. Incidentally, this procedure also demonstrates to the person that the interviewer is indeed trying to understand his problem. We generally use "mini-summary probes"—echo questions—all the way through an interview:

RESPONDENT:    After my husband's stroke, my whole world collapsed.
INTERVIEWER:   You were overwhelmed by the sudden change in your life.
RESPONDENT:    Yes, one day he was happily planning our trip to Sanibel Island . . . and then, in just a moment, he was paralyzed and couldn't talk. Now all our plans are up in the air . . . the new car, the checking account, he took care of all that.

The *stumbling probe* is a variation of the summary probe; we have found it helpful, especially with the reticent respondent. The interviewer rephrases a portion of the respondent's communication and then, attempting to interpret or comment upon it, he pretends to halt or stumble. For example, when interviewing the mother of a child allegedly beginning to stutter, the clinician might say: "Now, you were saying that Bruce first started to repeat and hesitate after he caught his finger in the car door. Under these conditions, it would be natural for you to . . . ah . . . ." This really works. The respondent's need for closure will precipitate significant information and, perhaps more important, significant insights.

Finally, there is the *assuming probe*. (This stems from the old incriminating question, "Have you stopped beating your wife yet?") Such a technique should, of course, be used sparingly and only after some interviewing experience; at times, however, it is the only way to get information out in the open. If the client has avoided an important area, if he has left much unsaid regarding his speech or hearing problem and what it means to him, then it is up to the interviewer to bring this out. One adolescent boy who had been vehemently denying that his stuttering bothered him, unburdened himself when we said, "It bothers you so much that you don't want anybody to know, do you?"

10. Avoid letting the client reveal too much in one interview. You may have had similar experiences: A good friend encounters severe trouble and you come to his aid, helping him through the crisis. A curious thing often happens when your friend recovers his equilibrium. He feels obligated to you; he felt exposed to you as a raw human being during the crisis, and now he is embarrassed, somewhat resentful, and perhaps even hostile. It is as if you are now an outward and visible sign of his former debacle. Sometimes a beginning interviewer makes the mistake of trying to get everything in one sitting. The client, sensing perhaps his first really understanding listener, may want to pour out his whole sad tale of woe. Later, however, the individual will feel embarrassed and foolish, perhaps even exposed and guilty at revealing so much of himself to this comparative stranger.

Bringing an interview to a graceful close can sometimes be more difficult than getting it started. In our experience, an interview is most effectively terminated by summarizing what has been discussed and reviewing the specific actions to be taken.

It is probably best not to consider new material at this time when neither the interviewer nor the client can devote sufficient attention to it. It is always important, however, to leave the door open for future contacts (see Stewart and Cash, 1974: 197-201, and Kadushin, 1972: 207-214, for more information on leave-taking).

11. Avoid trusting to memory. Record the information as the interview progresses. Tell the client that you will take some notes during the interview so that you can plan her treatment program more effectively and make recommendations for other services. Such note taking, or even recording devices, are rarely questioned. Indeed, we have found that clients expect you to write down some of the information they are giving you; they doubt that you would be able to remember all of their answers. You obviously would lose your relationship, however, if you scribbled furiously while the client was revealing some sensitive information. It is axiomatic that the respondent's confidence will be respected, but we have mixed feelings about mentioning this explicitly to the client. The clinician's manner should suggest that all information received is to be held strictly confidential. At times, the clinician can suggest the possibility that he might listen and tell others, and this had never entered the respondent's mind.

Prepare a report of the interview as soon as possible. Commit your observations to paper while the encounter with the respondent is still fresh in your mind (see Chapter 9 for information on writing reports).

### Goal Two: Give Information

The most common complaint of patients in hospitals and clinics is that they have not been kept informed of their condition and progress. Interviewing 214 patients, Pratt, Seligman, and Reader report (1958: 229): "Patients who were given more thorough explanations were found to participate somewhat more effectively with the physician and were more likely to accept completely the doctor's formulation than were the patients who received very little information." We have formulated a fundamental principle is this regard: *There is never too little information, there is instead misinformation.* Not one of us can stand uncertainty. All too frequently the information, if not supplied by the professional worker, will come distorted from other sources. When not correctly informed, parents become misinformed and this leads to confusion, misunderstanding, and further compounding of the problem. It is our responsibility, therefore, to provide accurate, unemotional, objective information on the status of the individual's speech and hearing problem. This is generally accomplished during the postdiagnostic conference (Martin, 1977).

Summarize the findings of the clinical examination in simple, nontechnical language; use common terms compatible with the person's background. We prefer to commence, if possible, with results that show a client's area of normal functioning, to review findings that indicate what is good before describing deficiencies. It is good technique to proceed by a review of the support systems for oral language—auditory, sensory, motor, psychosocial—and then describe the findings of language, voice, articulation, and fluency assessments. Relate comments to normative values whenever possible. Clarify and help the respondent to ask questions by using examples and simple analogies. If the interviewer is in doubt concerning the client's understanding of the diagnostic material (clients will rarely ask if they don't understand), he should talk more slowly, employ longer descriptions, and use more redundant language (Longhurst and Siegel, 1973). Recapitulation of a conference, by audio- or videotape playback fosters even greater understanding (Marshall and Goldstein, 1969).

HIGHLIGHT    *The Questions Clients Ask*

An interview is much more than a clinician posing questions and recording the client's answers. It is an important forum for *exchange,* a reflexive, dynamic experience of sharing between the diagnostician and the informant. Indeed, we find that a client—especially a parent of a young child being evaluated—frequently is eager to probe the worker's expertise.

But often the questions she asks may have a hidden meaning or purpose. The clinician must evaluate the informant's inquiries and decide: What is the person *really* asking? Is there an unstated concern behind the questions? Luterman (1979) distinguishes the questions clients ask into three categories: *content, opinion,* and *affect.* We will describe and illustrate these three types of inquiries with excerpts from an initial interview with the mother of a three-year-old child brought to the speech clinic as a beginning stutterer.

1. *Questions dealing with information or content.* In this instance, the client seeks an informative or factual response from the clinician. The question usually takes the form, "I want to know about something and I hope you have the right information."

MRS. BELL:    The type of choppy speech [disfluency] Jesse has—is it common among children his age?

CLINICIAN:    It sure is. Most children between the ages of two and a half and five do a lot of repeating and hesitating.

2. *Questions with predetermined opinions.* Here the client has an opinion regarding a particular subject and wants to determine if the clinician agrees with it. The clinician must be careful not to merely demolish the client's opinion until she understands *why* and *how strongly* the client holds it.

MRS. BELL:    Um, on TV a couple of times, I've seen a demonstration of the airflow technique for stuttering. What do you think of it?

CLINICIAN:    Those demonstrations are very dramatic, aren't they? What's your impression of the technique as it applies to Jesse?

3. *Questions that are "faint knocking on the door."* In this case, the client is not asking for information, or to determine the clinician's opinion, but rather for emotional support and reassurance. The question conceals a feeling the individual either is unaware of or is reluctant to reveal.

> MRS. BELL:    Do you think my divorce and remarriage had anything to do
> with Jesse's speech problem?
> CLINICIAN:    It's pretty easy for parents to feel guilty about something they
> might have done to cause their child to begin stuttering.

No doubt the reader has already detected a flaw in the triad: On the surface, each question posed by Mrs. Bell could be classified in any of the three categories. How does a clinician know *what* the client means? The clinician doesn't know in every case, but she tries to determine the purpose of a question by scrutinizing *how* a client asks it—by vocal inflection and body language—and by the context in which the inquiry appears. Interestingly, as long as the clinician is *trying to understand,* a client will not be alienated by an inaccurate interpretation (Chinn, Winn, and Walters, 1978).

In our experience, speech clinicians, probably because the bulk of their training focuses on information, do a good job of responding to content questions. However, many beginning clinicians find it difficult to respond appropriately to a client's expression of emotion. Although Luterman (1979: 48) is discussing clinical audiologists, his remarks pertain to many speech clinicians as well:

> Professional training programs rarely provide any information or experience for the student in how to deal with parents. They concentrate instead on providing considerable information and practicum experience with the handicapped child. As a result of that imbalance in emphasis, the young therapist feels very insecure in dealing with parents, who may be older and more experienced in the care of children. So the therapist begins to adopt defensive strategies to "distance" the parents, the most common one being to impart information. The content-based relationship is completely controlled by the teacher and subtly puts the parents down by increasing their feelings of inadequacy. That one-sided way of dealing with parents becomes habitual with time, and older teachers rely on content strategy almost exclusively. In some circles that approach is considered very professional. It is only when professionals feel secure as people that they can allow more intimacy and more freedom in their relationship with parents.

Avoid superficial statements of reassurance. Most people can see through this sort of sham. The individual's anxiety and uncertainty will be better relieved once he begins to understand his particular speech problem; the best antidote to fear and uncertainty is knowledge. Be sure, however, to avoid iatrogenic errors. Do not use terms or suggest consequences that will precipitate more stress for the client. One parent was told his child's hearing problem was caused by atrophy of the hearing nerve. It is difficult enough to have a hard-of-hearing child without worry about mysterious nerves atrophying, something about which the parent can do very little. Do not communicate your negative expectations regarding the outcome of therapy to the client. We are convinced that what the clinician thinks a client can do, that he shall do. In other words, after Parkinson, the client's behavior expands to fit the clinician's concept of his potential. Do we precondition our own therapeutic behavior when we make a prognosis? Is this communicated to the client and his relatives in some manner and on some level? We think it often is.

Below are six basic principles for imparting information to clients that we have found useful:

1. Emotional confusion may, and often does, inhibit the person's ability to understand cognitively what you are trying to say. Just because you have once reviewed the steps of articulation therapy is no reason to expect that its importance will be grasped.

2. Refrain from being didactic; do not lecture your clients. Focus on sharing options rather than on giving advice.

3. Use simple language with many examples and illustrations. If you must err, err in the direction of being too simple rather than complex. And repeat, repeat, repeat the important points—rephrasing each time.

4. Try to provide something that the client—especially a parent—*can do.* Action reduces the feelings of futility and anxiety. The activity should be direct, simple, and require some kind of reporting to the clinician.

5. Say what needs to be said pleasantly—but frankly. Do not avoid saying something that must be said on the assumption that the client cannot take it or that you will be rejected. People often display an amazing reserve of courage in difficult situations (Buscaglia, 1975).

6. Remember, however, that the one who finally communicates what the client may have been dreading to hear is often hated and maligned. If you are the first to say the feared words, you may become the focus for all the hostile, negative feelings thus aroused. As a professional worker, you will have to be strong enough to be the lightning rod for these emotions.

Clients and their parents expect to receive help from the clinician but often will resist change. No matter how maladaptive a client's behavior may seem from an objective point of view, it represents his best solution; in fact, he will often resist attempts to alter his equilibrium, precarious as it may appear to others. Change is stressful; diagnosis and treatment imply change; therefore, assessment and therapy are stressful.

According to Carkhuff and Berenson (1967) and others (Ginott, 1965; Gordon, 1970), the key feature of *creative listening* is the ability to scan a client's comments and respond in a way that fosters understanding and releases the potential for growth. Creative listening represents empathy in action: Before anyone can or will listen, he must first be listened to.

The particular kind of understanding we are referring to involves two facets, a *cognitive* aspect (the content) and an *affective* aspect (the feelings). In order for genuine understanding to take place, both must be included in the interviewer's response to the client's statement. If the clinician is successful in crystallizing both aspects of her response, she has provided an *interchangeable base* that allows the interview to move forward to levels of helping that involve direct action. Here are some examples taken from diagnostic interviews:

CLIENT:    (in response to a query regarding his marital status): No, I'm single
. . . who would want to marry a clod who stutters like me?

CLINICIAN:    You feel rejected because of your speech problem, is that right?

PARENT:    We tried to be good parents, we really did . . . but somehow we
messed up in helping Peter learn to talk.

CLINICIAN:    You feel a sense of failure, perhaps even guilt, that your child has
a speech problem.

CLIENT:    I stutter so badly that life is worthless . . . I can't get a job . . . the
business of living just doesn't seem to meet expenses.

CLINICIAN:    You feel thwarted and frustrated by your speech problem; sometimes you wonder if you can go on . . . .

Note the clinician's responses carefully. She does not simply repeat the client's comment; she attempts to restate it in clarified form. Observe that the interviewer used the second-person singular "you" in referring to the client's affect. Feelings are commonly stated first, since they are more important than content. We sometimes add a tag question ("Is that right?") to check on the client's intake of our responses.

### Goal Three: Provide Release and Support

The clinician does not, of course, wait until the end of the interview to provide release for the frustrations and fears of the client. Most of the parts of the interview already discussed will serve this purpose. By helping the individual talk out his problems, the worker is providing an excellent escape for pent-up feelings. We maintain that our purpose is not just to remove discomfort but also to promote a state of comfort and well-being.

More than advice is needed during interviews for the purpose of helping clients take some specific action or move in a particular direction. They need help in sorting out the confusing choices before them. To support a respondent's real strengths, we need to make it clear that we understand what the situation means to him and that we uncritically sympathize with his feelings and attitudes. We can restore the client's self-esteem and his ability to function more appropriately if we convey our interest in him as a person and our solid acceptance of his importance. If the client feels appreciated and understood, he can sometimes drop his self-protective behavior and see how the experience will eventually benefit him.

There is an unfortunate tradition of "sweetness and light" in client counseling. A person has a problem. She is sad and depressed, and we try to cheer her up. Sometimes this degenerates into a debate, with the interviewer attempting to persuade the person that she should not feel miserable. When a person feels depressed, anxious, and fearful, he does not want to count his blessings. He wants you to feel miserable, too. He wants you to share and identify with him on his own level. Thus, the interviewer is given a basis for communication with the person. We start where he is, accept it as the proper place to start, and tell him that it is a sad state of affairs that would make anyone sad and depressed. Then, using this bond of identification, which becomes a basis for communication, we can assist him in solving the problem. The main ingredient is *empathy,* the capacity to identify oneself with another's feelings and actions. The best way to demonstrate our attempt to understand a client's point of view is by listening creatively.[5]

How does one handle emotional scenes? They are bound to arise at some point in your interviewing experience. Some clinicians excuse themselves from the room and allow the respondent to recover his dignity alone. Others try to change the subject to something less emotional. Both of these approaches may, with certain clients, give the impression that the clinician is rejecting their feelings. It is more effective to indicate one's understanding of the feelings that are being expressed and accept them as natural human reactions. For example: "That's okay to let it come out, Mrs. Moody; you have been holding it back too long. Sometimes it helps to get it out in the open."

Not all clients seen by the speech clinician will need or even want extensive supportive interviewing. In some cases, the procedures discussed here would be grossly inappropriate. Visualize an interview as ranging along a continuum from affective concern such as feelings and attitudes to objective matters such as goals and advice. Some respondents simply need objective information so that they can do the job; others require considerable support and succor before they can take over and modify their behavior. The clinician's role in some interviews may consist of simply listening to and supporting a client.[6]

## IMPROVING INTERVIEWING SKILLS

We hope the material in this chapter will be useful to students majoring in clinical speech pathology and to our colleagues working in various settings. However, no one ever became proficient in interviewing solely by reading about it. Nor, it seems, are interviewing skills enhanced by increasing knowledge about communication disorders (Janz, 1982; Wolraich et al., 1982). It took us many years of constant searching and experimenting to evolve the interviewing approach presented here. And, by the indulgence of our clients and many long-suffering parents, we continue to explore for better ways.

We have included below a series of activities and projects for your own practice. Let them serve as the beginning steps in a continual learning effort toward improved interviewing. You will find that the time devoted to such training exer-

---

[5] In our judgment, of all the skills inherent in effective interviewing, the most important is the ability to listen carefully and empathically. This skill can be learned, although beginning clinicians find it difficult to employ remarks that facilitate a client's expression of feelings (Volz et al., 1978).

[6] We quite agree that love alone is not enough in a helping transaction; a good relationship is a *necessary* but not a *sufficient* condition for good interviewing. However, it may sound trite, but it is true that the secret of care *of* a client is caring *for* the client. The sense of being understood by a helping professional is a powerful stimulant to the client's growth (Llewelyn and Hume, 1979; Sherman and Fields, 1982).

cises is well spent. Now, consider these steps on how to improve your interviewing skills:

1. Read widely from a variety of sources. We have included a list of selected references to get you started. Find out what people are like by reading in sociology, psychology, anthropology, and philosophy. This is, of course, a lifetime project, which we feel is delightful since there is always a new frontier, an open horizon on which we can set our sails. Our profession has arisen so abruptly, grown so rapidly, and been so concerned with the urgent scientific and clinical issues that it has ignored the important issue—the development of a philosophical basis for our work. A speech and hearing clinician without a rationale is like a ship without a rudder. The fundamental and mandatory basis for sound, purposeful therapy is an overall point of view, a workable theory that does not necessarily include the specific activities that will be used to carry it out. Nothing is so pathetic as the clinician who, in a willy-nilly manner, empties a bag of therapeutic homilies on the client's lap, hoping somehow that one of them will work. Only a sequential system of logically interrelated theorems will enable us to evaluate our clinical effectiveness.

2. Listen to all sorts of people, to their dreams, their rationalizations, their insights—or lack of them—and their gripes. Get acquainted with the way common people think and talk, by following the example of Caldwell (1976) and others (Steinbeck, 1961; Walters, 1970; Coleman, 1974; Morris, 1972; Terkel, 1980; Least-Heat-Moon, 1982).

3. Form small heterogeneous groups of students majoring in speech pathology and audiology. Conduct some sensitivity and values clarification training, particularly as it relates to your self-concept, your assets and liabilities, your responses to people, and your relationship with your own parents and other older adults (Kaplan and Dreyer, 1974). The senior author finds, as a stutterer, that each time he works with parents of children beginning to stutter, he has a distinct tendency to summon up the "ghosts of his stuttering past." He must monitor his behavior by listening to recordings and scrutinizing interviewing protocols. In order to provide assistance to others, we must know our own foibles and potential blind spots and have them under reasonable control. Remember, too, that the way our academic preparation teaches us to explain a situation will tend to determine the way we perceive it. No one has immaculate perception.

4. Role playing is still one of the best methods to prepare for interviewing (White, 1982; Finn and Rose, 1982). Set up several typical interview situations in front of a class and play, for example, the roles of the reluctant parent, the spouse of an aphasic patient, or the hostile father. Discuss the interaction, and replay the situations with others assuming the roles. Write out interview purposes prior to the role playing and determine, or have the class determine, how effectively the interviewer accomplished his avowed purposes. Whenever the viewers feel that the interview went wrong or the responses were ineffective, see how many different ways it could have been handled. This builds up the beginning interviewer's repertoire of adaptive responses. You can do a surprising amount of intrapersonal role playing in your spare time. While we are waiting for a class to begin, for a light to change, or for our father-in-law to cease talking, we frequently imagine ourselves in various

interviewing situations and then explore alternate statements, probes, and so forth. Successful interviewing is largely a matter of attitude (Nideffer, 1976):

> Borrowing from a method of solitary practice devised by successful athletes, we use a simple technique to help students build clear cognitive maps of the clinical encounter. The prospective interviewer first assumes a comfortable posture, and breathes deeply for a few moments to induce a feeling of relaxation. Then, step-by-step, the individual mentally rehearses the interview: he pictures himself successfully orienting the client, encouraging communication by attending and responding in an emphatic manner; he tries to visualize the scene as vividly as possible—even to the point of feeling the satisfaction of accomplishing the interview in an easy, efficient manner.

5. Make recordings of your first few interviews, then analyze them carefully with your clinical supervisor or a colleague (Adler and Enelow, 1966; Cannell, Lawson, and Hausser, 1975; Irwin, 1975). We believe that multiple interviewers simply do not work (although seeing multiple interviewees—such as a mother and father at the same time—can be useful and productive); hence, we would suggest that your supervisor not observe your performance in the same room, especially for your first ventures.[7] We have found that when the supervisor stays in the room, the student has a tendency to seduce her into taking over the role of interviewer; and if she refuses to assume the mantle, she can only sit there looking at the clients as if they were bugs in an insect collection. We have no role sanction in our social structure for the silent scrutinizer, and his presence can seriously impair the effectiveness of the interview.

Play back your interview again and again, revising statements, underscoring errors, and scanning for the good parts. Have typed protocols prepared from some of these tapes—the errors really leap out at you from the printed page—and discuss them with your instructors, fellow students, or colleagues. We find this simple format useful:

| TOPIC | MESSAGE | INTERVIEWER'S RESPONSE |
|-------|---------|------------------------|
| Child's disfluency | Parent: "Billy gets worse in the evening." | "Is there more confusion at that time?" (Used a yes-no question instead of open-ended) |
| Spouse's intake history for adult aphasic | "Stanley was such a gentleman. Now he swears and curses. I just can't stand it." | "This sudden change in your husband's behavior is hard for you to accept." (Good use of empathy statement) |

[7]In a dyadic interview there are only two possible directions for communication ($1 \times 2 = 2$). When a third party is added it increases the potential interaction to six ($1 \times 2 \times 3 = 6$). Add yet another person and the possibilities for communicative exchange reach unwieldy proportions ($1 \times 2 \times 3 \times 4 = 24$).

**FIGURE 2.2   Checklist of interviewing competencies.**

Interviewer:_____ Date:_____

Client/Respondent:_____

    I.  *Orienting the Respondent*
        A.  Attends to comfort (coats, seating, and so on)
        B.  Engages in appropriate "flow" talk
        C.  Explains purposes, procedures
        D.  Structures roles

   II.  *Engendering Communication*
        A.  Attending behaviors (demonstrating receptiveness)
           1.  Relaxed, natural posture
           2.  Appropriate eye contact
           3.  Responses that follow the client's comments (restating, overlapping the client's message)
        B.  Open invitation to share (open-end questions)
        C.  Nondistracting encouragement to continue talking
           1.  Verbal ("Yes," "I see," and the like)
           2.  Nonverbal (nodding, shifting posture toward client)
        D.  Obtains an overview of the presenting problem

  III.  *Use of Questions and Recording*
        A.  Orderly, sequential questions
        B.  Nondistracting note taking

  IV.  *Active Listening*
        A.  Reflects feelings (empathic statements)
           1.  Matches affect
           2.  Matches content
        B.  Periodic summarizing of affect and content messages

   V.  *Monitoring Nonverbal Clues*
        A.  The diagnostician's
        B.  The respondent's

  VI.  *Skills in Presenting Information*
        A.  Transmission of information
           1.  Content
           2.  Style and language
        B.  Responds to questions appropriately
        C.  Appropriate use of humor, "flow" talk

 VII.  *Closing the Interview*
        A.  Summary, review of findings
        B.  Recommendations
        C.  Supportive comments

VIII.  *Analysis of Information*
        A.  Major themes in the client's presentation, association of ideas, inconsistencies and omissions
        B.  Descriptive report

Note: This checklist is designed to help monitor the performance of beginning interviewers. It can be used as a self-rating device or a format for supervisory feedback. (See also Enelow and Swisher, 1972; Garrett, 1972; and Maier, 1976.)

Use the set of questions devised by Stewart and Cash (1974: 201-202) as a guideline for evaluating your performance. Explore also the methods prepared by Iwata et al. (1982) and Molyneaux and Lane (1982) for the assessment and training of clinical interviewing skills. Finally, we suggest you evaluate your diagnostic interviews using the Checklist of Interviewing Competencies (Figure 2.2). Obviously, no beginning clinician will remember, let alone exhibit, all the skills delineated in the checklist; practice only a few at a time, and provide constructive feedback for each other.

We would like to end this chapter with a challenge to the reader. We challenge you to utilize the interviewing approach delineated above, find the errors, the things that just don't work for you, and then develop your own methods. We have given you the foundation blocks. Can you use them to make stepping-stones?

## BIBLIOGRAPHY

ADLER, L., and A. ENELOW (1966). "An Instrument to Measure Skill in Diagnostic Interviewing: A Teaching and Evaluation Tool." *Journal of Medical Education,* 41: 281-288.

ARGYLE, M., and M. COOK (1976). *Gaze and Mutual Gaze.* London: Cambridge University Press.

BENJAMIN, A. (1974). *The Helping Interview.* 2nd ed. Boston: Houghton Mifflin.

BIRDWHISTLE, R. (1970). *Kinesics and Context.* Philadelphia: University of Pennsylvania Press.

BOSMAJIAN, H., ed. (1971). *The Rhetoric of Nonverbal Communication.* Glenview, Ill.: Scott, Foresman.

BUSCAGLIA, L. (1975). *The Disabled and Their Parents: A Counseling Challenge.* Thorofare, N.J.: Charles B. Slack.

CALDWELL, E. (1976). *Afternoons in Mid-America.* New York: Dodd, Mead.

CANNELL, C., S. LAWSON, and D. HAUSSER (1975). *A Technique for Evaluating Interviewer Performance.* Ann Arbor, Mich.: Institute for Social Research.

CARKHUFF, R., and B. BERENSON (1967). *Beyond Counseling and Therapy.* New York: Holt, Rinehart & Winston.

CHINN, P., J. WINN, and R. WALTERS (1978). *Two-Way Talking with Parents of Special Children.* St. Louis: C. V. Mosby.

COLEMAN, R. (1974). *Blue-Collar Journal: A College President's Sabbatical.* New York: Lippincott.

CZIKSZENTMIHALYI, M. (1975). *Beyond Boredom and Anxiety.* San Francisco: Jossey-Bass.

DUNCAN, S., and D. FISKE (1977). *Face-to-Face Interaction: Research, Methods and Theory.* Hillsdale, N.J.: Lawrence Erlbaum Associates.

EGOLF, D., and S. CHESTER (1973). "Nonverbal Communication and the Disorders of Speech and Language." *Journal of American Speech and Hearing Association,* 15: 511-518.

EISENBERG, A., and R. SMITH (1971). *Nonverbal Communication.* New York: Bobbs-Merrill.

EKMAN, P. (1980). *The Faces of Man.* New York: Garland Press.

ENELOW, A., and S. SWISHER (1972). *Interviewing and Patient Care.* New York: Oxford University Press.

FEATHERSTONE, H. (1980). *A Difference in the Family: Life with a Disabled Child.* New York: Basic Books.

FELDMAN, S. (1973). *Mannerisms of Speech and Gesture in Everyday Life.* New York: International Universities Press.

FINN, J., and S. ROSE (1982). "Development and Validation of the Interview Skills Role-Playing Test." *Social Work Research Abstracts,* 18: 21-27.

GARRETT, A. (1972). *Interviewing: Its Principles and Methods.* 2nd ed. New York: Family Service Association.

GINOTT, H. (1965). *Between Parent and Child.* New York: Macmillan.

GOFFMAN, E. (1959). *The Presentation of Self in Everyday Life.* Garden City, N.Y.: Doubleday.

—— (1963). *Stigma: Notes on the Management of Spoiled Identity.* Englewood Cliffs, N.J.: Prentice-Hall, Inc.

GORDON, T. (1970). *Parent Effectiveness Training.* New York: Peter H. Wyden.

HARRISON, R. (1974). *Beyond Words: An Introduction to Nonverbal Communication.* Englewood Cliffs, N.J.: Prentice-Hall, Inc.

HINDE, R. (1972). *Nonverbal Communication.* New York: Cambridge University Press.

HODGES, K., et al. (1982). "The Development of a Child Assessment Interview for Research and Clinical Use." *Journal of Abnormal Child Psychology,* 10: 173–189.

IRWIN, R. B. (1975). "Micro-Counseling Interviewing Skills of Supervisors of Speech Clinicians." *Human Communication,* 4: 5–9.

IWATA, B., et al. (1982). "Assessment and Training of Clinical Interviewing Skills: Analogue Analysis and Field Replication." *Journal of Applied Behavior Analysis,* 15: 191–203.

JANZ, T. (1982). "Initial Comparisons of Patterned-Behavior Description Interviews vs Unstructured Interviews." *Journal of Applied Psychology,* 67: 577–580.

KADUSHIN, A. (1972). *The Social Work Interview.* New York: Columbia University Press.

KAPLAN, N., and D. DREYER (1974). "The Effect of Self-Awareness Training on Student Speech Pathologist-Client Relationships." *Journal of Communication Disorders,* 7: 329–342.

KNAPP, M. (1972). *Nonverbal Communication in Human Interaction.* New York: Holt, Rinehart & Winston.

LEAST-HEAT-MOON, W. (1982). *Blue Highways: A Journey into America.* Boston: Atlantic-Little, Brown.

LEATHERS, D. (1976). *Nonverbal Communication Systems.* Boston: Allyn & Bacon.

LLEWELYN, S., and W. HUME (1979). "The Patient's View of Therapy." *British Journal of Medical Psychology,* 52: 29–35.

LONGHURST, T., and G. SIEGEL (1973). "Effects of Communication Failure on Speaker and Listener Behavior." *Journal of Speech and Hearing Research,* 16:128–140.

LUTERMAN, D. (1979). *Counseling Parents of Hearing-Impaired Children.* Boston: Little, Brown.

McQUIRE, M., and S. LORCH (1968). "A Model for the Study of Dyadic Communication." *Journal of Nervous and Mental Disease,* 146: 221–229.

MAIER, N. (1976). *Appraising Performance: An Interview Skills Course.* La Jolla, Calif.: University Associates.

MARSHALL, N. and S. GOLDSTEIN (1969). "Imparting Diagnostic Information to Mothers: A Comparison of Methodologies." *Journal of Speech and Hearing Research,* 12: 65–72.

MARTIN, A. (1977). "Post-Diagnostic Parent Counseling by a Speech Pathologist and a Social Worker." *Journal of American Speech and Hearing Association,* 19: 67–68.

MATARAZZO, J., and A. WIENS (1972). *The Interview: Research on Its Anatomy and Structure.* Chicago: Aldine-Atherton.

MEHRABIAN, A. (1972). *Nonverbal Communication.* Chicago: Aldine-Atherton.

MOLYNEAUX, D., and V. LANE (1982). *Effective Interviewing: Techniques and Analysis.* Boston: Allyn & Bacon.

MORGAN, H., and J. COGGER (1973). *The Interviewer's Manual.* New York: Psychological Corp.

MORRIS, T. (1972). *The Walk of the Conscious Ants.* New York: Knopf.

MORSBACH, H. (1973). "Aspects of Nonverbal Communication in Japan." *Journal of Nervous and Mental Disorders,* 157: 262–277.

NIDEFFER, R. (1976). *The Inner Athlete.* New York: Crowell.

PRATT, L., A. SELIGMAN, and G. READER (1958). "Physicians' Views on the Medical Information Among Patients." In *Patients, Physicians and Illness,* ed. E. Jaco. New York: Free Press.

RICHARDSON, S., B. DOHRENWEND, and D. KLEIN (1965). *Interviewing: Its Forms and Functions.* New York: Basic Books.

ROSENTHAL, R., et al. (1974). "Body Talk and the Tone of Voice: The Language Without Words." *Psychology Today,* 8: 64–68.

SCHEFLEN, A. (1972). *Body Language and Social Order.* Englewood Cliffs, N.J.: Prentice-Hall, Inc.

SHERMAN, J., and S. FIELDS (1982). *Guide to Patient Evaluation.* 4th ed. Garden City, N.Y.: Medical Examination Publishing Co.

SIGELMAN, C. K. (1982). "Evaluating Alternative Techniques of Questioning Mentally Retarded Persons." *American Journal of Mental Deficiency,* 86: 511–518.

SPIEGEL, J., and P. MACHOTKA (1974). *Messages of the Body.* New York: Free Press.

STAPLES, F., and R. SLOANE (1976). "Truax Factors, Speech Characteristics and Therapy Outcome." *Journal of Nervous and Mental Disorders,* 163: 135–140.

STEINBECK, J. (1961). *Travels with Charley.* New York: Viking.

STEWART, C., and W. CASH (1974). *Interviewing: Principles and Practices.* Dubuque, Iowa: W. C. Brown.

TERKEL, S. (1980). *American Dreams: Lost and Found.* New York: Pantheon.

VOLZ, H., et al. (1978). "Interpersonal Communication Skills of Speech-Language Pathology Undergraduates: The Effects of Training." *Journal of Speech and Hearing Disorders,* 43: 524–542.

WALTERS, B. (1970). *How to Talk with Practically Anybody About Practically Anything.* Garden City, N.Y.: Doubleday.

WEITZ, S., ed. (1974). *Nonverbal Communication: Readings with Commentary.* New York: Oxford University Press.

WHITE, R. (1982). "Observer's Presence and Self-Focused Attention in Role-Rehearsal Activities." *Perceptual and Motor Skills,* 54: 839–842.

WOLRAICH, M., et al. (1982). "Factors Affecting Physician Communication and Parent-Physician Dialogues." *Journal of Medical Education,* 57: 621–625.

WOOLF, G. (1971). "Informational Specificity: A Correlate of Verbal Output in Diagnostic Interview." *Journal of Speech and Hearing Disorders,* 36:518–526.

# CHAPTER THREE
# THE CLINICAL
# EXAMINATION

We gain an understanding of a client and his communication disorder by two basic means: asking and testing. The interview provides us with a view of the presenting problem as the client or his parents perceive it; it also allows the clinician to observe the client's behavior and formulate hypotheses that can then be evaluated in a more structured form of interaction. In this chapter we present an overview of the clinical examination, a procedure for inspecting and testing the impressions generated during the intake interview.

The overall purpose of the clinical examination is to assemble sufficient information to provide a working image of the client. More specifically, the clinical examination is guided by the following interrelated purposes:

1. To describe the problem—What are the dimensions of the communicative disturbance with respect to voice, fluency, language, and articulation?
2. To estimate its severity—How large a problem is it?
3. To identify factors that are related to the problem—What are the antecedents and consequences of it?
4. To estimate prospects for improvement—What estimate can we make of the extent of possible recovery and the time frame of treatment?
5. To derive a plan of treatment—What are the specific targets for therapy, and how can the client best be approached?

Thus, we are concerned with the systematic collection, organization, and interpretation of information regarding an individual and his particular communication disorder. All of this activity is carried out to provide a basis for predicting the outcome of treatment and to guide the nature and scope of the therapeutic regimen. Repeated testing during therapy will also enable the clinician to judge the efficacy of the plan of treatment. Moreover, testing may be helpful for appropriate placement in group therapy. Finally, some workers urge more extensive testing of each client in order to provide additional scientific information on the various communication impairments.

## ASPECTS OF THE CLINICAL EXAMINATION

There are several important aspects of the clinical examination with which the beginning clinician should be acquainted. We have selected the most salient factors for discussion; all are potential pitfalls for the unwary.

### The Interpersonal Context

We see three major constituents in any clinical transaction: interpersonal dynamics, the sequence of goals, and the activities (see Figure 3.1). The most crucial factor in conducting a successful diagnostic session is the client-clinician relationship. When a person works with another, there is always human impact; even when clients are treated by computers, they come to accord human attributes to the machines. No matter how well prepared and rehearsed an examiner may be, if his approach to people is poor, he is bound to experience failure. All tests, all examinations, all so-called objective diagnostic procedures are mediated by person-to-person contact.

We can be seduced into grave errors by test norms, percentile scores, and standard examination procedures: A human being is a total functioning unit, and the various tests are multiple and fragmented. The instruments we use are relatively precise, and we are often deluded into thinking that the client is functioning with the same degree of precision in the testing situation. But human elements may disturb the validity of the tests no matter how refined the scoring procedures or how calibrated the machines.

**FIGURE 3.1    Basic constituents of the clinical transaction.**

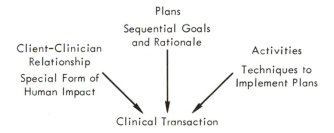

Plans
Sequential Goals
and Rationale

Client-Clinician
Relationship

Activities

Special Form of
Human Impact

Techniques to
Implement Plans

Clinical Transaction

Impersonal, test-oriented clinical examination sessions can also make treatment more difficult since there is no absolute division between diagnosis and therapy. The first contact with a client initiates treatment. During a diagnostic session he is forming opinions and conceptions about the clinician and the total clinical situation. Barker and his colleagues (1953: 310) have warned that "while to the medical practitioner, diagnosis and therapy are often routine technical jobs, to the patient the situation never has such limited personal meaning. To him diagnosis and therapy are a route to highly important life conditions."

Not all clients will require the full impact of this interpersonal dimension. Indeed, some individuals simply want to find out what is wrong and then rectify the situation. The point is, however, that the clinician should be able to discern what the client needs and then adjust her style appropriately.

*Age factors.* Although all age levels present unique diagnostic problems, three groups in particular—young children, adolescents, and to a lesser extent, older or aged clients—require special effort and expertise.

Young Children.  Preschool (and kindergarten) children are often difficult to test and examine. Unlike most older children and adults, they just don't see the payoff for all the questioning and prodding. The main problem is dealing with the child's fear of the clinical situation. This apprehension may stem from one or more of the following related factors: (1) inadequate preparation for the examination, which produces, (2) uncertainty as to what will be done to or with him by the clinician, (3) vivid memories of trauma during visits to dentists and physicians, (4) the contagious anxieties and uncertainties experienced by the parents, and (5) stress and conflicts engendered by past listener reactions to the speech impairment. Children confront the speech examination in a variety of ways, but the two most trying responses are shyness and withdrawal and, at the other extreme, aggressiveness and hyperactivity.

The shy ones are the most difficult to deal with clinically because there is no output—no speech or language to evaluate. The lack of response, per se, is behavior, too, however, and has meaning we must judge; the child is always telling us something even when he isn't talking. If he cannot or will not respond to our attempts to discern his capabilities, we have to employ special procedures to get him involved with the tasks. It is fascinating to witness how our students and colleagues attempt to deal with the reticent child:

> The impulse is to swarm the child's defenses with instant rapport, superficial bonhomie, or glib reassurance that everything is going to be all right. But youngsters don't want to be overwhelmed any more than adults do. One clinician, who claims to be able to obtain all manner of information from shy children, swoops down upon a youngster, holds him on her lap, fondles him, and chatters incessantly, repeating questions over and over at close range. Emerging from these somewhat explosive sessions, she is able to detail behavioral responses that equally competent clinicians cannot confirm. We

finally discovered how she does it when we videotaped her during a diagnostic session. She is simply receiving her own stimuli as reflected by the bewildered child and is mistaking these images for the youngster's responses. She is literally answering her own questions; small wonder she confirms her own predictions.

Most clinicians advocate a low key, easy-does-it approach with shy children, who must see that the diagnostician is not a threat and can be trusted. But that does not mean adopting a coy, childlike demeanor:

> One speech pathologist of our acquaintance adopts a vocal pitch at least a half octave above his normal pitch level and correspondingly childish inflections and immature motor behavior when he works with preschoolers. It was sometimes difficult to tell who was the client, and even the children seemed annoyed, bemused, or embarrassed by this cloying cuteness.

How *do* you get a small child to talk? Questioning is a common procedure but we must agree with Van Riper:

> Questions are demands. They immediately place the child in a subservient role, with the questioner in the position of power. Even when the child responds appropriately, the resulting relationship is one which immediately puts the questioner into the same category with other authority figures who have been controllers, a relationship which often regenerates the conflicts the child has previously experienced in threatening communication. If you ask what something is called and the child cooperates, he must either think that you must be stupid not to know its name or that you suspect he doesn't know it (which implies stupidity), or that you must want him to do a little verbal dance for your pleasure. . . . Moreover, the eliciting of speech by questions often yields very impoverished samples. At best, you'll get just a vocabulary item, not a good speech sample. Or, if you ask him a yes-no question, you'll get a yes or no answer, often the latter. Like a marriage, we do not feel that a therapeutic relationship should start with an invitation to say no. If the question is more elaborate ("What did you have for breakfast this morning?" "What did you do in school today?") the child has probably forgotten or finds it difficult to formulate, or feels that it is none of your business, anyway. Especially with children for whom the acquisition of speech has been no easy accomplishment, any question tends to pose some threat. They have been bedevilled by too many questions from too many questioners and, when they have answered, their listeners have not always understood them or have rejected them. For these children, the interrogative inflection is almost as potent a signal as the tone that makes the rat jump in expectation of shock.[1]

Eschewing questions, then, we recommend a simple play activity—a box of common farm animals or a doll house with miniature furniture is excellent—and the use of *self-* and *parallel-talk.*

---

[1] Charles Van Riper, *Speech Correction: Principles and Methods,* 5th ed. ©1972, pp. 108–110. Reprinted by permission of Prentice-Hall, Inc., Englewood Cliffs, N.J.

How then should one begin? We suggest that you should simply greet the child, then do some simple self-talk, commenting on what you are doing, or perceiving, and with plenty of moments of comfortable silence interspersed, until you have him playing with his box of toys. And then, in the role of the adult playmate, you can play with those in your own box—silently at first. No questions. No demands. *Solo play!* Once the child is comfortable in this activity, you should begin to put some self-talk into your own solo play; first noises (those of trucks, animals, etc.), then single words, then short phrases and simple sentences. All of these refer to what you are experiencing at the moment. Usually the child will begin to follow suit. His noises and his self-talk begin to flow. Next you should shift to contact play very gradually. Let your toy truck occasionally touch his fire engine, or help him find a block, or put another one on his toppling pile, or straighten it up a bit so he can make it higher. When you feel the time is ripe in this *tangential contact play,* begin to accompany it with some noises or commentary, using *parallel talk,* telling him what he is doing, perceiving, or feeling, again making sure you have more silence than speech. From tangential play, you can often proceed rapidly to *intersecting play* in which your activity becomes a part of his. (Let your truck go over the bridge he has built or feed your doll or toy dog a piece of the play fruit he has put on the play-house table.) Verbalize what you are doing. Next seek to achieve *cooperative play,* assisting him in what he is doing. (Have your truck bring him the blocks he needs to build his tower.) Usually by this time, the child is speaking very easily and often copiously, your own verbalizations primarily confined to reflecting what he has said. From this point onward, the communication can proceed fairly normally and naturally. We hope we have not given the impression that this process is too time-consuming. Often we can accomplish all the progressive interaction in a single session and build a very warm communicative relationship in less than an hour. There are, of course, many children for whom such a careful approach may not be vitally necessary, children who have learned that big people always seem to have to ask stupid questions, children who are willing to dance when the interrogative strings are pulled, children who relate easily. Yet even with these children this approach seems to work very well. The relationship established is less superficial, more satisfying. We do not meet with as many moments of resistance or negativism later on in therapy. (Van Riper, 1972: 108–110)

But what do you do with the aggressive, active ones, the children who cannot or will not sit still, who demand to structure the situation in the way they desire?

FIGURE 3.2    Diagram of interaction between clinician and child. (Van Riper, 1972; reprinted with permission.)

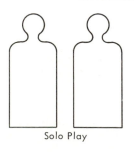
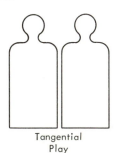
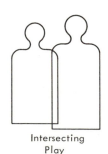
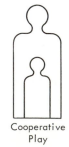

Solo Play                Tangential              Intersecting            Cooperative
                            Play                      Play                    Play

First, and most important, the clinician must retain control of the situation. She does this, basically, by defining the limits for the child and by a firm, but accepting manner. The child must see clearly that he cannot test the examiner, that the examiner is not threatened and has no intention of acquiescing. We do not mean a rigid intransigence, for it is often desirable to alter the testing situation to fit the child. To be sure, much of the behavior manifested by these children is for testing the limits of the situation; they want to know the rules of the game before they will cooperate. On some occasions, with a highly distractible child, we have had to reduce the stimuli in the room; we may have the child sit facing a plain wall, draw the window shade, and keep all test materials out of sight until used. We have even turned off lights in a room to force the child to focus on us. In a few instances we have found it necessary to take the child out of the testing situation and go for a walk before returning to the clinical tasks:

> Tim migrated restlessly from the window to the door of the examining room, whining belligerently. When an item was presented to him, he either threw it away or ignored it. We then took the child for a walk about the clinic; we looked into each room while carrying on a running commentary about what was going on. Then Tim was able to return to the examining room and was content to move through the various tasks we had planned.

With a few genuinely hyperkinetic children we have resorted to mild physical restraint, generally holding them close to us (Baxley and LeBlanc, 1976). They seemed to need and actually like external controls on their flighty behavior that they could not control from within. Although we don't recommend the procedure, we know one highly successful clinical audiologist who, when confronted with a recalcitrant child, firmly squeezes the youngster's trapezius muscle as he guides him toward the examining booth.

Second, don't plead or cajole the obstreperous child. If she ducks beneath the table and announces she will not cooperate, we go ahead with the various tasks, using self-talk. Don't reinforce crying or whining by soothing or placating. It is, however, a good practice to distract the child with some interesting task and then praise her attentiveness (Hubbell, 1977).

There are obviously many other considerations that could be discussed; additional suggestions will be offered in the several chapters concerning various disorders. But, for the present, here are several basic precepts on the management of children in a clinical examination:

1. Help the parents prepare the child for the diagnostic session. It is a good idea to call prior to the date of the examination and provide the parents with information about the experience. Suggest that they tell the child he will be going to a special school where he will look at pictures and play games of various sorts. If the parents report that their child is particularly shy, ask them to bring along his favorite toy or stuffed animal.
2. Play, rather than small talk, is the natural medium of expression for children. Try to arrange the diagnostic tasks with this in mind.

3. As a general rule, ask less and observe more. Children usually lack the insight and cooperation necessary to analyze their problem rationally and objectively. Naturalistic observations—assessing a child's behavior in his own environment—yields more useful information.[2]

4. The prospective diagnostician should learn everything possible about normal children in order to provide a baseline for observations of youngsters presenting problems. This can be done by taking courses, studying relevant norms, but most of all by extensive scrutiny of children in nursery schools and other settings. The prospective diagnostician should have a good idea of the typical or modal behavior for children at various age levels. One student claimed that a four-year-old client was in grave need of psychiatric appraisal and treatment. We remembered the child and were somewhat puzzled by this recommendation. We demanded a rationale. It seems that the child had an imaginary companion, a wrinkled green elephant that served as a scapegoat and alter ego. We chuckled and then sent the student scurrying to the Gesell profiles to see how common such fantasies are in four-year-olds.

5. Limit the choices you offer a child. Don't ask if he would like to go with you, do this or that, unless the alternatives do not conflict with the examiner's goals. He will invariably say no and you will be left with egg on your face.

6. Be flexible in your use of tests and examinations. If you cannot employ the rigid standardized format for administration, use the test to obtain all the data you can. If the child refuses to name the pictures and objects, you might be able to get a language sample from the items he has in his pockets.

7. Absolute honesty and candor is important in working with children. Don't make promises unless you can keep them. Children function better knowing the truth than they do with mystery, dread, or uncertainty. For obvious reasons, the examiner should avoid sarcasm, idiomatic expressions, ambiguous statements, and indirect requests (Blue, 1981).

8. Children relate very well to animals, and the clinician might consider having a hamster, rabbit, or an affectionate dog in the examining room. Puppets—or better, Muppets from "Sesame Street"—are also very useful in establishing a relationship with a young child.

9. The whole assessment does not have to be done in one session; marathon diagnostics tend to be counterproductive. Remember that all we can hope to obtain in one time frame is a sample of a child's behaviors. It is better to terminate (if possible, on a light, pleasant note) than to continue an unproductive session.

10. You should keep in mind that parents are people, too, not just vehicles to assist diagnosis or carry out therapy.

Adolescents. Experienced clinicians frequently report that adolescents—the classical teenagers, especially in grades 7 through 11—are often difficult to examine and resistant to therapy. The main problem seems to be getting through to the person. There is no magic formula for this, but we would like to make some suggestions that we have found helpful in guiding our work with adolescent clients:

1. Acquire an understanding of the myriad pressures and changes the teenager is experiencing: rapid physical growth, sexual maturity, conflicts between

[2] The observation tool prepared by Russo and Owens (1982) is useful for charting ongoing parent-child interaction.

dependence and independence, the development of self-confidence and inter-personal skills necessary to make decisions, definition of a new ego ideal, a search for identity and life work, intense group loyalty and identification, and many more. It is a turbulent, trying period of behavioral extravagance and excess. Small wonder that teenagers are often overloaded with personal concerns and do not always welcome an overture of clinical assistance. Empathy that flows from understanding is a powerful force in establishing a working relationship.

2.  There is an intense desire to be like others, not to stand out from the group in any way that would suggest frailty. Hence the adolescent will find it extremely difficult to reveal a speech impairment, even if he does want help. Often he is simply *sent* to treatment. In some instances, the teenager with a chronic problem may have been in therapy for a long time and is weary of continued treatment. He will tend to cover up his true feelings with a sullen bravado or a dense "it-doesn't-bother-me" shell. Denial is his particular forte. "Coolness" and image are very important. You can neither beat this down nor simply dismiss the individual with a shrug. Nor is silence a particularly effective tool in dealing with adolescent resistance. We advocate a straightforward approach: acknowledge the forces that are bearing on the individual; point up objectively the paths that others have taken; provide information about the economic and social penalties that accrue to the speech-defective person (have him talk to older clients). The young client may need more time to become accustomed to the idea of therapy. Basically, try to demonstrate by your demeanor and what you say that you care about him: A growing ego needs lots of nourishment; personal involvement and commitment are key factors.[3]

3.  Don't try to "swing" with teenage clients; empathy is not identification. Don't abandon your professional role for that of a teenager. Be yourself. As Will Rogers pointed out, if they don't like you the way you are, they are sure not going to like you the way you are trying to be:

    One public school clinician had a painful experience in learning to maintain her role and status as adult therapist. While waiting one day for a fourth member of a therapy group to arrive, she attempted to enter a rap session with three teenage males. She wanted to know the meanings of several "in" words, but the boys demurred and looked rather curiously at her. She responded by saying, "Look, teenagers want to know all about the adult world, right? So, turnabout is fair play, why shouldn't I learn about yours?" One of the bolder adolescents suggested that they were becoming adults and thus they needed to know—but was the clinician going to be a teen?

4.  Approach adolescents with tolerance and good humor. Don't be shocked or annoyed by their overstatements and superlatives; don't overreact to expressions of hostility or tempests of other emotions. Sometimes they will, in order to uphold their protective armor, resort to all sorts of strategies to confuse, defeat, or anger the clinician. The ability to laugh at yourself and to use humor in a gentle, needling manner is an asset. Remember, though, to always treat the adolescent with dignity—don't make fun of his intense and idealistic views. Young people typically are hopeful that they can change the world for the better: How could you use this trait in treatment?

5.  Talk person-to-person, not station-to-station (Ginott, 1969). Respond to the *individual,* not to the *group* of which he is a member. Try to describe rather

---

[3]The bibliography of juvenile literature depicting the communicatively impaired individual prepared by Tatelbaum (1984) may be useful dealing with adolescent resistance.

than judge. Avoid commenting about long hair, (sometimes outrageous) costumes, slouching posture, and so forth.

6. Demonstrate your competence and confidence to deal with the person and his problem. We like to do this by explaining what we are about, the reasons for the various tests and examinations, how we will use the information, and the process of checking out our hypotheses. However, don't be a know-it-all or talk about the obvious in the voice of adult mystery. We encourage the adolescent to challenge and question what we are doing. Finally, we usually give him an idea of the route we would follow when therapy commences; we enumerate the steps and even do some trial therapy.

7. Avoid the teacher image as much as you can. Unfortunately, many of our schools are more concerned with keeping order than with learning or with human relationships. Teacher is always right in some schools. We eschew this image by our style of interaction, by keeping the person's confidences, by listening to him when he complains about a teacher or a course. We don't enter into the criticism or side with the client against the school, nor do we try to defend the institution or retreat to moralisms.

8. When praise is offered, make it specific rather than general. Tell him that you like how he persisted on a particular diagnostic task rather than simply saying he is a good worker.

9. Discuss the results of the evaluation with the client before talking with the parents or school personnel. Be sure to let him know exactly what you intend to tell his parents and teachers (we sometimes make audiotapes of parents' conferences so the teenage client can check on our veracity).

These recommendations have been distilled from our clinical experience and are not presented as magical touchstones for all diagnosticians or all clients; nor do they represent the full range of possibilities for successful interaction with teenage clients. We present them here to provoke other workers to develop clinical generalizations on the basis of their experience (O'Connor and Eldredge, 1981).

HIGHLIGHT   *The Elderly Client*

Older clients present some rather special problems for the diagnostician. Although the concept of "elderly" is relative, we refer here to persons in their sixties or older. A word of caution: Although there are certain generalizations that are useful for planning and conducting evaluations, elderly people are not any more "all alike" than are children or adolescents.

The clinician should be alert to fatigue, disorientation, failing eyesight, and hearing loss. With advanced age, the person may find it more difficult to focus his attention on a task, and he generally has trouble remembering directions because of short-term memory decline. We need, therefore, to explain each step of our clinical procedures at greater length and repeat instructions several times to insure understanding. Our pace should be geared down, if necessary, to the client's slower level. Organize the testing sequence carefully to reduce distractions, noise, or interference. Older people are more cautious and have a greater need to be certain before they respond, so adapt the tasks with this in mind; following standard procedure may not be as important as providing an environment in which the person is able to perform at his optimum level. Since many older clients tend to feel useless and discarded in our youth-oriented culture, and resentful that their bodies are betraying them, we may find it important to spend some time listening to their memories of past achievements.

As with children and adolescents, the diagnostician should know as much as possible about aging. Here are a few references to help you begin a study of communication disorders in the elderly:

BEASLEY, D., and G. DAVIS, eds. (1981). *Aging and Communication.* Baltimore: University Park Press.
COWLEY, M. (1980). *The View from 80.* New York: Viking.
DANCER, J., and W. THOMAS (1983). "Beyond the Boundaries." *Journal of the American Speech and Hearing Association,* 25: 25-30.
LEUTENEGGER, R. (1975). *Patient Care and Rehabilitation of Communication-Impaired Adults.* Springfield, Ill.: Chas. C Thomas.
MOORE, J., and D. SHERMAN (1981). "Special Considerations with the Elderly Patient." *Journal of Communication Disorders,* 14: 299-309.
MUELLER, R., and T. PETERS (1981). "Needs and Services in Geriatric Speech-Language Pathology and Audiology." *Journal of the American Speech and Hearing Association,* 23:627-632.
NATIONAL COUNCIL ON AGING (1982). *Service-Learning in Aging: Implications for Speech, Language and Hearing.* Washington, D.C.: National Council on Aging.
OYER, H., and E. OYER, eds. (1976). *Aging and Communication.* Baltimore: University Park Press.
SCHOW, R., et al. (1979). *Communication Disorders of the Aged.* Baltimore: University Park Press.
WALKER, S., and B. WILLIAMS (1980). "The Response of a Disabled Elderly Population to Speech Therapy." *British Journal of Disorders of Communication,* 15: 19-29.

For additional information concerning aging, write to these agencies:

Communication Disorders of the Aging
American Speech-Language-Hearing Association
10801 Rockville Pike
Rockville, Md. 20852

National Council on Aging, Inc.
600 Maryland Avenue S.W.
Washington, D.C. 20024

The clinician should recognize and have under control her own ambivalence toward growing old. Let us state it more forcefully: The number of people over sixty composes a significant proportion of the population, and we cannot afford to perpetuate the stereotype that old people are expendable, that they should be relegated to demeaning idleness. In fact, the diagnostician must often determine the attitudes and opportunities existing in the elderly person's environment, whether it is an institution or a personal residence, and the possibility that the person may live in a communication-impaired environment (Lubinski, Morrison, and Rigrodsky, 1981).

*The factor of sex.*   In what manner does the sex of the diagnostician influence the clinicial examination and testing situation? Do young children relate better to female clinicians? Do adolescent boys feel more comfortable, and hence more able to reveal information about themselves, with male diagnosticians? We know of no scientific basis on which we can answer these questions, and no doubt it is often a highly individual matter. However, in our own practice, in the supervision of student clinicians and extensive consultation with colleagues working in various settings, we have observed several principles at work:

1. Female clients of all ages, with the possible exception of adolescents, seem to experience little difficulty with a male diagnostician. This might be the product of countless experiences with male dentists and physicians.
2. Adolescent females, girls in the process of becoming women physically and psychologically, seem to be more comfortable and open with a female clinician; likewise, male adolescents seem to work better with male clinicians.
3. Female clinicians of college age sometimes find it difficult to maintain a clinicial context when performing diagnostic examinations on men of the same age level. College-level male clinicians may experience some of the same difficulties in diagnosis with female students.

Obviously, the factors of age and sex are interrelated in a complex manner in the clinical relationship. We do know that the interpersonal context does influence the *kinds* of responses clients will give to various tasks; it also may influence the *amount* and *style* of response. Men talking together assume a rather distinct verbal style (the "locker room" set) as do women (the "bridge club" set). Since clinicians can do little about their sex at this point, they should inspect their value systems to see that this particular facet does not become obtrusive in the clinical setting.

*The work setting.*   Ideally, the speech clinician performs her professional role as she has been trained to do, regardless of where she works. However, diagnosticians working in schools often report several difficulties: (1) The speech clinician is identified in the child's mind with the teachers, some of whom may be penalizing or disturbing listeners. In addition, the clinician may find herself identified with authority figures, and this hampers the development of a clinical relationship. (2) The type of diagnostic regimen best suited for the client may be difficult to implement within the school. (3) The child usually has no choice about entering the examining situation; he is brought for diagnosis by his parents, referred by a teacher, or is "screened out" by the speech clinician. (4) It seems more difficult to secure active parental participation when children are seen in school. Some parents are suspicious of the authority that a school represents; they may harbor resentment for alleged bad treatment when they attended school. Inherent in this is the natural resistance manifested by many persons toward official institutions of government. The clinician may find that she has been tarred by the same brush and may be unable to obtain the cooperation of some parents.

Some clinicians, however, give up too easily; with a resigned shrug, they suggest that it is impossible to do careful, thorough diagnostics in the schools with the heavy caseload requirements. But *the nature of the child's problem, not the characteristics of the work setting,* dictates the nature of the clinician's responsibility. The needs of the client, not the arbitrary and often antiquated state codes or educational policies of the school, should and must determine the scope of the speech clinician's professional activities. To be accorded professional treatment, one must behave as a professional. The hallmark of professionalism is doing what needs to be done for the good of the client. A clinician's responsibilities do not end when the last school bell rings.

The ideal (seldom achieved) setting for conducting an evaluation is, most importantly, physically and psychologically comfortable. Many examining facilities we have seen unfortunately reflect an austere, clinical aura—banks of fluorescent lights, large mirrors, microphones, videotape cameras, sterile decor. In our experience, rooms furnished with soft chairs, end tables, table lamps, and tastefully decorated create a zone of comfort and safety; thus, they are conducive to self-revelation and exploration. The rooms should be free of distractions—noise, clutter, intrusions—and the diagnostic facility should provide an efficient working space for the clinician.

We have attempted to show how three factors—age, sex, and work setting—influence the clinical examination. There are no doubt many other conditions that also impinge: the timing of the diagnostic examination should coincide with the individual's readiness for help; the manner of referral; and idiosyncratic aspects such as the motives and fantasies of some clients. Additional comments will be presented in the discussion on test selection.

## THE SELECTION OF TESTS

There are many diagnostic instruments to assess all aspects of a client and his communication abilities. Thus, it becomes a matter of critical selection among the diverse tests available. What factors are employed in making a selection? In addition to such obvious criteria as the purposes of the evaluation, the amount of time available, the nature of the client's presenting problem, the client's age and level of intelligence, the constraints of the setting, and the diagnostician's training, the following factors should be considered:

1. Does the test provide information that cannot be obtained by interviewing or by less structured observation? All diagnostic instruments cause a certain amount of stress to the client; if it is feasible within reasonable time limits to obtain data by indirect means, then the clinician should be wary of using the test. We find that observation of ongoing behavior affords us a better idea of a child's typical behavior (what he usually does) than do many formal tests that assess abilities (what he can do in maximum performance). It must be stressed, however, that both observation and test information are hypothetical constructs that provide only samples of the client's total repertoire.

2. Is it possible to convey the instructions without lengthy and complicated explanations? The more intricate the introduction to a task, the greater the possibility that a client's errors in performance are an artifact of the instructions.

3. Is the test relatively easy to administer and score? Some diagnostic instruments are so complicated that unless used daily, the clinician may forget how to administer them. Complexity in a diagnostic tool does not necessarily correlate with precision or validity. Further, it is important to keep in mind the purpose of testing: Beyond a certain point, precision is meaningless and clinically irrelevant.

4. Is the test economical in terms of the client's time and energy? Is it efficient? How much time does it consume relative to the quality and quantity of data obtained?

5. Are the theoretical constructs upon which the test is constructed congruent with the examiner's beliefs? It is difficult to use an instrument clinically unless the examiner is convinced of its explanatory adequacy.

6. Does the test permit objective scoring? Although the important decisions, clinically as well as scientifically, are judgmental, the basis for making the judgments is sounder to the degree that human bias is at least identified and, hopefully, limited. Is the test standardized—are the procedures and materials fixed so that, regardless of where or by whom a client is evaluated, the same methodology can be employed?

7. Will the test actually make a difference in solving the person's problem? Is it practical in the sense that the results lead logically to a program of treatment?

8. Does the test suggest to the client that he might have additional problems? A diagnostic procedure should not be iatrogenic. The inadequacy of some attitude scales and personality inventory scales is such that the respondent can recognize the acceptable and the nonacceptable answers.

9. Does the test violate the client's integrity? We would not use a picture-naming test of articulation with adult clients; some violations are less obvious: Perhaps there should be a bill of rights for adult aphasics; more ill-considered activities have been used with them than with almost any other group of persons with communication handicaps. Many of the tasks on widely used language inventories are patently infantilizing—they rather blatantly impugn the client's mental status.

10. Does the diagnostic instrument permit the development of clearly defined and reportable concepts regarding the client and his communication disability? Does the test yield clinically relevant descriptive information about the person's problem?

11. Is the instrument reliable? Does it give consistent measures when administered repeatedly to the same client? Do separate examiners arrive at the same conclusions from this instrument when making independent judgments?

12. Is the test valid? Does it test what it says it does? Obviously, an instrument must be reliable—you must evoke the same "something" each time—before it can be valid; for example, if every time we said "corn" a client responded "tree," he would be reliable but consistently wrong. There are several types of validity: content validity (how well does the test *sample*—all tests obtain only a sample, not a parameter or whole—the particular aspect in which we are interested?); predictive validity (how well does the test predict performance?); concurrent validity (how well does the test data we have check with other evidence available?); and construct validity (how well does the test

show or reflect some trait, quality, or construct presumed to underlie perfor-mance on the test?).

13. In what manner was the test standardized? What types of norms are set forth and on what population are they based? Is it "fair" to give a measure of ver-bal intelligence, based on suburban, middle-class vocabulary, to an Ojibway Indian child? *Norm-referenced* tests compare an individual's behavior to that of others of the same age, sex, socioeconomic level, etc. *Criterion-referenced* tests, on the other hand, delineate the contents of an individual's perfor-mance. How well established is a particular behavior?

Space limitations do not permit a review and analysis of the many diagnostic instruments available. The reader will want to consult the work of Cronbach (1960) and that of others (Buros, 1978; Darley, 1979; Salvia and Ysseldyke, 1981; Barnes, 1982; McCauley and Swisher, 1984) for a comprehensive discussion of psychometric testing and a compendium of measurement devices in print. We now turn to a review of possible dangers involved in testing persons with communication disorders.

## DANGERS IN TESTING

At some point in the future, the speech and hearing clinician might have a massive diagnostic computer system for rapidly assessing speech and language disorders. Into the maw of this marvelous machine, the diagnostician will feed certain key signs, and error-free diagnosis, with suggestions for remediation, will emerge follow-ing a short wait. But, alas, this is a mythical beast, at least for the present. We must rely on the fragile magic of human perception.

It is axiomatic that no testing device or examination procedure is any better than the person who administers it. *The efficacy of an evaluation rests on the calibration of the diagnostician.* A test is merely a systematic way for obtaining, describing, and comparing a sample of behavior under rather structured conditions; every test was once a system for observing clients that one person had in mind. Tests are tools, after all, and can be used wisely or foolishly. In this section, we focus on some of the dangers involved in using tests: overtesting, undertesting, and other assorted dangers.

### Overtesting

Many clinicians employ a shotgun approach to diagnosis. They administer several tests and collect a plethora of data on the assumption that quantity is the key issue—the more information they have, the more likely they are to have some-thing relevant. This type of procedure is especially evident in some training pro-grams where the unfortunate client is poked and prodded in the interest of clinical experience. We do not favor the battery concept of assessment: Each diagnostic procedure should have a rationale, a clearly stated goal or hypothesis.

The worst aspect of overtesting is the tendency to fragment the patient into a series of clinical artifacts and, in the process of sorting out the scores and profiles, to lose his unique wholeness. It is possible to become engrossed in test scores and forget our mission. A test score is simply an estimate of a client's performance under a particular set of conditions—it is not a fixed trait. *We may overlook the person for the percentiles.*

Overdependence on the process of testing and test scores may prevent us from seeing important clues about the person and her life situation. By placing too much emphasis on the formal diagnostic instruments we can ignore how the client and her family see the problem.

Another danger, also a form of overtesting, is delaying treatment. The structure afforded by the administration of various diagnostic instruments does provide a sense of security to the clinician.

Finally, because diagnosis and treatment are part of the same continuous process, we should carefully consider how tests may structure relationships in an undesirable way. Extensive test batteries may lead the client to suspect that his problem will be handled in a detached and authoritative manner.

### Undertesting

We certainly do not mean to imply that testing is bad or has only a minor role in the diagnostic encounter. In fact, we advocate the judicious use of diagnostic instruments to help determine *if* a problem exists and the *extent* of the problem. When a clinician employs a standardized test, it enhances the precision and reliability of the findings.

Grave errors may also be committed by not having sufficient information on a given client. Many clinicians who work in schools operate as if they have made a diagnosis when they state that a child has a frontal lisp; this is a description—and a superficial one at that—not a diagnosis. It is certainly not the basis for a therapeutic program.

Consider the child who was enrolled in speech therapy year after year for a "simple" functional disorder of articulation. More extensive assessments revealed sensory problems, mild motor impairments, psychological conflicts, and other learning disabilities—all hiding behind the "simple lisp" label. The ubiquitous diagnosis of "functional articulation problem" may result from insufficient scrutiny of the client. Obviously, then, a very real danger in undertesting is the fact that you may well overlook something serious if you do not investigate beneath the obvious. Also, you will not have enough information to convey in reports to experts in the field when you want to refer a client; perhaps you may not even know when there is a need for referral.

### Assorted Dangers

In addition to the polar dangers of over- and undertesting, there are several other possible risks involved in the use of tests. They are all interrelated:

*The client's participation.* No diagnostic procedure is a one-way street; if the client cannot or does not participate in the testing to the level required—because of attitudes, moods, personal background—the results may be spurious. We are, in a very real sense, at the mercy of the respondent's cooperation. The relationship with the client is critical. What is the client's frame of reference for the testing situation? Does he consider it a threat, a challenge, a silly adult game? Does he feel anxious or manipulated? Some highly structured tests are so formal that a clinical relationship is strained; the style in which the tasks are administered tend to make the client feel uncomfortable, inhibited, even ridiculous. We must remember always to consider the test results in light of the person's total behavior.

*The competence of the examiner.* The prospective diagnostician should be thoroughly familiar with a diagnostic instrument before she attempts to administer it. The test manual should be carefully studied and several trial attempts with normal-speaking individuals completed before assessing a client.

*The magic of tests.* Some clients feel that a test will do something for them; once the test has been administered, someone will be able to figure out the exact cause of their problem and pinpoint a solution. Tests, thus, often raise false hopes.

*The mean scores.* Most diagnostic instruments have tables for interpreting given scores obtained; these norms are generally based on the average performance of a large number of subjects. Hence, their application to a given individual is problematical.[4]

*The presumption of the test.* Some tests are contraindicated because they presume normal speech and hearing. Their application to clients with communication problems is suspect:

> Our favorite aphasic client, perhaps our all-time favorite client, was Charles S. Hanford. Following a thrombotic stroke, with resultant auditory aphasia, his employer demanded a psychological appraisal, fearful of the possibility of brain damage. Mr. Hanford was taken by his wife to a local clinical psychologist, who gave him a comprehensive intelligence measure. The psychologist, although noting the aphasia, did not modify the test instrument. He made recommendations on the basis of the test results, including an IQ score of 54, which was remarkable in terms of Mr. Hanford's degree of auditory aphasia at the time. The client's wife was told that "he had suffered extensive brain damage, would be unable to work or drive again [he had no paralysis] and would not be able to make judgments with regard to family finances, etc." When Mr. Hanford eventually learned of this, he was furious. In retribution for the psychologist's actions, he paid the twenty-five dollar fee in quarters and other small change over an interval of eighteen months, always demanding a receipt and always indicating that if the psychologist left town he would immediately pay his bill in full.

[4] Gutnick and St. John (1982) offer a model for predicting when average or mean differences meet the minimum requirements for generalization to individual clients.

*Looking where the light is.*   The joke about the drunken man looking for his lost watch under the bright illumination of a street light rather than in the darkened alley where it was lost applies to the way some clinicians use tests. They have a pet instrument that they apply willy-nilly to each client without regard to his particular needs.

*Following the fads.*   It is very difficult to identify the beginning and end of a particular fad or intellectual *Zeitgeist* when you are in the middle of it. There are some workers who make a total commitment to one way of assessing and talking about a particular communication impairment and cannot change to meet the needs of a client who does not fit the mold of the test in vogue. In fact, some clinicians focus narrowly on a particular test, not on the client; instead of using the instrument as a tool, they defer to it as their master. We urge you not to abrogate your responsibility for exercising clinical judgment with respect to test results. A test *describes* certain aspects of behavior, but it does not *explain* the level of performance.

*Hardening of the categories.*   Following the fads can easily lead to that dread clinical disorder "hardening of the categories." This involves being able to see behavior only through well-worn perceptual grooves with regard to identification and classification of clients and their responses.

With all these possible pitfalls it is easy to see why some impressionistic diagnosticians, the artisans described in Chapter 1, eschew formal tests. Many of these individuals feel that tests tend to traumatize clients. There is little hard evidence that this has to be true. Indeed, Schuell, Jenkins, and Jimenez-Pabon (1964: 159–176) observe that when the tasks are presented in the spirit of mutual exploration, they can be factors in correcting misapprehensions and misinformation. This is to say that a diagnostic session can be therapeutic; the client explores himself and the dimensions of his problem with the objective support of the clinician. The unknown begins to take on limits and definition; the client is no longer faced with a global failure. Testing can and should reveal the client's strengths as well as weaknesses.

## PROGNOSIS

Prognosis may be defined as a prediction of the outcome of a proposed course of treatment for a given client: how effective therapy will be, how far we can expect the client to progress, and perhaps, how long it will take. Inasmuch as diagnosis is a continuing process, prognosis should, like therapy planning, have both long-range and immediate facets. Immediate prognosis covers what the person can do now, what steps in therapy are possible, what is the best route to take. Prognosis for specific communication disorders will be discussed in subsequent chapters; in this section we will present some generic purposes and a possible danger involved in predicting a client's response to therapy.

The basic purpose in making a prognosis is to economize our therapeutic efforts. There is only so much time and energy, and we must focus it on those clients who show the greatest promise of improvement. This seems to be difficult for speech clinicians to do. Perhaps because we are such a young profession, we feel we must help all clients; we try too hard and hate to give up even when the client is plainly signaling that he has had enough:

> Mrs. Bachman was sixty-nine and had global aphasia. In addition to a severe cerebral vascular episode, she was hypertensive and diabetic. The speech clinician had been seeing the client for several weeks before she asked for our consultation. We examined the individual thoroughly and, in our judgment, decided that it would be better to work out patterns of communication with her environment (the end result of therapy is not always speech). We advised that Mrs. Bachman's husband should be shown how to provide language stimulation and that the medical social worker should be consulted with regard to family readjustment. The clinician demurred and continued to work with the client, maintaining that she saw a certain something in Mrs. Bachman's eyes that would not allow her to "give up." One later session which we observed entailed the repetition of the phrase, "I wear a size 34C bra" at least twenty-three times by actual count. Not only is that a phrase that would be rather difficult to fit into a conversation, its use suggested to the physician and other members of the treatment team that the clinician was not employing good professional judgment in her insistence on not terminating therapy.

Prognosis also provides direction for treatment; we must know where we are going so that we will know when we have arrived. Some predictive factors are specific to a particular speech or language disability and will be discussed in the appropriate chapters. There are, however, a number of general factors that the clinician must consider when making predictions: the client's age, habit-strength, the existence of other problems, the type and intensity of reactions from significant persons in the client's environment, the client's motivation, and secondary gains the client may derive from the problem.

Accurate prognoses can help establish our credibility with other professions. The ability to predict with reasonable precision is perhaps the highest form of scientific achievement. Needless to say, however, these predictions should be based on something more than clinical intuition. Impressionistic conclusions, especially when made by experienced workers, can often be startlingly accurate, but they should always be labeled as impressionistic: A prognosis should be supported by a substantial amount of information.

In what sense might a prognosis be dangerous? We have become suspicious of what these predictions can do to our therapeutic interaction with the client; we are becoming increasingly convinced that the clinician's expectations regarding the case's potential influence the treatment program. It is certainly possible that our negative prognoses can be communicated to a client and affect the course of therapy.

## SOME TESTS AND EXAMINATION PROCEDURES
## COMMON TO MANY DIAGNOSTIC UNDERTAKINGS

A number of tests and examination procedures are clinically useful regardless of the client's particular communication impairment. In order to avoid repetition in the chapters that follow, these commonly utilized assessment techniques are discussed here; in the chapters dealing with the various disorders, we shall present diagnostic procedures that are pertinent to the specific speech problem.

### The Oral Peripheral Examination

It is a common practice to inspect a client's oral structures to determine their structural and functional adequacy for speech. To provide an example of typical data gathered during an oral peripheral examination, we have included notes hastily scribbled during an evaluation of a nine-year-old boy with a hoarse voice and several articulation errors:

> Lips look okay. No asymmetry of face. Slight open bite; poor dental hygiene (lots of cavities and tarter buildup). Tongue has good mobility, no paralysis or sluggishness; can protrude, wiggle from side to side swiftly, and touch the alveolar ridge; can even curl and groove. Hard palate seems OK, no scars. Soft palate has good tissue supply; elevates fine, no asymmetry. Palatine tonsils are *really* enlarged, filling the whole isthmus between the fauces. Pharynx looks inflamed (possible postnasal drip?). Good gag reflex. Wonder why he has mandible thrust to left side on /sh/ and /ch/?

Note the systematic nature of the inspection. Although the period of observation was relatively brief—an oral examination is generally completed in less than two minutes—the clinician has a sound basis for making a referral to a laryngologist. Now we shall present a rather detailed procedure for conducting an oral examination.

*Tools you will need.*    You will need a light source; a small flashlight is good (we avoid the head mirror because it make us look like a physician). Next, obtain a supply of plain applicator sticks. We dislike tongue depressors because of their association with doctors; in addition they are so blunt they do not permit evaluation of point-to-point sensitivity in the oral area. If you do use tongue depressors, the individually wrapped ones are best for sanitary purposes (it is curious that no one has yet invented a flavored tongue blade). Finally, your kit might include several pads of cotton gauze (for holding onto tongues), a few candy suckers, and a mirror.

*How to get into a small child's mouth.*    Most older children and adults will open their mouths on request. Small children, however, are sometimes rather reluctant to let the clinician examine their tongue and teeth:

Jimmy cooperated, cautiously but willingly, in all the diagnostic tasks until the clinician brought out a tongue depressor. He clamped his little jaw shut in bulldog fashion and tears began to form in the corners of his huge brown eyes. The clinician unwrapped the wooden blade and produced a small pen light, chatting amiably all the time. "Let me see, here is my mirror. I wonder if that little black dot is still on the back of my tongue. Hmmmm. Only three boys have ever seen it. . . ." (The clinician opened his mouth and looked intently with light and mirror.) Then, turning to Jimmy, the clinician requested, "Say, can you help me find that black dot? It's way on the back of my tongue. That's right, here's the flashlight." Jimmy, curious now, looked cautiously into the clinician's mouth. The clinician giggled and suggested he look further back. "I taw it, I taw it," Jimmy said triumphantly. "Hmm. You did? Say, I wonder if . . . no, I bet you don't . . . but maybe you do, maybe you have a black dot, too?" suggested the clinician. The child handed the light to the clinician and opened his mouth, erasing a small grin.

There is another method we have used, which, although slightly indelicate, is more universally effective:

Children are engrossed with magic and guessing games. We make a wager—some small token will do—that he cannot guess what we had for breakfast (or lunch). Then, after he scrutinizes our oral cavity and makes a guess, we agree, with shocked surprise at his wizardry. Now we ponder aloud what he might have had for the most recent meal. Generally, their mouths pop open like baby starlings. Our first guess is usually something outlandish (like sardines and Bermuda onions) which provokes much mirth and a chance to look and guess again.

With some especially shy children or those for whom the oral examination conjures vivid memories of past trauma, we have used another technique. It may take more time, but children almost always like to play follow-the-leader games. Using a large mirror so that we can see each other, we go through a series of comical movements of our arms, legs, and torso. Gradually we shift the focus of movement to our head, using our eyes and lips. Finally, we open our mouths and make weird movements with our tongue. The children usually follow in this "play," and we end up peering into each other's mouth before the glass.

*What to look for.*  It is important to be *systematic* and *swift* when conducting an oral examination. This demands considerable practice. Use every opportunity to scrutinize normal-speaking persons, not only to perfect your technique and observational skills but also to establish a frame of reference on the range of structural and functional variation. The following outline is presented as a guide for conducting oral peripheral examinations:[5]

[5]Laryngoscopic examination is the professional responsibility of the physician. The speech pathologist usually describes breathing patterns and examines the external musculature of the larynx for tension, but an assessment of the vocal folds must be undertaken by a laryngologist.

1. Lips and lip movement: Inspect the lips first for relative size, symmetry, and scars. Can the client smile, pucker his lips, and retract them? Can he close his lips tightly for the sounds /p/, /b/, and /m/? Can he utter the nonsense syllable "puh" at least once per second (Fletcher, 1972)?

2. Jaws: Scrutinize the client's jaws in a state of rest; observe for symmetry. Can he open and close his mandible at least once per second? Does his mandible deviate to the right or left on opening? Assess mandibular strength by having him attempt to open or move his jaw laterally against resistance.

3. Teeth: Inspect the client's bite during a state of rest. A normal dental bite is characterized by the upper incisors overlapping the lower incisors by not more than one half of their vertical dimension. Is there an open, under-, or overbite? Does the client have cavities, jumbled teeth, gaps between teeth, or more than the normal complement of teeth? Does he wear a dental prosthesis?

4. The tongue: Note the size of the tongue relative to the oral cavity. Observe for symmetry in structure and during movement. Is there scarring, atrophy, or fasiculations? Can the client protrude and retract his tongue, wiggle it from side to side, and touch the alveolar ridge without random movement or extraordinary effort? Inspect the tip of tongue and the frenulum for any evidence of tongue tie. Some children, especially those presenting neuro-muscular problems, may find it difficult to elevate the tip of their tongue to the alveolar ridge on command. We use a sucker, placing the moistened candy behind the upper incisors and encouraging the child to go after it. A spot of peanut butter or a tiny paper wedged high between the central incisors can also be used. Can he trill his tongue when the mandible is stabilized? Test for diadochokinesis by having him utter "tuh"; can he say one per second? Norms for diadochokinesis may be found in Fletcher (1972) and elsewhere (Bloomquist, 1950; Canning and Rose, 1974). Be sure to look for regularity as well as rate in any tongue movement task. Is there any evidence of tongue thrust? (An open bite might alert you to this possibility.) When he swallows does he have an exaggerated lip seal? Does his tongue protrude beyond the incisors? Is there no apparent bunching in the masseter? If the answers to these last three queries are positive, then the client may be a tongue thruster.

5. Hard palate: Note the shape (is it flat? high and arched?) and width of the hard palate. Are there any scars present? Can the client produce /r/ and /l/? One public school clinician noted that three of his cases with persistent /r/ defects had rather high and arched hard palates. He experimented with several materials (bubble gum and peanut butter were consumed too swiftly) to re-duce the palatal height; finally, in cooperation with a local dentist, he made prosthetic devices of denture material. All three children began to make the elusive /r/ with their devices. The dentist gradually shaved off the structures. The cases' tongues were thus coaxed higher and higher until they were making the /r/ on their own hard palates.

6. Soft palate and velopharyngeal closure: Inspect the velum for size, scars, and symmetry. Look carefully for any variations in color, such as bluish borders or striations. Does the soft palate move back and up toward the posterior pharyngeal wall? What is the size of the velum relative to the depth of the pharynx? Can you visualize lateral movement of the velum? Can the client whistle or puff up her cheeks?[6]

---

[6]Individuals presenting nasal vocal quality or nasal emission will require more extensive evaluation of their velopharyngeal competency. See Chapter 8.

7. Fauces: Inspect the pillars for scars, the status of the palatine tonsils, and the width of the isthmus. Check the general condition of the oropharynx.
8. Others: Observe the client's breathing during speech and at rest. Is there an obstruction of the nasal passages? Is the client a mouth breather? Observe the facial muscles: Is a nasolabial fold flattened; does an eyelid droop (ptosis); is one side of the face smooth and devoid of normal creases? Is there anything unusual about the appearance of the individual's head?

For further information regarding the oral peripheral examination, consult the work of Mason and Simon (1977) and others (Dworkin and Culatta, 1980; St. Louis and Ruscello, 1981; Siegel and Hanlon, 1983). At some point in the not too distant future, the diagnostician may have instruments that measure tongue and lip movements very precisely (Porter and Lubka, 1980; Barlow and Abbs, 1983). Remember, though, one swallow does not make a summer, and one deviancy in the oral area does not necessarily cause disordered speech.

### Motor Abilities

During the oral examination the diagnostician may observe disturbances in the client's gross and fine motor abilities that suggest possible neurological dysfunction. Although the diagnostic appraisal of motor dysfunction is the responsibility of the neurologist, the speech clinician should have a basis for making intelligent referrals. This can be accomplished by comparing various facets of the client's motor performance with norms corresponding to his age level.

A public school clinician referred Steve Munroe to us with the following note:

"Steve is almost unintelligible. . . . His whole pattern of articulation seems uncontrolled and bizarre. Although he is nearly thirteen, he is only in the sixth grade and that's where the problem lies. Unless we can show, somehow, that he belongs in the orthopedically handicapped room—where he could stay through high school—they will put him in a junior high class for the trainable retarded. Why? Solely on the basis of his score on the Wechsler; although he obtained an IQ of 62, I don't think he is retarded. His articulation is so bad I'm sure he failed the verbal items because the psychometrician could not understand him; and I think his incoordination shot him down on the motor tasks. Anyway, I need help. The physician at the public medical clinic refuses to refer him for a neurological examination; he claims that Steve is clearly retarded and belongs in the trainable room."

We decided to examine Steve in two sessions. We first wanted a global impression of his motor abilities, following the format presented by Wood (1964: 64–71). Here are our notes:

1. General body description. Steve is thin and wiry, has a slightly stooped posture. He appears on the small end of normal in height and weight.
2. Locomotor. His gait is characterized by a slight shuffle, and he seems to drag his right foot slightly. His stance is not broad-based (not wider than his shoulders). Speed and range (distance or extent of excursion) seem restricted and "jerky"; they lack synergy.

3. Balance. He can stand for three seconds on one foot (left) with both arms extended and his eyes closed; he refused to attempt the task with his right foot. He tried to walk forward with one foot directly ahead of another but failed after three steps and refused to try again.

4. Manual dexterity. His copying and drawing attempts are jerky, and he must exert great effort to control a slight intentional tremor in his right arm and hand. He picked up eleven small buttons and put them in a box in seventeen seconds, using his left hand for the task after fumbling for a few seconds with his right.

5. Psychomotor. The tremor in Steve's right hand was more noticeable when we asked him to place a knitting needle through a small plastic loop suspended on a string. There was overflow of movement in the shoulder and upper chest area while he attempted this task. His speech efforts are often grotesque when he attempts to produce certain phonemes, particularly /r/ and /l/; some drooling was observed.

At the end of our first session we tape-recorded Steve reading a standard passage ("My Grandfather"). Later, using the procedures detailed in articles by Darley, Aronson, and Brown (1969a, 1969b), we rated the speech sample on the several dimensions provided by the authors. Our clinical hunch was confirmed; the ratings showed that Steve's performance was startingly identical to the several clusters associated with pseudobulbar palsy (Darley, Aronson, and Brown, 1969b: 483). We are now certain that we had sufficient ammunition to insist upon a neurological referral but, knowing we had to work through the obdurate institutional physician, we wanted our case to be overwhelming. Well aware that medical practitioners are impressed by percentiles and normative comparisons, we administered the Oseretsky Test (Doll, 1964) during our second diagnostic session with Steve. This instrument evaluates motor proficiency by means of age-graded tasks and yields six measures. Here are the results we obtained:

1. General static coordination. Steve failed at the seven-year-old level (he could not balance on tiptoe, bending forward from the hips for ten seconds).

2. Dynamic coordination. He performed at the eight-year level. (This test requires the subject to touch all the fingertips of one hand successively with the thumb of the same hand, beginning with the little finger; it took him five seconds with his left hand and nine seconds with his right.)

3. General dynamic coordination. Steve passed all the items up to the ten-year level on this subtest. (Ten-year test task: given three trials to jump and clap his hands three times while in the air, Steve was successful on his third attempt.)

4. Motor speed. Steve also passed all the age-graded tasks up to the ten-year level. (He was required to make four piles with forty matchsticks in thirty-five seconds for the right hand and forty-five seconds for the left.) He took almost two minutes to complete the task with his right hand but finished in less than forty-five seconds with the left.

5. Simultaneous voluntary movements. Steve had trouble with this subtest, a task that requires simultaneous movements with both limbs. He got up to the eight-year level (tapping the floor rhythmically with his feet, alternating right and left, while at the same time tapping the table

with his fingers in the same rhythm.) He became upset and confused, pounded on the table in anger, and refused to continue.

6. Synkinesis. This subtest requires the subject to perform muscle movements without overflow such as wrinkling the forehead without any other movements at the eight-year level. Steve was tired and refused to do any of the tasks.

We held a formal conference with the physician, reviewed our findings and suggested politely but strongly that, since Steve had never been evaluated by a neurologist, we were sure that the doctor would certainly want conclusive evidence beyond a reasonable doubt before relegating the child to the irreversible category of "trainable." Somewhat defensive at first, the physician eventually concurred and expedited the referral; he even went one step further and enlisted the professional counsel of a physiatrist to direct the planning for a comprehensive, long-range program of rehabilitation for Steve.

Obviously not all of our clients will require such extensive investigation of their motor abilities. The point is, however, that the clinician must be capable of supporting his convictions with data. An emotional appeal—which the public school therapist had tried unsuccessfully in the case of Steve—without carefully prepared evidence serves only to create a rather unprofessional image.

There does seem to be a parallel course of development between acquisition of language and growth of motor skills. For further information concerning the evaluation of motor abilities, see the work of Berry (1980) and Riley (1972). Bruininks (1977) has revised the Oseretsky Test of Motor Proficiency to include a screening battery for children from the ages of four to eighteen; the revised instrument was standardized on 892 subjects and yields age equivalent scores and percentile ranks. Grinker and Sahs (1966), Chusid and McDonald (1967), and Rutter, Graham, and Yule (1976) present extended discussions of the neurological examination.

### Estimates of Development

Experienced clinicians recognize that in order to understand handicapped children, it is absolutely essential to have a thorough working knowledge of normal patterns of growth and behavior. What is typical or modal behavior for a four-year-old? What should he be able to do at this age level? It is possible, of course, to answer these questions in an impressionistic manner *if* the diagnostician has a clear idea of what is normal for various age levels. However, standardized scales devised on the basis of extensive observation of many children provide greater reliability and objectivity. Knobloch and Pasamanick (1974) have prepared a very useful guide for comparing behavior patterns at various age levels, based on the exhaustive research of the Gesell Institute for Child Behavior. When preparing for a diagnostic session with a child, we review the descriptions of characteristic behaviors for that particular age level.

Several checklists and interviewing guides have been devised from the data gathered at the Gesell Institute and from other research dealing with child development. Many clinicians find the Vineland Social Maturity Scale (Doll, 1964) a useful device for assembling information on a child's maturity; the diagnostician does not observe the child directly but rather queries the parents on the youngster's ability to dress and feed himself, his social interaction, and daily activities. The items on the scale are arranged in age categories. For example, here are the six items at the three- to four-year-old level:

1. Walks down stairs one step per tread.
2. Plays cooperatively at the kindergarten level.
3. Buttons coat or dress.
4. Helps at little household tasks.
5. "Performs" for others.
6. Washes hands unaided.

Although it is possible to derive a social age and social quotient on the basis of the information obtained in an interview, we often prefer to use the Vineland as a screening device, which affords a way to compare the child's development—at least as perceived by her parents—against normative expectations.

There are several distinct advantages to observing directly the child's perfor-mance instead of relying on an informer. At present several tests (actually checklists for recording behavior, which allow comparison with established norms) are avail-able that permit the clinician to chart the development of a child in age-graded tasks. The *Communicative Evaluation Chart* (Anderson, Miles, and Matheny, 1963), *Verbal Language Development Scale* (Mecham, 1971), and *Sequenced Inventory of Communication Development* (Hedrick, Prather, and Tobin, 1975) concentrate on assessing language development; they are easy to use and do provide the clinician with an objective means of evaluating expressive and receptive verbal language skills. The *Developmental Activities Screening Inventory* (DuBose and Langley, 1977), *Inventory of Early Development* (Brigance, 1978), and a recently developed test, *Assessment in Infancy* (Uzgiris and Hunt, 1983), also include items that assess physical well-being, motor coordination, normal growth and development, visuo-motor perception, and general knowledge and comprehension.

For a practical, clinically useful tool to help detect children with serious developmental delay, we prefer the Denver Developmental Screening Test (Frankenburg and Dodds, 1969). The Denver instrument is very simple to adminis-ter, takes less than twenty minutes to finish, and in its published version, comes complete with all the forms and materials needed. It permits evaluation of the following aspects of a child's functioning: gross motor abilities, fine motor coordi-nation, language development, and personal-social maturation (the ability to perform tasks of self-care and relate to others). Here is a portion of a report we submitted to a family physician regarding Robbie O'Neill, a three-year-old child tentatively diagnosed as autistic:

> The vertical line drawn through the four dimensions represents the child's chronological age (see Figure 3.3). We administered the items through which

FIGURE 3.3 Score sheet for Denver Developmental/Screening Test. (W. Frankenburn and J. Dodds, *Denver Developmental Screening Test.* Copyright 1969; reprinted by permission.)

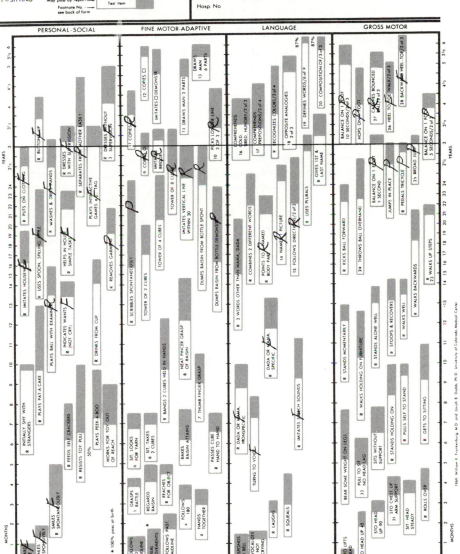

DENVER DEVELOPMENTAL SCREENING TEST

Date 4/27/69
Name Robbie ONeill
Birthdate 2/10/66
Hosp. No.

this line passes in each dimension. On those items Robbie passed, we placed a large letter "P" on the horizontal bar at the midpoint; "F" indicates a failure and an "R" stands for refused. In order to assist you in interpreting the scale, we quote from the Manual (Frankenburg and Dodds, 1969: 7): "Each of the test items is designated by a bar which is so located under the age scale as to indicate clearly the ages at which 25%, 50%, 75%, and 90% of the standardization population could perform the particular test item. The left end of the bar designates the age at which 25% of the standardization population could perform the item; the hatch mark at the top of the bar 50%; the left end of the shaded area 75%; and the right end of the bar the age at which 90% of the standardization population could perform the item. Normal children will generally show a fair amount of scattered successes and failures on items within one area and between the four areas. A *delay* is defined as any failure by a child on an item if he is older than the age at which 90% of the children pass that item. In other words, his vertical chronological age line is to the right of the right end of the bar representing the items he fails."

Robbie appears to be well coordinated in gross motor functioning; even though he refused most of the fine motor tasks, we noted a great degree of manual dexterity (he played almost continually with baby food jars filled with small nails, transferring the nails from one to another). Note that he does not use language in a meaningful way; his parents report only "compulsive" laughter, but no speech per se. Consider also Robbie's responses on the personal-social dimension: he refuses to associate with others and is operating in a very delayed fashion.

Although the speech pathologist is concerned with developmental milestones and patterns of maturation, we quite agree with Berelson and Steiner (1964: 55): "Maturation, by definition, is always a *necessary* condition, but it is not always (strictly speaking, never) a *sufficient* condition; no child can do anything he is not biologically equipped to do, but no child can do everything he *is* biologically capable of."

### Intelligence and Educational Performance

Since the development of speech and language is dependent, in part, on the child's capacity to learn, the speech pathologist is interested in her client's intelligence; many disorders of oral communication stem from low intelligence or inability to utilize an existing level of intelligence. A client's intelligence is also an important consideration in planning therapy.

We like to obtain a general impression of a client's intelligence and, if further testing is indicated, we refer him to a qualified psychometrician. The two most comprehensive measures of intelligence are the *Stanford-Binet Intelligence Scale* (Terman and Merrill, 1960) and the *Wechsler scales* for children (1949, 1967) and adults (1955). These instruments provide a multidimensional profile of an individual's intellectual abilities. The Leiter (1948) and Raven (1948) scales assess only mechanical or performance abilities. Unless the clinician is qualified to administer these tests, he will generally rely on some screening device such as the *Goodenough Draw-a-Man Test* (1926), the *Ammons Full Range Picture Vocabulary Test*

(Ammons and Ammons, 1948), the *Van Alstyne Picture Vocabulary Test* (1960), or the *Peabody Picture Vocabulary Test* (Dunn, 1980). We prefer the latter test because of its ease of scoring and interpretation and the modern stimulus pictures provided. The Peabody Test is really a measure of recognition vocabulary, but it correlates highly with the more comprehensive instruments cited above (Taylor, 1963; Blatt, 1959).

We do not generally report a percentile if the client's performance is within normal limits. If a client's performance is not within normal limits, we usually cite the age level at which he responds:

> Conrad's recognition vocabulary was evaluated with the Peabody Picture Vocabulary Test (Form A). His performance on this scale was characteristic of children two years younger; in terms of auditory recognition, then, Conrad appears to be functioning at a level of six years, or two years below his chronological age.

The Peabody Test is also useful because it allows the examiner to observe the client's behavior on a structured task and to get a feel for how he uses language. We can scrutinize his style of responding, how long he takes to complete the items (latency of response), and how he reacts to failure. Many children comment about the pictures, and the task thus provides another sample of their language output.

We should not give undue importance to one measure of intelligence. This is especially important in dealing with youngsters, as the younger the child, the less reliable is any intellectual assessment. We have also seen wide fluctuations in the tested intelligence of older children that seemed to stem from environmental events. Finally, IQ scores, like all test data, should be related to other sources of information, such as case histories, interviews, direct observation, and, when possible, school performance.

A child's school folder can be a rich source of information regarding her ability to learn and adjust. What scores did she obtain on various achievement tests? How does she go about learning? What are her attitudes toward success and failure in school? What about her abilities in problem solving, reasoning, and identifying relationships? How does she perform in the language skills—spelling and reading in particular? What kinds of things does she perceive as worth working for in the classroom?

### Motivation

Motivation is a critical variable in speech therapy, particularly at the outset of treatment and again during the carry-over phase of therapy. People learn basically what they want to learn. When an individual undertakes to make a significant change in himself, questions regarding desire and drive often emerge. Is change needed? Is it possible? In what direction? To what degree? Will the work and discomfort be worth it? In order to endure the uncertainties of behavioral shift, a client must have positive expectations—hope—that a favorable outcome is likely. A

person's level of motivation obviously is not constant; it will rise and ebb throughout the course of treatment. The assessment of a client's motivation, by means of
testing or impressionistic observation, is then a very useful clinical procedure.

> What is motivation? A motive may be defined as: . . . an inner state that
> energizes, activates, or moves (hence "motivation"), and that directs or chan-
> nels behavior toward goals. (Berelson and Steiner, 1964: 240)

Motivation arouses a person to strive, perform, do better; it also provides
direction and persistence to behavior. Motives may be classified as primary (hunger,
thirst, etc.) or secondary (need for social stimulation or recognition). Maslow
(1943) proposed a hierarchy of human motives ranging from physiological (sleep,
hunger) to psychosocial (love, esteem) and to personal (self-actualization). In his
view, deprivation of motives at the bottom of the scale will dominate the individual's behavior and prevent activity based on motives farther along the hierarchy.
The speech clinician is generally interested in the relative strength of various
secondary or social motives; as an agent or catalyst of change, she is concerned with
how to release the potential for growth. Low motivation is commonly regarded
as a poor prognostic sign; however, if the individual is highly aroused, if he mani-
fests very high motivation, he may not be able to concentrate on the sequence of
treatment. Unfortunately, a client's level of motivation is very difficult to measure
directly.

One widely used means of assessing a client's motivation is to measure his
level of aspiration:

> Bill said he wanted to work on his lateral lisp, but his laconic nature and
> scholastic underachievement belied the fact. In order to assist him in gaining
> insight and provide us with some examples of his typical goal-setting
> behavior, we administered the Cassell Test (1957). This instrument measures
> goal-setting behavior by means of a graphomotor task: The client draws
> squares around circles as swiftly as he can. A four-page booklet consisting of
> eight units with three rows of twenty small squares each is provided. Within a
> specified limit—thirty seconds—Bill attempted to draw the squares. Prior to
> each trial, he was requested to estimate or predict the number of squares he
> felt he could complete in thirty seconds. The Cassell Test yields a "D" score,
> which is the average of the difference between performance and subsequent
> estimate for all test trials. When a client consistently bids higher than his pre-
> vious performance, his "D" score is positive. When he bids lower than his
> previous performance, his "D" score is negative. Here are Bill's scores:

| PREDICTION | PERFORMANCE |
|:---:|:---:|
| 10 | 12 |
| 11 | 14 |
| 12 | 16 |
| 12 | 16 |
| 13 | 16 |

"D" score $= -3.2$. Divide 5 (the number of trials) into 16 (the total discrepancy between prediction and performance).

Normally, individuals tend to have slightly positive discrepancy scores because they balance their idealistic aspirations against realistic expectations of attainment. As a group, handicapped persons, as well as persons with a long history of failure, manifest "D" scores that are lower than those obtained by normal groups. We have also noted that some handicapped individuals react to failure with very high shifts in their goal settings; by so doing, they put the attainment of their goal out of reach and thus insulate themselves from failure. An individual's level of aspiration—the strength of his achievement motive—is influenced by several factors: the difficulty of the task; felt competence; the degree of satiation or deprivation; recent experience with success and failure; perception of the payoff. An individual's belief concerning the cause of a particular outcome—how much she attributes the outcome to internal (ability, effort) or external (difficulty of the task, luck)—is an important predictor of how she will behave (Weiner, 1974).

There are other ways of assessing a client's motivation. McClelland (McClelland and Steele, 1972, 1973) has devised an intriguing system for determining the strength of an individual's "achievement motive" by analyzing thematic content in stories they write and by scrutinizing their doodling. A client's autobiography is another means of evaluating long-range themes regarding his motivation.

> We have also used an informal "test" of motivation in our work with young stutterers. It is based on the observation that highly driven persons tend to feel uncomfortable if they are interrupted while completing a task and will tend to return to it as soon as they are permitted. We have used various activities—arithmetic problems, classifying and sorting objects, puzzles; when the youngster is well into the task, we interrupt him and then record the time elapsed until he resumes the activity. Although lacking sufficient data to present norms, we have found that children with high motivation—those who strive for success—tend to return to the task more swiftly than those with low motivation—those who avoid the threat of failure. The former also do better in treatment. Persistence is essential to success in therapy as well as in life.

McDaniels (1969: 139) presents a provocative formula for analyzing the potential motivation of a handicapped individual:

$$\text{Motivation} = \frac{P(Os) \times U}{C}$$

where:

$P(Os)$ = the probability of a *successful outcome* of treatment (based on the client's and clinician's judgment)

$U$ = the meaning or value (*utility*) the client places on the particular performance to be acquired

$C$ = the expense (*cost*) in money and the physical and mental effort required

For extended discussions of motivation, consult the work of McClelland and Steele (1973) and others (Atkinson and Raynor, 1974; Weiner, 1974; Bolles, 1975; Deci, 1975; Lepper and Greene, 1978; McMillan, 1980).

### Audiometric Evaluation

Because of the close relationship between auditory sensitivity and speech and language development, we generally perform an audiometric assessment on each client. We often do this simply by combining informal, nonaudiometric testing with an audiometric screening procedure. Individuals manifesting abnormality on these tests should receive more complete audiological evaluation. For a discussion of hearing loss and assessment, consult the work of Emerick (1971) and others (Davis and Silverman, 1970; Martin, 1975; Northern, 1976; Newby, 1979).

### Socioeconomic Status

Speech clinicians do not routinely obtain a measure of socioeconomic status on each client. However, social class may have a bearing on the assessment and management of an individual's communication problem in one or more of the following ways: (1) Parental attitudes toward clinical assistance may differ between classes (lower-class parents are more distrustful of authority); (2) child-rearing practices—including the amount and type of speech stimulation—seem to differ between lower and middle classes; (3) the economic position of the parents will influence the recommendations made; and (4) some types of speech differences, rather than being regarded as speech defects, may more appropriately be designated as subculture dialects.

There are several measures of social class; the scales devised by Hollingshead and Redlich (1958: 387-397) and Warner, Meeker, and Ells (1960: 139-142) are representative, and we have found them useful for conducting research or for an extensive study of a particular child:

> Social class alone may not be as important clinically as the identification of discrepancies between the elements (occupation, source of income, place of residence, amount of income) used in ranking. When there are gaps between these elements—for example, high-prestige occupation but low salary—it can provoke intense striving behavior and subsequent pressure upon children. Social mobility can produce stresses and strains that the clinician may wish to identify.

The occupation of the head of the household is the most reliable index of social status, and many clinicians find the Minnesota Scale for Parental Occupations (1950) a useful tool for ranking various jobs. We prefer, however, the North-Hatt Scale of Occupations (Reissman, 1959: 401-404); the authors present an alphabetical listing of various occupations and, on the basis of empirical research, assign a prestige or ranking score to each job.

### Personality

Although the evidence suggests no systematic causal relationship between personality disturbances and speech defects, clinicians recognize that many clients present varying degrees of emotional reaction to their impaired communication.[7] Speech is perhaps people's most human attribute, and when a person cannot talk well, it affects him in a most profound way. However, a few speech impairments are a direct result of psychological conflict:

> Hugh did not seem like other stutterers we had seen: he was so calm, so relaxed, with a perpetual bittersweet smile on his face as he discussed his problem. His stuttering had started suddenly in his junior year at a religious college where he was studying to be a minister. His blocks were long, silent vigils during which he assumed a posture startlingly like one being crucified. He talked at great length, revealing sadly that now he could obviously not be a clergyman. Stuttering, he said, was a sign from the Almighty, a cross to bear. For Hugh, it seemed to us, stuttering, rather than *being* a problem, was a *solution* to a problem. The psychiatrist to whom we referred him confirmed our hunch: Hugh had made a dramatic emotional commitment during a religious revival meeting when he was an impressionable teenager. His decision had been vividly reinforced by his relatives who scrimped and saved to send him to college to be a minister. As he proceeded through school he began to realize that the church was not "his thing" but could find no face-saving way out of his commitment—until he began to stutter.

A speech clinician should not play psychologist unless he is qualified by virtue of training and experience to administer and interpret psychodiagnostic tests. He should, however, be able to recognize the difference between good mental hygiene and psychopathology. Persons who are psychologically healthy manifest most of the following characteristics (Rubin and McNeil, 1981):

> They are oriented by and large to reality and derive most of their satisfaction in that arena.
> They display adaptive or coping behavior in a sensitive way to environmental demands.
> They perceive the difference between socially acceptable and nonacceptable goals.
> They most often select socially acceptable goals for themselves.
> They select a variety of goals rather than just one or two.
> They select goals that are within their power to achieve.
> They tolerate a reasonable amount of frustration.
> They tolerate a reasonable amount of anxiety.
> They are able to deny immediate gratification.
> They establish warm relationships with others.
> They are reasonably consistent in their behavior.
> They accept the outcome of their behavior.

---

[7]A series of studies in California (Waller et al., 1983) shows a rather high prevalence of psychological problems among children with articulation and language disorders. The authors recommend using screening devices, parent-teacher questionnaires, and child performance measures with school-aged populations.

Not even the most well-balanced individual displays all those attributes all the time. In fact, as many as one-quarter of the "normal" population have incidents that might be described as aberrant in their life histories (Sunberg and Tyler, 1962). After two decades of working with speech-handicapped individuals and their relatives, it is sobering to reflect on how relatively fragile are most persons' adjustments. There are signs of obvious psychopathology, however, which a diagnostician should be able to recognize (Page, 1975). Here are a few:

> Excessive readiness to react to stimuli, lability, and mood swings
> Chronic fatigue or psychosomatic ailments
> Anxiety, guilt, or hostility that is out of proportion to objective circumstances
> Phobias or obsessions that limit work or avocations
> Overuse of common defense mechanisms such as denial, rationalization, projection
> Chronic discrepancy between intent and outcome of actions

When a diagnostician identifies these characteristics of a client, she should make a referral that is humane and appropriate. It may still be difficult to determine, however, if the client possesses a primary emotional problem or a secondary, psychological reaction to the communication disorder (Darby, 1981).

It is important, when we first set out to examine a client, that we let him know it may be necessary to look at his problem from many aspects, including psychological. We should not pop out of a box at the end of a diagnostic session and recommend that the client see a psychiatrist. Nor, in our judgment, is it clinically wise to make a psychological referral (without prior indication that a referral may be necessary) when the client is not responding to therapy. Such a referral is basically assaultive. We are saying, in effect, that if you don't respond to our treatment you must "have your head examined."

We prefer, in the case of an adult or adolescent, to help the client see his need for psychological evaluation. Generally, we do this by pointing out that the themes arising in his discussions with us are problem areas with which we are not professionally equipped to deal. The referral is then very specific—to a particular agency or even to a particular person. Most individuals with speech disorders will not need psychiatric or psychological appraisal and treatment (Bloch and Goodstein, 1971), but we might have to adapt our remedial procedures to fit the needs of particular clients.

One of the most useful procedures in clinical work is the information contained in Hahn's (1961) classic article on direct, nondirect, and indirect methods in speech correction.

> We made a grave mistake with Ricky: we assumed that he could profit from the same kind of direct therapy the other children were receiving. From the start he tried to show us that he needed something different; despite our best efforts he persisted in his misarticulations. Recalling Hahn's article we decided to make a change. We assigned a senior student to work with Ricky, a

student who by his appearance and manner was childlike and "simple." His job was simply to do things *with* Ricky such as making airplanes, taking him for Cokes, and so on. After they had done this for a time, the senior author entered the scene and accused the student therapist, in front of Ricky, of wasting time and goofing off. The child did more work in the remaining six weeks of the school year than he had ever done; he had to achieve to protect the student, his friend.

## PRECEPTS REGARDING THE CLINICAL EXAMINATION

In this chapter we have presented rather explicit methods for conducting the clinical examination. We dislike diagnostic formulas, and our purpose has not been to give out recipes but rather to describe some way of approaching various problems without going too far astray. By way of summary, we now present a list of interrelated and overlapping precepts regarding the clinical examination.

1. We examine persons, not speech defects or speech defectives. Our primary concern is with communicators, not communication.
2. The clinical examination is conducted interpersonally; the catalyst of a diagnostic session is the person-to-person relationship between therapist and client.
3. There is an element of magic in every transaction between people. A diagnostic session can, in some instances, ameliorate a problem situation by engendering hope or be deeply disappointing to a client who hopes that a test or examination will resolve his difficulty.
4. A most important requisite for conducting a clinical examination is a thorough understanding of normalcy.
5. Diagnosis is the initial phase of treatment. The very first contact with a client—the manner in which she is treated during a clinical examination—is a crucial determining factor in her response to therapy.
6. The clinical examination, or more broadly, diagnosis, is not necessarily confined to a single session.
7. Treatment is often diagnostic; we often discover the nature of a client's problem during therapy.
8. The clinical examination is performed to provide a working image of the individual; it is accomplished by interviewing, examining, and testing.
9. An important aspect in acquiring a working image of an individual is determining how he perceives himself and his situation.
10. An individual makes certain adjustments to his problem; his attempts to solve his difficulty—which may include a protective cover of defenses—may be a part of the problem but must not be confused with it.
11. Behavior is a function of the individual and the situation. We should be aware that our test results reflect not just the client's abilities but also his performance *in* the diagnostic setting.
12. Our diagnostic activities should include an assessment of a client's larger social context; the younger the individual, the more important this aspect of the evaluation becomes.

13. Tests are only tools to provide a systematic guide for our observations. They enable the clinician to scrutinize a client in a structured manner.

14. Although for the examiner the testing situation may be very familiar and routine, for the client it is a novel experience.

15. Examination and testing can be iatrogenic. It can suggest problems to the client that she had not considered.

    It is remarkable that those who live around the social sciences have so quickly become comfortable in using the term *deviant,* as if those to whom the term is applied have enough in common that significant things can be said about them as a whole. Just as there are iatrogenic disorders caused by the work that physicians do (which gives them still more work to do), so there are categories of persons who are created by students of society and then studied by them (Goffman, 1963: 140). Do we create problem children by labeling them "tongue thrusters," "culturally deprived," "learning disabled"?

16. Simply because a testing device is made up of a series of precisely defined tasks, administered and scored in a rigidly structured manner, this does not mean that a client's responses are similarly precise.

17. It is as important to observe *how* the client responds during a testing procedure as it is to obtain a score.

18. There is a distinct tendency for students to be caught up in diagnostic fads—the "recent article" syndrome.

19. It is very easy to reify a particular testing instrument, to endow a scale or diagnostic concept with a special form of reality independent of its creator. Some clinicians embrace a diagnostic device with militant enthusiasm and attack all intellectual queries or criticism with apostolic zeal.

20. An intellectual awareness of the nature of his problem, or the factors causing it, will not guarantee insight, acceptance, or remission by the client.

21. Impressions formed on the basis of the first careful evaluation of a client are generally accurate. There is a distinct tendency to discount or deny our findings especially, for example, if they suggest a child is mentally retarded or that an adult aphasic is not capable of further improvement.

22. A professional works when and where she is needed. The needs of the client, not the setting in which the clinician works, determines the scope of her professional activities.

## BIBLIOGRAPHY

AMMONS, R., and H. AMMONS (1948). *Ammons Full-Range Picture Vocabulary Test.* Missoula, Mont.: Psychological Test Specialists.

ANDERSON, R., M. MILES, and P. MATHENY (1963). *Communicative Evaluation Chart.* Golden, Colo.: Business Forms, Inc.

ATKINSON, J., and J. RAYNOR, eds. (1974). *Motivation and Achievement.* Washington, D.C.: V. H. Winston & Sons.

BARKER, R., et al. (1953). *Adjustment to Physical Handicap and Illness: A Survey of the Social Psychology of Physique and Disability.* Bulletin 55. New York: Social Science Research Council.

BARLOW, S., and J. ABBS (1983). "Force Transducers for the Evaluation of Labial, Lingual, and Mandibular Motor Impairments." *Journal of Speech and Hearing Research,* 26: 616–621.

BARNES, K. (1982). *Preschool Screening.* Springfield, Ill.: Chas. C Thomas.

BAXLEY, G., and J. LeBLANC (1976). "The Hyperactive Child: Characteristics, Treatment and Evaluation of Research Design," in *Advances in Child Development and Behavior*. New York: Academic Press.

BERELSON, B., and G. STEINER (1964). *Human Behavior*. New York: Harcourt, Brace and World.

BERRY, M. (1980). *Teaching Linguistically Handicapped Children*. Englewood Cliffs, N.J.: Prentice-Hall, Inc.

BLATT, S. (1959). "Recall and Recognition Vocabulary." *Archives of General Psychiatry,* 1: 473–476.

BLOCH, E., and L. GOODSTEIN (1971). "Functional Speech Disorders and Personality: A Decade of Research." *Journal of Speech and Hearing Disorders,* 36: 295–314.

BLOOMQUIST, B. (1950). "Diadochokinetic Movements of Nine-, Ten-, and Eleven-Year-Old Children." *Journal of Speech and Hearing Disorders,* 15: 159–164.

BLUE, C. (1981). "Types of Utterances to Avoid When Speaking to Language-Delayed Children." *Language, Speech and Hearing Services in Schools,* 12: 120–124.

BOLLES, R. (1975). *Theory of Motivation*. New York: Harper & Row.

BRIGANCE, A. (1978). *Inventory of Early Development*. North Billerica, Mass.: Curriculum Associates.

BRUININKS, R. (1977). *Bruininks-Oseretsky Test of Motor Proficiency*. Circle Pines, Minn.: American Guidance Service.

BUROS, O. (1978). *The Mental Measurement Yearbook*. Highland Park, N.J.: Gryphon Press.

CANNING, B., and M. ROSE (1974). "Clinical Measurements of the Speed of Tongue and Lip Movements in British Children with Normal Speech." *British Journal of Disorders of Communication,* 9: 45–50.

CASSELL, R. (1957). *The Cassell Group Level of Aspiration Test*. Beverly Hills, Calif.: Western Psychological Services.

CHUSID, J., and J. McDONALD (1967). *Correlative Neuroanatomy and Functional Neurology*. 13th ed. Los Altos, Calif.: Lange Medical Publications.

CRONBACH, L. (1960). *Essentials of Psychological Testing*. 2nd ed. New York: Harper & Row.

DARBY, J., ed. (1981). *Speech Evaluation in Psychiatry*. New York: Grune & Stratton.

DARLEY, F. (1979). *Evaluation of Appraisal Techniques in Speech and Language Pathology*. Reading, Mass.: Addison-Wesley.

DARLEY, F., A. ARONSON, and J. BROWN (1969a). "Differential Diagnostic Patterns of Dysarthria." *Journal of Speech and Hearing Research,* 12: 246–269.

—— (1969b). "Clusters of Deviant Speech Dimensions in the Dysarthrias." *Journal of Speech and Hearing Research,* 12: 462–496.

DAVIS, H., and S. SILVERMAN (1970). *Hearing and Deafness*. 3rd ed. New York: Holt, Rinehart & Winston.

DECI, E. (1975). *Intrinsic Motivation*. New York: Plenum.

DOLL, E. (1964). *Vineland Social Maturity Scale*. Circle Pines, Minn.: American Guidance Service.

DuBOSE, R., and M. LANGLEY (1977). *Developmental Screening Inventory*. Boston: Teaching Resources Corp.

DUNN, L. (1980). *Expanded Manual for the Peabody Picture Vocabulary Test*. Circle Pines, Minn.: American Guidance Service.

DWORKIN, J., and R. CULATTA (1980). *Dworkin-Culatta Oral Mechanism Examination*. Nicholasville, Ky.: Edgewood Press.

EMERICK, L. (1971). *A Workbook in Clinical Audiometry*. Springfield, Ill.: Chas. C Thomas.

FLETCHER, S. (1972). "Time-by-Count Measurement of Diadochokinetic Syllable Rate." *Journal of Speech and Hearing Research,* 15: 763–770.

FRANKENBURG, W., and J. DODDS (1969). *Denver Developmental Screening Test*. Denver: University of Colorado Medical Center.

GINOTT, H. (1969). *Between Parent and Teenager*. New York: Avon.

GOFFMAN, E. (1963). *Stigma: Notes on the Management of Spoiled Identity*. Englewood Cliffs, N.J.: Prentice-Hall, Inc.

GOODENOUGH, F. L. (1926). *Measurement of Intelligence by Drawings*. Yonkers, N.Y.: World Book.

GRINKER, R., and A. SAHS (1966). *Neurology*. 6th ed. Springfield, Ill.: Chas. C Thomas.

GUTNICK, H., and R. St. JOHN (1982). "A Model for Predicting Clinically Relevant Group Differences of Open-Response Tests." *Journal of Speech and Hearing Research,* 25: 468–472.

HAHN, E. (1961). "Indicators for Direct, Nondirect, and Indirect Methods in Speech Correction." *Journal of Speech and Hearing Disorders,* 26: 230–236.

HEDRICK., D., E. PRATHER, and A. TOBIN (1975). *Sequenced Inventory of Communicative Development.* Seattle: University of Washington Press.

HOLLINGSHEAD, A., and F. REDLICH (1958). *Social Class and Mental Illness.* New York: John Wiley.

HUBBELL, R. (1977). "On Facilitating Spontaneous Talking in Young Children." *Journal of Speech and Hearing Disorders,* 42: 216–231.

KNOBLOCH, H., and B. PASAMANICK (1974). *Developmental Diagnosis.* 3rd ed. New York: Harper & Row.

LEITER, R. (1948). *International Performance Scale.* Chicago: Stoelting.

LEPPER, M., and D. GREENE (1978). *The Hidden Cost of Reward: New Perspectives on the Psychology of Human Motivation.* Hillsdale, N.J.: Lawrence Erlbaum Associates.

LUBINSKI, R., E. MORRISON, and S. RIGRODSKY (1981). "Perception of Spoken Communication by Elderly Chronically Ill Patients in an Institutional Setting. *Journal of Speech and Hearing Disorders,* 46: 405–412.

McCAULEY, R., and L. SWISHER (1984). "Psychometric Review of Language and Articulation Tests for Preschool Children." *Journal of Speech and Hearing Disorders,* 49: 34–42.

McCLELLAND, D., and R. STEELE (1972). *Motivation Workshops.* New York: General Learning Press.

—— (1973). *Human Motivation: A Book of Readings.* New York: General Learning Press.

McDANIELS, J. (1969). *Physical Disability and Human Behavior.* New York: Pergamon Press.

McMILLAN, J. (1980). *The Social Psychology of School Learning.* New York: Academic Press.

MARTIN, F. (1975). *Introduction to Audiology.* Englewood Cliffs, N.J.: Prentice-Hall, Inc.

MASLOW, A. (1943). "A Theory of Human Motivation." *Psychological Review,* 50: 370–396.

MASON, R., and C. SIMON (1977). "The Orofacial Examination Checklist." *Language, Speech and Hearing Services in Schools,* 8: 155–163.

MECHAM, M. (1971). *Verbal Language Development Scale.* Circle Pines, Minn.: American Guidance Service.

*Minnesota Scale for Parental Occupations* (1950). Minneapolis: Institute of Child Welfare, University of Minnesota.

NEWBY, H. (1979). *Audiology.* Englewood Cliffs, N.J.: Prentice-Hall, Inc.

NORTHERN, J., ed. (1976). *Hearing Disorders.* Boston: Little, Brown.

O'CONNOR, L., and P. ELDREDGE (1981). *Communication Disorders in Adolescence.* Springfield, Ill: Chas. C Thomas.

PAGE, J. (1975). *Psychopathology.* New York: Aldine.

PORTER, R., and J. LUBKA (1980). "The Linguameter: A Device for Investigating Tongue-Muscle Control." *Journal of Speech and Hearing Research,* 23: 490–494.

RAVEN, J. (1948). *Progressive Matrices.* New York: Psychological Corp.

REISSMAN, L. (1959). *Class in American Society.* New York: Free Press.

RILEY, G. (1972). *Motor Problems Inventory.* Los Angeles: Western Psychological Services.

RUBIN, Z., and E. McNEIL (1981). *The Psychology of Being Human.* New York: Harper & Row.

RUSSO, J., and R. OWENS (1982). "The Development of an Objective Observation Tool for Parent-Child Interaction." *Journal of Speech and Hearing Disorders,* 47: 165–173.

RUTTER, M., P. GRAHAM, and W. YULE (1976). *A Neuropsychiatric Study in Childhood.* Philadelphia: Lippincott.

St. LOUIS, K., and D. RUSCELLO (1981). *The Oral Speech Mechanism Screening Examination.* Baltimore: University Park Press.

SALVIA, J., and J. YSSELDYKE (1981). *Assessment in Special and Remedial Education.* 2nd ed. Boston: Houghton Mifflin.

SCHUELL, H., J. JENKINS, and E. JIMENEZ-PABON (1964). *Aphasia in Adults.* New York: Harper & Row.

SIEGEL, G., and J. HANLON (1983). "Magnitude Estimation of Oral Cavity Distances." *Journal of Speech and Hearing Research,* 26: 574–578.

SUNBERG, N., and L. TYLER (1962). *Clinical Psychology.* New York: Appleton-Century-Crofts.

TATELBAUM, B. (1984). "Contemporary Juvenile Literature Depicting the Communicatively Impaired Individual: A Bibliography and Implications for Therapy." *Language, Speech and Hearing Services in Schools,* 15: 137–139.

TAYLOR, J. (1963). "Screening Intelligence." *Journal of Speech and Hearing Disorders,* 28: 90–91.

TERMAN, L., and M. MERRILL (1960). *Stanford-Binet Intelligence Scale: Manual for the Third Revision* (Form L-M). Boston: Houghton Mifflin.

UZGIRIS, I., and J. HUNT (1983). *Assessment in Infancy.* Champaign: University of Illinois Press.

VAN ALSTYNE, D. (1960). *Van Alstyne Picture Vocabulary Test.* New York: Harcourt, Brace & World.

VAN RIPER, C. (1972). *Speech Correction: Principles and Methods.* 4th ed. Englewood Cliffs, N.J.: Prentice-Hall, Inc.

WALLER, M., et al. (1983). "Psychological Assessment of Speech- and Language-Disordered Children." *Language, Speech and Hearing Services in Schools,* 14: 92–98.

WARNER, W., M. MEEKER, and K. ELLS (1960). *Social Class in America.* New York: Harper & Row.

WECHSLER, P. (1949). *Manual for the Wechsler Intelligence Scale for Children.* New York: Psychological Corp.

—— (1955). *Manual for the Wechsler Adult Intelligence Scale.* New York: Psychological Corp.

—— (1967). *Preschool and Primary Scale of Intelligence.* New York: Psychological Corp.

WEINER, B. (1974). *Achievement Motivation and Attribution Theory.* Morristown, N.J.: General Learning Press.

WOOD, N. (1964). *Delayed Speech and Language Development.* Englewood Cliffs, N.J.: Prentice-Hall, Inc.

# CHAPTER FOUR
# LANGUAGE DISORDERS IN CHILDREN

If we were to travel around the country and peer through the one-way mirrors of language treatment rooms, we would find a confusing conglomeration of activities being performed under the aegis of linguistic assessment. Come, let us look through the windows:

—A clinician has a child repeat sentences.

—A child plays silently while the clinician takes notes.

—A child is trying to obtain a toy and the clinician resists.

—A clinician is having a child point to one of three pictures.

—A clinician is giving instructions telling a child to act out a scene with dolls.

—A child is trying to get a piece of candy with a string tied around it by pulling the string. The clinician is scribbling on a clipboard.

—A clinician is watching a child and the parents play.

—A clinician is pushing a car back and forth with a child and suddenly pushes a horse on wheels back to the child instead of the car.

—A child is trying to complete open-ended sentences presented by the clinician.

—A child is describing pictures for a clinician behind a cardboard barrier.

Note: This chapter is lengthy because language is an area of study that is large and complex. Basically the chapter has a background portion (pp. 88-109) and a section that addresses specific assessment techniques (pp. 109-143). Teachers and/or students may wish to divide the chapter into these sections for reading assignments.

What does it all mean? Are all these clinicians really performing language assessments? How does a clinician know what to do with a particular child?

If one thing is clear today, it is that language assessment requires more varied skills and more diversity of educational background on the part of the clinician than ever before. In this chapter we hope to provide some guidelines for those who are charged with the task of assessing the language of children.


## GENERAL BACKGROUND INFORMATION

When one contemplates language assessment or acquisition in the 1980s, it is not enough to consider structural components (semantics, syntax, and the like) alone. Conceptions of language have changed considerably since the 1950s, when in some quarters the syntactic component was the primary emphasis (Chomsky, 1957). Behavioristic thought in the 1950s and 1960s viewed language as just another behavior. Also, in the 1960s, Osgood's model of language was applied in a "specific abilities" orientation (Bloom and Lahey, 1978). Tests and language training programs were developed that emphasized specific psycholinguistic abilities such as auditory memory span and auditory sequencing. Thus, language has traditionally been "fractionalized" in one way or another since theorists first began to theorize about it.

One can see this isolation of components in society as a whole with the specialization of workers after the Industrial Revolution, the rise of medical specialties, and the institution of particular designations in the behavioral sciences (Toffler, 1981). The decade of the 1970s, however, brought with it a larger view. In society as a whole, the emphasis on ecology was in full flower, and people began to talk about the reciprocal influence of different components formerly thought to be isolatable. We began to consider the far-reaching effects of a single act toward one element in the ecology on the entire ecosystem. A movement toward holistic medicine was observed, and inter-multidisciplinary team evaluations of exceptional children attempted to view "the whole child." After years of fractionalizing the world—and language along with it—into "little boxes," we began to put it together again.

It is not realistic to assess or train only isolated components of the total communication process. An analogy to fragmenting the communication process is to conceptualize an automobile as individual parts and systems. For instance, one can assess the fuel system of a car, but from that evaluation the functioning of the car will not be known until it is driven in real conditions. So when someone begins to think of language as just linguistic elements, or worse, one type of linguistic structure, some very important aspects of the process are being ignored. Language does not exist in a vacuum. It occurs when humans who possess a reasonable amount of symbolic ability (intelligence) use a communication system in a social environment.

Thankfully, in the late 1970s the language area called pragmatics received renewed emphasis. The focus on pragmatics has had far-reaching implications for assessment and treatment of both child and adult language disorders. It has also influenced the study of child language acquisition. Although pragmatics is an area of language, it permeates all the other areas of linguistics, and the authors view it as somewhat of a unifying force. That is, pragmatics deals with the use of language in context and all of the changes in the structure of an utterance in response to differing communication situations.

Most current conceptualizations of language are more integrative than linguistic models of the past three decades. By integrative, we mean that language depends on biological, cognitive, and social variables that are both prerequisite to communication and significant determiners of how linguistic structures are used in day-to-day situations (McClean and Snyder-McClean, 1978; Carrow-Woolfolk and Lynch, 1982; Bloom and Lahey, 1978; Muma, 1978; Hubbell, 1981). The present chapter will also take this integrative point of view because it helps to make language acquisition and assessment more understandable.

### What Makes Language Assessment Difficult?

Language assessment in children is one of the most difficult and challenging tasks faced by the speech pathologist, and many clinicians are insecure about their diagnostic ability in this area.

One complicating factor for the diagnostician is that the population exhibiting a language disorder is extremely heterogeneous (Aram and Nation, 1975; Wolfus, Moscovitch, and Kinsbourne, 1980). Also, children from a wide spectrum of etiological groups manifest language impairment, and thus the practitioner is faced with youngsters who are mentally retarded, autistic, hearing-impaired, learning-disabled, or who exhibit a variety of other organically based conditions. This heterogeneity makes diagnosis appear to be quite difficult for the clinician who knows only one approach to language assessment.

A second variable that makes language diagnosis difficult is the difference in the degree of severity found in the language-impaired population. The children can range from nonverbal with a lack of social and cognitive bases for language to youngsters who inconsistently omit or misuse grammatical morphemes. Thus, for each evaluation the clinician must be prepared to assess the broad representation of linguistic and prelinguistic behaviors.

A third factor that makes language assessment confusing is the complex nature of language itself. Most introductory courses discuss language as an area that comprises various domains. In fact, many textbooks are organized in terms of language areas, such as semantics, syntax, morphology, phonology, and more recently, pragmatics. If we consider these areas for language expression alone, much time would be spent researching the literature. If language comprehension is added to the equation, even more effort would be required to understand the nature of language. Complicating the problem further is the fact that authorities in the area of linguistics are not in total agreement regarding certain aspects of these domains of language.

Still another difficulty in language evaluation is the proliferation of assessment devices and procedures available on the market. We are inundated with fliers and catalogs, many reputed to offer "the best language assessment device." How does one select a test? Is one test enough? The fact that people have designed tests of language for children, oftentimes with very inclusive titles, suggests that it is possible to find out all one needs to know from a single test. Unfortunately, the disclaimers that some authors place in their test manuals regarding the shortcomings of the instruments are forgotten and the perhaps overly ambitious title remains in the mind of clinicians and parents. Tests, also, are based on different theoretical points of view or models. The differing theoretical underpinnings result in dramatically different types of tasks and areas of emphasis on tests. The plethora of tests, then, is a source of confusion to many clinicians.

It is also difficult to know what to do in language assessment because language development and disorders encompass so much more than just linguistic ability. In the literature on language acquisition, for instance, one routinely reads about cognitive development, neurolinguistics, linguistic theory, adaptive behavior, play development, social development, self-help skills, phonology, motor ability, caretaker-child interaction, and other areas that may not appear to be directly related to linguistic symbols. Because language itself has many domains (semantics, syntax, phonology, morphology, pragmatics, and so on) and the related areas mentioned above are numerous, language assessment may take on quite different guises, depending on the focus of the evaluation. This is clearly a source of confusion for clinicians and requires a very broad base of skill and knowledge.

The writers are frequently asked by clinicians in the field to recommend a single best language assessment device or procedure. Quite simply, it is not possible to make such a recommendation in good conscience because of the variables discussed above. However, models, as we indicate in the following section, are sometimes helpful in reducing the difficulties in understanding an area and assisting diagnosticians in developing workable clinical procedures.

### Components to Consider in Language Assessment

In a language evaluation the clinician must have some framework upon which to gather and organize the data. For years, authorities have been "model building." Many people, however, tend to think that the models that are built in paneled dens across the country are exclusively the stuff of intellectualization and idle theorizing. There is a point, however, where some models begin to have clinical relevance. When a clinician has some sort of guiding principle to use in assessment and treatment, the model appears as a relevant clinical concept. As Nation and Aram (1977) indicate, you cannot operate effectively unless you have some organization of your data base. Models, then, are "organizing principles" that help to make the clinician more efficient.

The way that the clinician conceptualizes language and communication will largely dictate how language disorders are assessed and treated. For instance, a strict behavioral model of language and communication would not necessarily consider cognitive or social prerequisites. It does not deal with intent or other unobservable phenomena. If a clinician subscribed exclusively to this model, there may be no evaluation of these other areas. Models that emphasize modalities of input and output such as that of Kirk and Kirk (1971) do not focus particularly on such linguistic aspects as syntax, morphology, or pragmatics. Prerequisite areas (cognitive, social, biological) are also ignored. These are just two examples of how the model of language adopted can constrain a clinician's thinking and clinical behavior. Thus, all models are not equally useful to a clinician because certain important aspects of the language can be missed.

There are some cautions in the use of models. First, general semanticists have said for decades that the "map is not the territory." So it is with models. They are not the knowledge or behavior they represent. Clinicians should never forget that it is what they know that is important, far beyond any model. Models are perspectives and guides for organizing clinical information, nothing more. If the clinician is confronted with a real child who is performing at odds with a model's prediction, the validity of the child's behavior is not questionable, but the applicability of the model is certainly a bit dubious. Do not, as they say, let the tail wag the dog. A second caution is that at the present time no one knows for certain exactly how language is developed, processed, or most efficiently assessed. Thus, any model is likely to be inaccurate or, at least, incomplete. Clinicians, like theorists, must be open to change in their conceptualizations of language and its evaluation.

Before discussing assessment of language in children, it is important to review some aspects of language in a developmental perspective. Figure 4.1 lists some com-

**FIGURE 4.1**   **Selected components involved in language acquisition and use.**

*Biological*
Intact vocal tract
Intact sensory system
Intact motor system

*Cognitive*
Representation (symbolic ability)
Concepts underlying language

*Social*
Interaction with others
Stimulation with model by caretakers
Reasons to communicate with others
Joint referencing with caretakers

*Linguistic*
Structural aspects
—Semantics (word meaning)
—Syntax (word ordering)
—Morphology (word endings)
—Phonology (sound ordering)

Functional aspects
—Listener perspective
—Discourse rules
—Contingency

ponents of language development included in the integrative models of a number of authors (McClean and Snyder-McClean, 1978; Bloom and Lahey, 1978). No doubt there are additional processes that could be listed under each area. We will briefly expand on each domain in Figure 4.1.

As mentioned previously, language has some obvious biological prerequisites. A child must have an intact nervous system and be physiologically capable of using the auditory-vocal channel for speech output or gestures for nonspeech output of language. This prerequisite should not be overlooked, as cognitive, social, and linguistic development depend on it. The diagnostician will gain most of this information from parental interviews and from reports by physicians, neurologists, or other specialists. Some neurological and biological information may be gained by the speech pathologist through the oral peripheral examination. If the clinician has any doubts about the child's neurological, medical, or physical status, a referral should be made to the appropriate professional.

A highly important biological prerequisite to oral language learning is an intact auditory system. The writers have seen a significant number of children, referred for language delay, who were experiencing hearing impairment and had a history of middle ear involvement. This has also been reported by other professionals (Downs, 1981). It cannot be emphasized enough that any language assessment should include an audiometric evaluation to ensure that the child has the auditory-biological prerequisites for language. Nothing is more disheartening than to have performed language treatment for a long time and then discover that the child has a hearing loss. The auditory problem might have received early attention and resulted in greater treatment progress.

A second prerequisite area that is included in most integrative models is cognitive development. Cognitive prerequisites are important on at least two levels. First, because language is an abstract symbol system, the user must be capable of symbolic representation, which is a higher cortical function (Morehead and Morehead, 1974). Thus, just to appreciate language, a certain degree of cognitive attainment is necessary. On a second level, language has been said to "map" or "code" aspects of reality that the child understands (Brown, 1973; Bowerman, 1974; Nelson, 1974). The implications for assessment and treatment are (1) that a child who is not capable of symbolic/abstract representation is not likely to be as successful in learning a language, and (2) that the language a child is trained to use in treatment should reflect the youngster's cognitive holdings (that is, what he knows about the world). We talk about objects and relationships in the world that we "know." More will be mentioned about cognitive development when we talk briefly about language acquisition.

The social basis of linguistic acquisition is a third prerequisite area typically referred to in current models of language. The social area is important for two major reasons. First, language is learned in a social context. We learn it from our caretakers by (1) hearing a model of what the language sounds like, (2) seeing how the language is used by others in our environment, and (3) using the language ourselves as we learn it in real interactions with caretakers. If parents never talked to their child but constantly played the television so that he would be exposed to language, it would not be effective because the television is not relevant to the child's activity. It cannot comment contingently when the cat climbed the drapes or when mother inadvertently severed the power cord of the electric knife while carving the turkey at Thanksgiving dinner. Thus, socialization with caretakers is important in hearing what the language sounds like, seeing how it is used, and having the language presented in relevant contexts.

Another social aspect important to consider in a language model concerns the functions that language serves for the child. In essence, we want to know why the child speaks. What are the intents behind her communications? Is language used to regulate, inform, question? Also, joint referencing takes place when a child can identify which referent or event the caretaker is referring to in an utterance (McClean and Snyder-McClean, 1978). This joint referencing takes place socially when an adult directs a child's attention to utterances and events or when the caretaker becomes involved in an activity the child is already interested in. In an assessment, these social prerequisites can be evaluated by interviewing the caretakers, observing caretaker-child interactions, and simply taking a sample of the child's communication to determine why he talks. We will deal more specifically with these variables later.

The three prerequisite areas briefly discussed above are important both individually and interactively. One can readily see that if biological prerequisites are not attained, a child's cognitive and social development may be affected. Likewise, a child with no obvious biological abnormalities may not possess the cognitive prerequisites for language and the social behavior may be affected. Certainly, in cases where any of the three prerequisites, individually or interactively, are affected, language development has the strong possibility of being delayed.

It is interesting that, so far, we have not discussed language and its traditional areas of semantics, syntax, phonology, and pragmatics. Yet, in a nonverbal child, there is really no language to assess. It is not unusual to receive lengthy reports on nonverbal children that focus only on the cognitive, social, and biological prerequisites to language.

The portions of most integrative models that clinicians are most familiar and comfortable with are the linguistic-structural aspects. Many introductory textbooks provide a good review of these areas (for example, Dale, 1976; Bloom and Lahey, 1978; Devilliers and Devilliers, 1978; Brown, 1973; Carrow-Woolfolk and Lynch, 1982; Trantham and Pedersen, 1976; Wood, 1981), and we will not go into them here. It is enough to say very superficially that semantics deals with the meaning of lexical items in a child's vocabulary, syntax has to do with the rules for sentence construction, and phonology focuses on the rules for regulating the sound system of the language.

We have said before that language is used in a social context. The pragmatic influences on our utterances are many, and Figure 4.1 only mentions a few. For instance, our utterances are often contingent on the statements of others. That is, they stay on the same topic and provide more information. We must also take into account our listener's perspective when we select a sentence to say and consider such variables as age, sex, social status, and what the listener can see in the situation (for example, "Give me one of those"). There are also rules for conducting a conversation that most adults know and children must learn (Grice, 1975). These pragmatic aspects of language must be acquired by children just as surely as they must acquire the structural elements of syntax and semantics. Thus, an integrative model of language has as its base the biological, cognitive, and social prerequisites and these feed into the linguistic portions of the model.

Different authors arrange the model in slightly different ways, because they do not really know for certain how the language process works. We do suspect, however, that all the areas are involved, and they participate interactively in some fashion. We also can see some "primacy" in certain parts of the model, which is why some authorities call some sections (biological, cognitive, social) "prerequisite" for others. The model not only has to do with language production but with linguistic development as well. Essentially, if the prerequisite parts of the model are not in place for a particular child, the normal development process could be affected.

One final implication has been previously alluded to: The model is, by definition, integrative. This means that the language process cannot be fractionalized and retain its integrity. The only way the model can be fractionalized is by college professors when they attempt to explain language to classes of burgeoning speech pathologists. This fragmentation is acceptable for purposes of exposition of the model; however, it is critical to remember the importance of reintegrating the model after taking it apart. It is even more important to recall the integrative nature of language processes in assessment and treatment.

### Normal Language Development:
### A General Overview for Assessment

It is beyond the scope of this chapter to present a detailed view of the aspects of language acquisition. However, we would be remiss if we did not touch on some "highlights" of the process that are related to language assessment. The areas discussed are only suggestive of some linguistic and prelinguistic attainments of children between birth and age four. The particular achievements mentioned are discussed only to place in context the assessment suggestions that follow later in the chapter. Many fine textbooks are available that summarize research in language acquisition, and the reader should become familiar with this information before engaging in any language assessment (Bloom and Lahey, 1978; Devilliers and Devilliers, 1978; Muma, 1978; Brown, 1973; Dale, 1976; Hubbell, 1981; Carrow-Woolfolk and Lynch, 1982).

*Cognitive development.* Perhaps the most well-known researcher in the area of children's cognitive development has been Jean Piaget. A most significant period in language development occurs between birth and two years. By the age of two, a child is typically beginning to use multiword utterances and has clearly demonstrated the symbolic capacity for dealing with language. Piaget calls the period between birth and age two the sensorimotor stage of cognitive development because most learning takes place through active sensorimotor exploration of a child's environment. There are many sources available that describe this period of cognitive growth in detail (Ginsburg and Opper, 1969; Morehead and Morehead, 1974; Beard, 1969).

Here we hope to present a flavor for some of the developmental landmarks that a child is thought to pass on the way to becoming representational. The implication for the diagnostician is that these landmarks may be assessment targets for severely language-disordered children. It should be emphasized that not all of these "cognitive prerequisites" have been shown to correlate directly or strongly with language acquisition. However, many authorities have advocated the administration of Piagetian assessment batteries that examine cognitive attainments in the sensorimotor period (Newhoff and Leonard, 1983; Ruder and Smith, 1974; McClean and Snyder-McClean, 1978). Some skills examined on these scales seem to be "logically related" to language development, and others have been shown to have a statistical relationship to linguistic acquisition. There is, however, a difference between correlation and causation. Actually, the relationship between specific cognitive developments and specific language acquisitions has not been clearly shown (Leonard, 1978). In reviewing the cognitive development literature, however, there seem to be certain "skills" that are in cognitive assessment scales and often referred to by authorities as being potentially language related.

One cognitive skill that is "logically related" to language development is that of object permanence. At a certain point in development an infant will not be able to represent an object mentally when it is not in physical view. They seem to forget about the object, even if it is one that they desire. If you cover an object with a cloth, a child of a certain age and cognitive level may stop searching for it. Some studies, however, have not shown a strong relationship between language development and object permanence (Bates et al., 1979; Leonard, 1978), although it is included in many scales administered to language-developing children (Uzigiris and Hunt, 1975; Merhabian and Williams, 1971).

Another cognitive skill thought to be prerequisite to the acquisition of language is the ability to appreciate the means-end relationship (Morehead and Morehand, 1974; Bates et al., 1979). The idea that a particular process is a means to accomplishing an end is similar to the use of language in affecting the environment of the language user. Language is, in fact, a means to accomplishing a variety of ends, such as regulating the environment, obtaining information, or sharing information (Halliday, 1975). If the child does not have the basic means-end concept, it is doubtful that language will be used as a means to accomplish any purpose.

Another precursor for the development of language has been said to be the knowledge of functional object use (Steckol and Leonard, 1981). Using an object for its intended purpose (for example, combing hair with a comb) requires the mental representation of both the object and its use. Also, when a child begins to talk about basic relations in the environment, utterances typically concern objects, their functions, and all the relationships an object enters into (Nelson, 1974). Steckol and Leonard (1981) have found that training in the functional use of objects resulted in an increase of protoimperative responses (that is, nonverbally using adults to accomplish a task or manipulate objects) in nonverbal children.

Imitation and deferred (delayed) imitation have also been regarded as cognitive prerequisites of language (Bates et al., 1979). Imitation requires mental representation of an act for a short time period, and deferred imitation requires holding onto an event for a longer duration. Both suggest at least an ability to represent reality for a length of time without depending on immediate stimulus support.

Finally, the prerequisite of symbolic play (pretend behavior) is frequently regarded as evidence of a child's general symbolic capacity. One can think of symbolic play on a continuum from playing with exemplars of an object that are physically similar to the real object (for example, a box representing a car) to playing with exemplars that are dissimilar to the real object (a comb for a car) and finally to playing with no object at all (pantomime) (Elder and Pederson, 1978). The use of one object to stand for another is similar to the way that words represent objects in the real world. A basic symbolic capacity must be present in order to use a symbolic play routine, and these routines should be noted in a child's behavior as positive sign of increased symbolic capacity.

Thus far, the cognitive prerequisites of object permanence, means-end, functional use of objects, imitation and deferred imitation, and symbolic play have been suggested as possibly important to the development of language. Of course, no one knows how much each contributes or for certain even if each of them does contribute to the acquisition of language. They may only be correlated with language development (Newhoff and Leonard, 1983). Piaget has divided his sensorimotor period of cognitive development into six substages. Several investigators report that a child must have at least attained stage 4 to evidence expressive single-word utterances and stage 5 or 6 for multiword constructions. There are also studies that point out exceptions to this point of view (Leonard, 1978). Again, children exhibit individual variability in this cognitive-linguistic correspondence, thus attesting to a more general relationship between representational development and language acquisition. It is clear, though, that language development is related in very potent and complex ways to cognitive capacities.

*Social development.*    Language development takes place in a social context. From the moment of birth a child interacts with his caretakers and is bombarded with visual, auditory, and tactile stimuli in this relationship.

Various important dimensions must be considered in a discussion of social development. For example, there are the modifications that caretakers make in their behavior when confronted with the infant. Research has shown that caretakers alter many aspects of their communicative behavior. Suprasegmentally, they raise their fundamental frequency, increase their pitch range, speak more slowly, and use double primary stress patterns (Garnica, 1974). The caretaker is less disfluent when talking to an infant and pauses at major linguistic constituent bound-aries. Linguistically, the mean length of utterance is reduced, and the vocabulary and syntactic complexity are simplified (Snow, 1976).

Developing children, in addition to being exposed to a simpler language model, are given an introduction to the reciprocity of communicative interchange. Snow (1977) has shown that mothers engage in turn-taking reciprocal behavior with babies even as young as three months of age. Early on, the child's "turn" is a non-verbal action that is biologically programmed, such as a smile, sneeze, or burp. The mother simply responds to this with some sort of language response and oftentimes takes the child's turn for her linguistically. As the child develops, the caretaker de-mands that the youngster's turn more closely resemble the adult correct model.

Another aspect of caretaker-child interaction is attachment bonding (McClean and Snyder-McClean, 1978; Bates et al., 1979). The caretaker, in being sensitive, available, and responsive, develops an affective "bond" with the child that makes interacting enjoyable. This increases the number of interactions and opportunities for learning. The youngster also benefits cognitively from interacting with the care-taker. Mothers and fathers typically show the child "how the world works" in terms of demonstrating the functional use of objects, body parts, attributes of ob-jects, and many other conceptual aspects of the environment. Children have been shown how to follow their caretaker's line of visual regard—to look at objects their parent is focused on—very early in development (McClean and Snyder-McClean, 1978). Adults also show the child how to play with a variety of objects and even stimulate symbolic play.

We see, then, that caretakers demonstrate language structure, language use, concepts, and the reciprocity of communication. Children are highly sensitive to their social environment, and they learn that language is a tool to be used for a variety of social and nonsocial purposes (Halliday, 1975; Dore, 1975). With young children, it is clear that their early exposure to language and their early use of it are highly social. These various aspects of adult-child interaction should be assessed in the evaluation of nonverbal, single-word, and early multiword-level children, as these interactions may significantly influence language development.

*Communication development.* Thus far we have briefly sketched the de-velopment of cognitive and social prerequisites to language. This section deals with formation of the linguistic code in communication development. Our discussion will consider four general phases: nonverbal (prelinguistic), single word, early multi-word, and syntax. These stages are based on length of utterance, which, up to about age four, generally correlates with chronological age (Miller and Chapman, 1981) and linguistic attainment (Brown, 1973; Carrow-Woolfolk and Lynch, 1982; Lund and Duchan, 1983). Each stage has certain acquisitions associated with it that may indicate the child is ready to make the transition into the next stage.

As mentioned previously, a prelinguistic or nonverbal child has no expressive language. This does not imply, however, that the child does not communicate. Any parent of a prelinguistic child will attest that these children communicate profusely about their desires, moods, and a variety of pleasing or displeasing biological states.

Bates (1976) studied the sensorimotor performatives of young children and determined that they have primitive forms of imperatives or commands in which they use adults to obtain access to objects in their environment. Initially, the child physically manipulates the adult, as by putting the adult's hand on a jar to open it. Later, the child may use pointing coupled with vocalizations to indicate to the adult what he wants done. Bates (1976) also noted primitive forms of the declarative in which the child uses an object to gain adult attention as the goal. There appears to be a progression that begins with the child showing and giving objects to adults. Ultimately, the child exhibits the declarative by pointing toward an object with alternating gaze between the adult and the object. Bates et al. (1979) reported a "gestural complex" that, in part, may be related to language development. Thus, communication takes place quite vividly in the preverbal child.

There is also preverbal evidence of the "functions" of language alluded to by Halliday (1975) and Dore (1975). That is, children use the greeting function nonverbally by waving, question by exhibiting a quizzical look, and regulate adults physically before they use language for these purposes. In preverbal children, the primary evidence for their communication ability is found in gestures, facial expressions, and/or vocalizations. These phenomena can be observed by a clinician in a diagnostic session, or caretakers can be asked in an assessment interview about how the child makes his needs known at home and at school. A nonverbal child is also beginning to expand the phonetic inventory, and the clinician can transcribe the phonetic elements present in the child's system.

A possible diagnostic variable found in a prelinguistic child was contributed by Dore et al. (1976). Dore and his colleagues noted that a prelinguistic child is not simply uttering "jargon" vocalizations. At a certain point in development they noted the presence of phonetically consistent forms (PCFs), which they termed "transitional phenomena." PCFs are vocalizations that are stabilized around certain situations. They are not word approximations but are fairly stable phonetic productions typically consisting of vowel or consonant-vowel combinations. They are repeatedly associated with specific situations such as affect (emotion), indicating or pointing to aspects of the environment or expressing a desire to obtain an object or event. Dore and coworkers observed that these PCFs seem to act as a transition to words where certain phonetic elements must be stabilized around a specific referent.

After a period of using no real words and becoming more consistent in using vocalizations accompanied by gestures, the child begins to use single words to code objects and events. The words are not adult productions but typically consonant-vowel (CV) or CVCV approximations of the correct production (Nelson, 1973). Nelson has found that children's early lexicons represent specific categories. These one-word utterances were formerly called "holophrases," which means a single word referring to an entire thought—"cookie" may really mean "I want a cookie" (McNeill, 1970). Recent research has reported that subgroups of language-developing children are "referential" (word- and object-oriented) or "expressive" (social- and conversation-oriented). That is, the referential children use mostly nouns and refer to objects and events. They also like to play with objects and spend more time playing alone. The expressive children, on the other hand, enjoy talking to and being with people and use more personal-social words (Weiss et al., 1983). There are perhaps other ways to characterize early single-word productions, but the point is that children go through a period of talking, as Bloom says, using "one word at a time" (1973).

Toward the end of the single-word period, Nelson indicates that the child accrues an expressive lexicon of about fifty words and then begins to attempt word combinations. Prior to the first word combinations, however, Dore et al. (1976) noted another transitional phenomenon, the presyntactic device (PSD). They stated that a syntactic utterance is one in which two words that have a meaning relationship are combined under the same intonational pattern—"Mommy go." A presyntactic device, on the other hand, is the combination of two elements under an intonation contour that do not have a meaning relation because one element is not a real word or because the word combination is duplicated or a highly learned "rote production." Thus, a child who says /WI KITI/ is combining a real word (*KITI*) with a nonword (*WI*) under an intonation contour.

Another presyntactic transitional element that has been reported is empty forms, which are consistently used productions that appear to be nonsense words— "wida," "gocking" (Bloom, 1973; Leonard, 1975). Bloom (1970) reports also the use of two single words that have a meaning relationship with a pause inserted between the two elements—"car . . . go." All of these presyntactic devices prepare a child to combine two meaningful language elements under an intonation pattern, which is the essence of early multiword combinations.

Perhaps the most researched and reported period of language acquisition is the time when children begin to combine lexical items to form meaning relationships (semantic relations). There has been a long history of interpreting these early utterances as traditional parts of speech (noun, verb, and so on), telegraphic speech (Brown and Fraser, 1963), pivot/open classes (Braine, 1963), or underlying structures of transformational grammar (McNeill, 1970). Currently, many authorities support a semantic view of early multiword utterances using a case grammar (Fillmore, 1968) and have rendered interpretations of early utterances using semantic relations (Bowerman, 1973; Brown, 1973; Bloom and Lahey, 1978; Bloom, 1970; Leonard, 1976; Schlesinger, 1974).

Some of the basic early multiword constructions are composed of the semantic cases (Brown, 1973); see Figure 4.2. Note that these basic semantic relations code aspects of the world that the child has learned about during the sensorimotor period of cognitive development—one reason why some authorities have indicated the strong cross-cultural similarities in early utterances (Brown, 1973). There are many more "fine grained" analyses of children's early multiword utterances (Bloom, Lightbrown, and Hood, 1975; Braine, 1976; Leonard, 1976), and the basic relation types in Figure 4.2 are included in these analyses along with some other, more subtle distinctions. Semantic relations must always be interpreted in light of the nonverbal context surrounding the utterance.

The main point here is that children begin to use word combinations that code various common relationships in their environments. If we merely assign

| | |
|---|---|
| Nomination + X | "This ball" |
| Recurrence + X | "More milk" |
| Nonexistence + X | "Allgone egg" |
| Agent + action | "Mommy run" |
| Action + object | "Hit ball" |
| Agent + object | "Mommy shoe" |
| Action + locative | "Go outside" |
| Entity + locative | "Ball kitchen" |
| Possessor + possession | "Mommy skirt" |
| Entity + attribute | "Ball red" |
| | |
| Agent + action + object | "Mommy hit ball" |
| Agent + action + locative | "Mommy run outside" |

**FIGURE 4.2  Semantic relations reported by Brown (1973).**

adult, syntactic categories (noun, verb) to their utterances, we miss some of the skill that children have in coding rather subtle relations cognitively understood in the sensorimotor period. This has been termed a "rich interpretation" by Brown (1973) and gives the child credit for being able to talk about various relationships that syntactic metrics do not. As in the single-word period, these semantic relations are used for various functions. For example, agent + action can be used as a comment-label—"Mommy run," when a child points to mother jogging—or as a regulatory statement—"Mommy push," when the child is trying to get mother to push the wagon. According to authorities, it is wise always to consider both the structure (form) and use (function) of early multiword utterances (McClean and Snyder-McClean, 1978; Bloom and Lahey, 1978). There is a more recent move toward dropping a priori semantic relation categories and giving a child credit for a multiword relation only after he has demonstrated "productivity" of use (Leonard, Steckol, and Panther, 1983; Howe, 1976; Lund and Duchan, 1983).

When a child is leaving the early multiword period, she has acquired a mean length of utterance of more than 2.25 morphemes. At this point, the acquisition of a variety of syntactic conventions begins to emerge. Brown (1973) has indicated that after the basic building blocks of a sentence have been learned (semantic relations), grammatical morphemes and function words are learned. Figure 4.3 indicates some of the grammatical morphemes acquired after semantic relations are established, according to the longitudinal research of Brown (1973) and the cross-sectional research of Devilliers and Devilliers (1973). As the child increases his processing capacity for longer and longer utterances, more complex syntactic structures are acquired, and adult productions of questions, negatives, imperatives, and embedded and conjoined sentences are mastered. It is quite beyond the scope of this chapter to detail the course of complex syntactic development in young children. The reader is referred to the excellent sources on language acquisition suggested at the beginning of this section.

During the acquisition of syntax the child is also learning many of the subtle pragmatic skills necessary to carry on a conversation. She learns how to initiate, maintain, and change a topic. A child learns how to make relevant and efficiently presented contributions to a conversation. The child also learns to take into ac-

| | |
|---|---|
| Present progressive | -ing |
| Preposition | in |
| Preposition | on |
| Regular plural | -s, -z, -es |
| Past irregular | ran, came |
| Possessive | -s, -z |
| Uncontractible copula | is, am, are |
| Articles | a, the |
| Past regular | -ed |
| Third-person regular | -s, -z |
| Third-person irregular | does, goes |
| Uncontractible auxiliary | is, am, are |
| Contractible copula | is, am, are |
| Contractible auxiliary | is, am, are |

**FIGURE 4.3   Brown's fourteen grammatical morphemes in developmental order.**

count the physical context of conversation, the history, demography, and perspective of the listener, as well as the information that has been covered in the current discourse exchange. Later, in school, the child is faced with using language to solve many complicated problems and having to understand quite complex strings of linguistic material presented by teachers. These areas are just beginning to be understood by researchers.

Thus far we have presented brief sketches of language development in prelinguistic, single-word, early multiword, and syntax stages. They provide a broad overview of acquisition of language, and the reader should have an appreciation for the various "prerequisites" to language acquisition, as well as some of the milestones in linguistic development. The obvious implication is that, in assessment, we will look for certain manifestations of language development and try to locate a child in "developmental space." It is also important to note that more studies are emerging that point to individual language development strategies in the acquisition of both the structural and functional aspects of language. To attempt a language assessment without a thorough grounding in the normal acquisition literature is clinically irresponsible.

### Characteristics of Delayed- and Deviant-Language Children

One way to consider language-disordered children is to describe the language they use in comparison to that of younger, normal children in an effort to determine if their language is "delayed" (similar to younger children) or "deviant" (different from younger children). This difference has been referred to as "qualitative versus quantitative" by some (Menyuk, 1964). It is clear from the literature that language-disordered children can manifest problems with any or all aspects of language. There are frequent reports of difficulties with concepts, single-word onset, vocabulary, semantic relations, grammatical morphemes, syntax of more complex sentences, phonology, and pragmatics. Most authorities would not dispute the fact that language disorder can affect any or all facets of linguistic processing for communication.

Leonard (1979) has reviewed many studies of children with language disorder and no physical or cognitive abnormalities. The studies compared language-impaired and normal children balanced by mean length of utterance (MLU) to determine if the language of the disordered group was similar (delayed) or dissimilar (deviant) to that of younger, normal children. Much of the research reviewed by Leonard supports the notion that these language-impaired youngsters exhibited more of a delay than a deviance in their linguistic ability. That is, the language used by disordered children was similar to that used by younger, normal children. Leonard (1972: 1979) has also pointed out that often it is not the total absence of a structure but the less frequent use of the form that characterizes the language-impaired youngster.

This is not to say, however, that deviance is not reported in the language-impairment literature (Arwood, 1983; Trantham and Pedersen, 1976). The present authors have observed that many language cases exhibit symptoms of delayed language; however, it is not unusual to see children with some deviant characteristics. The clinician should expect to encounter both varieties of error in a given child. Also, until we are aware of the various strategies of language acquisition, it is difficult to confidently assign the designation "deviant" to a child. In relation to the general population of language-developing children, too few have been studied longitudinally to determine the variety of paths children from different social strata take to learning language. Finally, when children with cognitive and psychosocial deficits are included in the language-disordered population, there is increased potential that they will be acquiring language with a deviant processing system. Many studies have attested to the heterogeneity of the language-impaired population (Aram and Nation, 1975; Chapman and Nation, 1981; Wolfus, Moscovitch, and Kinsbourne, 1980).

Thus, it is difficult to address the issue of delay versus deviance in a confident manner because we still have so much to learn about the range of behavior in normally developing children. But why address the issue at all? Some researchers indicate that if language-disordered children are arrested in the normal developmental progression, then models based on normal development may be more easily applied to assessment and treatment. Others, however, indicate that even if language-disordered children are found to be delayed, these children are operating with a disordered language processing mechanism; the normal language development process has failed and may not be applicable to assessment and treatment (Arwood, 1983). The present authors find that most authorities come down on the side of considering a normal developmental model in assessment and remediation with the provision that clinicians can deviate from the model when their clinical judgment indicates it is appropriate to do so for functional purposes.

### Theoretical Considerations in Language Assessment

Following the lead of Muma (1973a, 1978, 1983) we would like to echo some basic diagnostic precepts that we feel should underpin language assessment. First, the best language assessment device, as Siegel (1975) stated, is a well-trained clinician who keeps up with current developments. There is no "best" language test, just as there is no ideal language treatment program.

Second, language is a multidimensional process that has many facets of structure and use. There are also the prerequisite areas discussed earlier to consider in evaluation. The existence of the multidimensional process makes it unrealistic to separate structure and function or syntax from semantics or pragmatics. The most ecologically valid methods of analyzing the process are preferable. Whenever we fractionalize the communication process, we are no longer really looking at it.

Third, Muma (1978) has reminded us that whatever we do in assessment must apply to treatment of the language disorder. If we administer tests and then do not consider their results in planning our treatment, the time spent in assessment is wasted. For instance, children with language disorders frequently score poorly on a comprehension test, yet clinicians often choose to begin their treatment with elicited imitation, ignoring the comprehension results. Either comprehension should be addressed in treatment or possibly the test should not have been administered in the first place. Our assessment and treatment procedures should also be based on similar assumptions about the communication process.

A fourth important concept was also articulated by Muma. He stated that the diagnostic paradigm seems to have two levels or issues associated with it. The most basic issue is the "problem/no problem" issue. Standardized tests help to solve the problem/no problem issue by comparing a child's test performance to that of other children. This type of testing emphasizes group similarity and minimizes individual variability. The "nature of the problem" issue, however, must be addressed through description of the individual child's communication performance. This is best accomplished through nonstandardized, descriptive techniques that are more ecologically valid. Fortunately, the problem/no problem issue is solved by many parents when they have referred their child for evaluation. Typically, they know something is wrong when they compare the communication of their youngster with his peers. A standardized test can confirm this, but it rarely can be prescriptive in terms of specifying treatment targets (Millen and Prutting, 1979).

A fifth important notion has to do with sampling. All we ever do in a diagnostic evaluation is obtain a sample of communication behavior. There are several important implications that stem from the sampling idea. First, the samples we obtain should be "representative" of the child's communication performance. The notion of representativeness has been with us for a long while, and we must not forget that a sample we obtain may or may not represent a child's typical or "best" performance. Second, speech pathologists have subscribed for years to the idea that an evaluation can and must take place within a two-hour block of time. This kind of thinking can result in frustrated clinicians when they do not obtain the data they need in the allotted time, or if the child is uncooperative. Evaluation is ongoing, and there should be no pressure to find out all there is to know in a limited time. The medical profession does not feel compelled to diagnose in a limited time with short, abbreviated procedures. Physicians order examinations that they feel are appropriate, and the diagnostic process takes place over as much time as is necessary.

This is not to say that we should emulate the lengthy testing procedures of the medical profession, but, on the other hand, we should not become like purveyors of fast food. Third, whenever possible, the clinician should attempt to obtain multiple samples. Many children behave differently in the clinical setting than they do at home or in preschool. There have not been many comparisons of language in preschool settings with clinical environments, but we suspect that there are important differences.

> Tyrone had said nothing during the two-hour evaluation session. He was brought to the clinic by a caseworker from the state pensions and securities office as a foster child. The caseworker said that Tyrone did talk and could not explain why he was so taciturn upon meeting us. He seemed shy and reluctant to participate even in play with the clinicians. We decided to make an observation the next week at Tyrone's day-care center. We sat unobtrusively in a corner and watched Tyrone carom off the walls like a buzz saw gone awry, pulling pigtails and spewing broken crayons. He yelled at his classmates, and when the teacher asked who wanted to play ball, Tyrone was one of the first to initiate his loud request. Lucas (1980) has observed that some preschoolers take on the role in the classroom of "stater of the rules." They tell other children, "You can't do that," "The paper has to be over here," etc. (We often wonder what types of people these children develop into when they become adults. Know any?) Tyrone frequently made rules statements to the other children. We half felt that we had seen a "medicated" Tyrone at our clinic. Our goals for treatment would have been far different had we not observed Tyrone in more than one setting. It may have been appropriate, based on our first impression, to begin work on increasing child-initiated language.

What we have described above is not an isolated case. We have often made the recommendation to clinicians in the field to observe children in other settings if possible before deciding on treatment goals. In many cases the feedback from these professionals has been, "I thought he was a different child when I saw him in the classroom."

A sixth basic premise of language assessment is that for every technique or test that the clinician uses, she must realize that certain assumptions are implied about child language. To use an instrument, you should "buy the assumptions" that underlie it. Whenever we receive the myriad fliers and announcements of new language assessment instruments, we should remember that each is based on assumptions. We should ask ourselves, "What do I have to believe about language to use this instrument?"

Finally, we feel compelled to say that the quality of the information obtained is proportional to the amount of time the well-trained clinician spends in evaluation. In short, there is no free lunch. A twenty-minute screening test that is easily administered and simply scored will not yield as much information as various analyses of a twenty-minute spontaneous interaction.

The above suggestions should not be taken to mean that we are opposed to the use of standardized tests. We do, in fact, recommend the use of such instruments for the purpose they are most able to accomplish: to determine if a child is performing similarly to other children of a particular age group. Standardized tests, however, cannot make a principled clinical judgment; clinicians make decisions. Assessment has aspects of both art and science (Allen, Bliss, and Timmons, 1981). We advocate the use of a combination of normative measures coupled with nonstandardized tests and more naturalistic sampling of communication behavior (Lund and Duchan, 1983). Reliance on one type of procedure will not provide as complete a picture of a child's performance as a combination. Additionally, school systems and other institutions often require some form of standardized testing.

The rest of this chapter is devoted to outlining some suggestions for the evaluation of cognitive, social, and linguistic aspects of child language. We provide guidelines and references for the clinician to use in learning about these various aspects of language assessment. In cases where we cannot adequately summarize a procedure (which is most of the time) we refer the reader to a primary source with the hope that she will critically evaluate and learn techniques that will be clinically useful.


## AN ORGANIZATION FOR LANGUAGE ASSESSMENT—
## FOUR BASIC CLINICAL TYPES
## AND RELATED ASSESSMENT TARGETS

For purposes of this chapter, we will segment the language-disordered population into four groups, based on their presenting linguistic development level. This is similar to an approach to assessment that was suggested by McClean and Snyder-McClean (1978) in which they recommended certain evaluation areas based on the child's utterance length. Carrow-Woolfolk and Lynch (1983) also recommended determining a child's mean length of utterance and then suggest specific analysis procedures for each level. Figure 4.4 describes four "types" of language-disordered children the clinician is likely to encounter and the high probability assessment targets associated with each type.

There are some children who are largely nonverbal. They use vocalizations and perhaps gestures, but their caretakers report no real use of language to control their environment. Obviously, in dealing with a nonverbal child, a test of language ability would be too advanced. Faced with the virtual elimination of the entire shelf of standardized tests, the clinician must focus on more informal assessment procedures. There will be no lengthy transcripts here, just assessment of more "primal" things like cognitive skills, caretaker-child interaction, adaptive behavior, social development, phonetically consistent forms, phonetic inventory, and other things not found in formal test batteries.

A second group of children are those who speak largely at the single-word level. The single-word stage has been reported in the developmental literature (Nelson, 1973), and according to some authorities, the child may accrue a lexicon of about fifty words before starting the use of word combinations for generative

*Nonverbal Level*
Biological prerequisites
Social prerequisites
Adaptive behavior
Caretaker-child interaction
Vocalization analysis
Communicative functions
Cognitive status
Comprehension testing
Phonetic inventory

*Single-Word Level*
Biological prerequisites
Social prerequisites
Adaptive behavior
Caretaker-child interaction
Single-word analysis
Communicative functions
Cognitive status
Comprehension testing
Phonetic inventory
Language sampling

*Early Multiword Level*
Biological prerequisites
Adaptive behavior
Caretaker-child interaction
Semantic relation analysis
Communicative functions
Comprehension testing
Cognitive status
Phonetic inventory
Phonological process analysis
Language sampling
Formal language tests

*Syntax Level*
Biological prerequisites
Language sampling
Formal language tests
Comprehension testing
Elicited imitation testing
Syntax analysis packages
Descriptive syntax analyses
Conversational pragmatic analysis
Cognitive status (IQ)
Phonetic inventory
Phonological process analysis

**FIGURE 4.4   Specific diagnostic procedures for four clinical types.**

language. Clearly, the assessment of a "single-word child" is different from dealing with a nonverbal one. We can look at the structure of the lexicon and we can search for some evidence of a transition into multiwords by watching for presyntactic devices (PSD) as reported by Dore et al. (1976). The clinician should also determine the functions behind these early single-word utterances, which are evident by interpreting the verbalizations in light of contextual and gestural cues (Halliday, 1975; Dore, 1975). Other areas in this category (see Figure 4.4) may also be evaluation targets.

A third type of child is one who is using early multiword combinations in what has been called "telegraphic speech." For this type of child, it is clear that the basic cognitive capacity for using a symbol system is present because he is, in fact, using one. It becomes more important with an early multiword child to focus on the types of word combinations used and the functions for which the child uses utterances. The phonetic inventory and phonological processes also become important for this type of case, because a child's language can only be functional if it is intelligible to listeners. Thus, for the child using early multiword utterances, we must examine the language used but not necessarily in the same way as we would in a child who has a longer length of utterance. Also, we must examine social, gestural, and contextual variables to determine what and why the child is attempting to communicate.

Finally, there is the child who is speaking in almost adult syntax, with the exception that certain elements are omitted, permuted, or misused in some manner. The "syntax-disordered" child is a bit easier for the diagnostician to describe because there is language to analyze and not so much emphasis needs to be placed on the cognitive and social prerequisites. One complication, however, is that we must still analyze this child's communication both in terms of structure and use. We must be prepared to make statements on communication effectiveness and the pragmatic aspects of language, as well as the structural form of the utterance.

We have seen that there are at least four categories into which we can place the language-disordered children whom we assess. Implied in the four categories are different assessment targets, many of which cannot be evaluated using formal test instruments. The clinician's first step is to determine which category the client's preponderant language behavior fits. The next step involves considering the high probability diagnostic areas associated with the category. Finally, the clinician can use procedures, referred to in the remainder of this chapter, to evaluate the pertinent areas.

Although we have characterized language-disordered children by their general linguistic development level, two other ways to describe language-impaired children have been reported. First, some authorities have classified language-disordered children by etiology (mental retardation, hearing impairment, and so forth). We agree with those who suggest that classification of language disorder by etiology does not relate productively to assessment (Bloom and Lahey, 1978; Newhoff and Leonard, 1983; Aram and Nation, 1975). The various etiological groups themselves are highly heterogeneous, and thus to refer to a "mentally retarded" child means little in terms of predicting what he might be like. Also, the language disorders manifested by these various groups frequently are very similar. Therefore, the language samples gathered from children who are hearing-impaired, mentally retarded, learning-disabled, autistic, or language-delayed with normal intelligence may be highly similar. In essence, there does not appear to be a "language of the mentally retarded" that is critically different from the language produced by members of other causation groups. Diagnostic grouping, then, does not necessarily provide the clinician with valid guidelines for assessment of language skills.

A second way of characterizing language disorder is to specify children's performance in many different areas of linguistic ability (Aram and Nation, 1975; Chapman and Nation, 1981). Researchers reported patterns of language disorder involving differing performance skills in comprehension, formulation, and imitation. They also demonstrated differing performance levels in the linguistic domains of syntax, semantics, and phonology in groups of language-impaired children. The acceptance of Aram and Nation's specific patterns of language disorder has not been widespread, perhaps because the measures they used to establish the patterns have been criticized in the literature and no pragmatic assessments were performed. To the present authors, however, the important contributions of this type of research are to (1) understand the fact that the language-impaired population is heterogeneous and (2) remind the diagnostician to examine a variety of language domains and performance areas. Because the patterns of language disorder are unknown, and many objective tests that establish these patterns lack ecological validity, the clinician is again faced with no real guideline for assessment, other than to examine a variety of behaviors.

A final observation in the area of establishing patterns of language impairment is that this enterprise may become of even greater interest in the next decade. With the proliferation of microcomputers and the computerization of clinical record keeping, it is possible that clinical data gathered on language-disordered children may be more easily analyzed for commonalities among clients. Analyses that were not possible prior to the advent of computers for record keeping can be done, not only to determine types of client historical and examination data, but also their response to treatment. Patterns of language performance among disordered children continue to be described and reported (Fey and Leonard, 1983; Bashir et al., 1983; Leonard, 1983).

## SPECIFIC ASSESSMENT AREAS— PROCEDURES, CONSIDERATIONS, AND DIRECTIONS FOR FURTHER STUDY

### The Parent Interview and Pertinent Historical Information

The information obtained from caretakers of language-impaired children is highly important. First of all, most of these children do not have the means or cognitive development to express themselves well, and the parent or guardian must be relied on to provide pertinent background details and estimations of present skill levels.

As mentioned in Chapter 2, on interviewing, we do not recommend that the diagnostician write down specific questions prior to the evaluation. Appendix A (see pp. 334–337) contains an interview protocol for children's language assessment. The protocol is divided into broad areas covering the prerequisites to language as well as linguistic development. The interviewer should ask questions in the broad areas, obtaining information in each subarea. The exact wording of questions is not provided due to the pragmatics of the interview situation. Parents represent differing levels of education, intelligence, socioeconomic status, and experience, and we have found it more feasible to tailor interview questions for each individual case.

The protocol is designed only to "jog the mind" of the clinician to ask questions in specific topic areas. When remarkable information is reported in any area, the interviewer should formulate appropriate follow-up questions to illuminate clearly the area of interest. The major interview areas represent biological, social, and cognitive prerequisites to language, as well as linguistic level, and were gleaned from a variety of child language-acquisition and language-impairment sources. The interviewer should especially focus the interview on the most applicable portion of the protocol and not ask unnecessary questions. For instance, if a child appears to exhibit a syntax problem, it would be inappropriate for the interviewer to spend inordinate time on cognitive and social prerequisites. This protocol is designed for the well-informed child language clinician. The question areas will mean nothing to the interviewer who does not know the relevance, rationale, and research that underpin each major area and subheading.

Finally, no single item on the protocol is significant in its own right. We are looking for patterns among the major areas. It should be remembered that the areas are divided in the protocol only for convenience and that in reality the domains are interrelated. In obtaining information the interviewer should:

1.   Tape-record the interview and take notes after obtaining permission.
2.   Frame questions on the correct level of abstraction for the parent.
3.   Use many examples when asking questions, and do not use frequent yes/no questions. For instance, we would ask such questions as "How does Randy let you know he wants something?" "Tell me what he likes to do when he plays." "What kinds of sentences have you heard him say?" "Under what circumstances does he try to communicate with you?" If the parent is not providing enough specific information, the clinician can ask some follow-up questions such as, "Does he seem to use objects for the purpose they were intended? For instance, does he use a comb to comb his hair?"
4.   Ask the parent to give you examples of behaviors and language you are interested in.
5.   Space is provided on the protocol for the interviewer to make a brief note as to remarkable findings in any area.

### Assessment of Social Prerequisites and Caretaker-Child Interaction

It is especially important in cases of nonverbal, single-word, and early multi-word-level children to observe them interacting with their caretaker. There are two reasons for this. First, we want to observe the child with someone that she is familiar with and comfortable being around. It is often the case that the best sample of the child's communication is obtained in this portion of an evaluation. When strange clinicians attempt to establish rapport with a child in unfamiliar surroundings it may be quite difficult to observe natural communication, especially in a limited time period.

Occasionally, we have seen children who refused to interact with us in an evaluation. In these cases the caretaker-child interaction is the only data base available. In the early years of speech pathology we were frequently told that the initial step in an evaluation was to separate the child from the mother. Often this resulted in a catastrophic reaction on the part of the child, and little information was gained from the evaluation (other than the fact that the child did not "separate well from the mother"). We must not lose sight of our goal, which is to observe the child's communicative and prelinguistic skills through talking and play. If the caretaker can provide a more effective demonstration of certain skills than the clinician, then we must take advantage of this opportunity and not feel that we have failed as clinicians. Rather, we have succeeded in getting the data we were after as the result of making a sound clinical judgment. Establishing a relationship with a child can always be accomplished in the initial treatment sessions where we are not under severe time constraints.

Thus, the caretaker-child interaction can provide a rich sampling of the child's communication. As we will soon indicate, however, it can also give the clinician a meager, constrained, and repetitive sample.

A second goal of the caretaker-child interaction is to observe the quality of the language model provided by the parent. Specifically, we examine the complexity, length, abstractness, rate, suprasegmentals, and content of the caretaker's utterances. As important as the model itself are the circumstances under which it is delivered. Does the caretaker talk about the "here and now" (Holland, 1975) or about things removed in time and space? What kind of joint referencing takes place in the interaction? Does the caretaker talk about and participate in things that the child appears to be interested in? Does the caretaker direct the child's play to things that he feels are significant, disregarding the child's preferences? More importantly, is there a balance between when the parent joint references with the child and other times when the child joint references with the parent? Regarding the use of language, does the parent force the child into limited or respondent modes of communication functions? It is not unusual to observe parents of early language-disordered children who ask incessant questions ("What's this?" "What color is this?") or require the child to imitate constantly ("Say ball.").

We are not intimating that the parent's interactive style is in any way causally related to the child's language disorder. In fact, a parent's way of talking to a child could be the result of the disorder rather than a cause. Whatever the relationship, the caretaker's model, as it presently exists, may not be conducive to language development and should be changed. The only way to determine this is through the observation of caretaker-child interaction.

Socially, the child's eye contact and willingness to participate in reciprocal nonverbal activities should be observed. A child who does not tolerate or seek out the participation of another person may not have any need for a communication system. Perhaps this child might need to work on some prelinguistic social skills prior to developing language. Language is, after all, a social tool, and a child who is not social has little need of a code to use with people he does not even communicate with nonverbally.

> Natalie entered the examination playroom and her attention settled on the juice. She ran to the table and tried to remove the top of the container. When she could not, she proceeded from item to item, pausing only a few seconds on each. When the clinician called her name loudly, she did not respond. Small noises in the hallway occurred several times and she paused, transfixed on the door with her head cocked to one side like a dog listening to a distant sound. The clinician physically caught her and tried to engage in reciprocal play with a car. Natalie would not look the clinician in the eye, and the car was thrown across the room behind her. Throughout the two-hour session, the child never maintained eye contact longer than two seconds and never participated cooperatively with the clinician. More important, even when it

was clear she wanted something out of reach, she never sought out help from the other human being in the room. The mother reported that Natalie plays alone most of the time and with animals outside in the rural farmyard. It is doubtful that this child has much need for social interaction, let alone a use for a communication system.

Adaptive behavior scales typically rate a child's development of motor skills, social behavior, self-help skills, and language ability. Children are either given tasks to perform or the parents are asked to respond to items on the protocol. The advantage of such scales is that they help to broaden the perspective of the speech pathologist beyond exclusively examining language ability. Although we will assess social cognitive development as it relates to language, much of a child's adaptive behavior depends on cognitive and social attainments. We can obtain a better overall picture of the child's level of functioning, and this information, when coupled with other assessment data, can be valuable. Also, many conditions (for example, mental retardation) may show a child to be generally low functioning in most areas and that language is only part of the problem. Knowledge of adaptive behavior will also be important to the clinician in making referrals. Language treatment activities can also be designed to incorporate motor, social, and self-help areas so that the child is learning a variety of needed skills plus the language associated with them. Several adaptive behavior scales are available (Balthazar, 1973; Lambert et al., 1981; Project RHISE, 1979).

### Assessment of Cognitive Prerequisites to Language

Conceptual holdings are thought to be important to linguistic acquisition, for several reasons. First, language is a representational act. It represents reality or stands for objects and relationships in the world. Second, language is an abstract symbol system. In order to appreciate abstract symbols, we must be able to represent them mentally. Third, language is a tool that we use in social interactions. Tool use implies certain conceptual underpinnings such as the apprehension of relationships like means-end. Fourth, language use involves telling about objects, events, and relationships in the world. It is necessary that one know the properties of these objects and relationships before talking about them coherently. As Nelson (1974) said, we use words as "tags" for the concepts that we have.

There appears to be some agreement that children prior to Piaget's sensorimotor stage 4 typically do not use language in a productive way. The present authors can find no report of a child in stage 3 using language normally. Thus, the diagnostician might find it useful to obtain at least a "ball park" estimate of a child's level of development in the sensorimotor period. A primary reason to do an assessment of cognitive level is to confirm or deny a child's ability to represent reality and deal with symbols. As we mentioned in an earlier section, some of the specific behaviors that have been associated with language development are imitation and deferred imitation, means-end, functional use of objects, and symbolic play (pretend). These "cognitive prerequisites" to language will be focused on here because they are the behaviors included in cognitive test batteries and have been referred to most often as being possibly related to language development.

An important notion to keep in mind is that when assessing cognitive prerequisites, we watch a child's behavior and infer conceptual holdings. As Lund and Duchan (1983) point out, it is often difficult to categorize a behavior as indicating knowledge of a concept because we have no history of how a child behaves. Lund and Duchan say, for example, that a child who tries to drink from an empty cup may not be exhibiting symbolic play by pretending to drink. Rather, the child may be trying to drink, which is a functional use of an object and not symbolic play. Thus, in cognitive assessment we only can make inferences about what a child knows, and we must bear this in mind as the assessment is completed. We should obtain as much information as possible about the child's typical play routines and object use. The parent interview is invaluable here. The failure of a child to perform a task that we set up to evaluate a particular cognitive prerequisite is not necessarily evidence of a lack of the concept. A child can "fail" a cognitive task due to inattention, disinterest, lack of familiarity with the task, or some other reason that has nothing to do with her cognitive status.

With the above admonitions in mind, how does one perform a cognitive assessment, and what type of child undergoes the evaluation? We have found it productive to take note of cognitive prerequisites in children who are nonverbal and those who are at the single-word level. Those children who are currently using productive early multiword utterances are evidencing some representational and symbolic abilities just by using language normally. Children who are using multiword utterances abnormally (echolalic or inappropriate) are candidates for further cognitive assessment. It is not useful to administer routinely a complex cognitive test battery initially. We recommend that the diagnostician move from general analyses to more specific ones. Figure 4.5 contains references for use in cognitive assessment.

The first level of analysis can be a lengthy behavioral observation of the child engaged in play. In our experience, children whose cognitive levels are low will exhibit primitive play routines and perseverative use of objects. Westby (1980) outlines some useful stages to use in assessing the developmental relationship among cognitive development, language, and play. The clinician can set up a play situation

---

FIGURE 4.5    Measures of cognitive development.

- The Ordinal Scales of Psychological Development (Uzigiris and Hunt, 1975)
- Albert Einstein Scales of Sensorimotor Development (Corman and Escalona, 1969)
- Infant Cognitive Development Scale (Merhabian and Williams, 1971)
- A Clinical and Educational Manual for Use with the Uzigiris and Hunt Scales of Psychological Development (Dunst, 1980)
- Beyond Sensorimotor Intelligence: Assessment of Symbolic Maturity Through Analysis of Pretend Play (Nicolich, 1977)
- The Symbolic Play Test (Lowe and Costello, 1976)
- Evaluation of Cognitive Behavior in Young Nonverbal Children (Chappel and Johnson, 1976)
- Assessment of Cognitive and Language Abilities Through Play (Westby, 1980)

and watch the child interact with objects and people. The examiner should be looking for behavior that suggests the specific cognitive prerequisites indicated above.
It is optimal to videotape the play interaction for later specific analysis (Lund and
Duchan, 1983). The clinician must always view the specific behaviors in terms of
the context in which they occur. For instance, pretending that a block is a car can
qualify as symbolic play only if the clinician did not demonstrate this activity
earlier in the sesson.

At any rate, it is important to view the child's nonverbal play behaviors contextually and, if possible, to obtain some historical data on the play routines. Sometimes there is a clear cognitive deficit:

> Ralph was enrolled in a preschool handicapped classroom. He was two years
> old and nonverbal. He seemed to enjoy imitating the clinician when she put
> blocks into a coffee can. When presented with other toys, however, Ralph
> just persisted in putting the blocks in the can and dumping them out again.
> The cycle continued, putting the blocks in and dumping them out. The other
> toys were immediately mouthed and banged on the floor. No matter what
> other toys Ralph had access to, he would put them in his mouth and/or bang
> them on the floor. When the clinician attempted to provide a model of func-
> tional use of objects or more productive play routines, Ralph would persist
> with his limited repertoire.

After observing play routines, the clinician should note whether a cognitive
delay is suspected based on the quality of play exhibited. Sometimes there will
clearly be no representational problem due to the sophistication of the play
routines observed. Other times, as depicted above, behavior will occur that strongly
suggests a rather primitive representational ability. Many cases fall between the two
ends of the cognitive continuum, and these children may require further testing to
determine which level of cognitive development they have attained. Again, we
recommend Westby (1980) for an account of "normal" play behavior. Sometimes,
in dealing with so many disordered clients, it is easy to forget that we must also be
familiar with normal behavior. Students should actively observe and play with normal children to learn what kinds of things they typically do at various ages.

The second level of analysis can involve the administration of cognitive
screening scales and specific tasks that more closely evaluate certain conceptual prerequisites. Chappel and Johnson (1976) and Merhabian and Williams (1971) have
devised rather simple scales that help the clinician to arrive at a general level of
cognitive development. These scales can be administered in a short time and involve
the clinician setting up task situations for the child to respond to. Again, we recommend proceeding to this second level of analysis primarily with children who are
clearly not playing normally or who are "suspicious" to the clinician because of
behavioral observation. If the child performs at a delayed level of cognitive development on the screening scale, then further testing might be undertaken.

A final level of analysis is to administer a more detailed scale, such as that
developed by Uzigiris and Hunt (1975). Dunst (1980) has developed some helpful
procedures for use with the Uzigiris and Hunt scales that make the clinical adminis-

tration of the tasks more streamlined. Such lengthy measures should be administered to a case who is strongly suspected of exhibiting cognitive deficits.

The speech pathologist should be careful, when assessing cognitive prerequisites for language, not to allow other professionals or parents to perceive this evaluation procedure as the testing of a child's intelligence. We should make no judgments about how "smart" a child is or necessarily even her potential for cognitive growth. If a child's play behavior and performance on cognitive scales indicate questionable cognitive development she should be referred to other professionals such as a psychologist for diagnosis of mental ability and potential for learning. It should be emphasized that we examine cognitive prerequisites only because they appear to be related to the acquisition and use of abstract language systems. If we determine that a child does not possess the cognitive holdings for acquiring the normally abstract and arbitrary symbol system, we then can consider attempting to train the child in cognitive prerequisites or in a communication system that is less abstract, such as simple signs that code concrete and frequently occurring activities.

### Assessment of Communication Intent and Function

Some authorities have indicated that a frequent manifestation of early language disorder in children is a difference in the use of language (Lucas, 1980). We can divide language use into a number of different levels of analysis (Chapman, 1981). As a child's MLU becomes longer, it is more difficult to discern a particular intent behind the utterance. Chapman (1981: 133) gives the example of a person saying, "Hey Jim, find the red ball, OK?" This, as Chapman points out, is a request for attention, a request for action, and a request for information about the listener's compliance. This same sentence could also be analyzed at the discourse level to determine the child's conversational competence.

We have found it useful to separate our thinking about the use of language into early language cases and older language cases. For instance, a child who is in the single-word or early multiword stage is most often reported to have difficulty with the number of uses he has for language. Frequently, children are referred because they do not initiate language enough. These children are typically not referred for being poor conversationalists. Indeed, Bloom, Roscissano, and Hood (1976) have reported that normal single-word and early multiword children are not very "contingent" in their conversations.

The point here is that when one considers disorders of communication intent and language function, it is often helpful to think separately about early language cases and later language cases. The early ones need to have an inventory taken of why they use language; the later ones need to be examined for the quality of their conversational participation. This portion of the chapter will focus only on assessment and communication intent in early language cases.

According to Chapman (1981), the clinician may adopt an existing classification scheme or change available systems so that functions that are of interest can be coded. The two most famous systems referring to children's use of language are the schemes developed by Halliday (1975) and Dore (1975). However, other systems might also be useful clinically (Lucas, 1980; Tough, 1977; Dore, 1978; Coggins and Carpenter, 1978; Folger and Chapman, 1978). From examining the categories in these systems, it is clear that many of the terms overlap regarding the functions they describe. McClean and Snyder-McClean (1978) have suggested that functions of language may be distilled down into two basic uses: one, to influence joint attention, and the other, to influence joint activity. These functions basically correspond to the imperative and the declarative in English. Thus, as Chapman (1981) suggests, it makes little difference exactly which system is used to assess function of language. The clinician should select a system, however, that at least contains some basic declarative and imperative operations so that the child's initiation of and response to communications can be coded.

As the clinician uses her chosen system of coding a child's communication intent, several issues should be considered. First, very little data are available on the reliability of the major coding schemes. Dale (1980) has found that clinicians can reliably code imperatives and declaratives; however, little information has appeared in the literature on the reliability of clinical judgments using the Dore or Halliday system. Reliability should be checked routinely because functions that are unreliably assigned are not useful to the clinician. Chapman (1981) provides some questions for troubleshooting when reliability is low:

1. Is sufficient information about the context available so a decision can be made about what the child "intended"?
2. Are the categories used in the coding scheme overlapping and clearly defined?
3. Are the categories too detailed for easy use by the clinician?
4. Are there too many categories?
5. Has the clinician practiced the system enough? Reliability is a function of practice.

Some additional general guidelines should be discussed. The assessment of communication function should be carried out in a natural situation. It is sometimes difficult to contrive situations in which a child will express a genuine communication intent. The clinician should have present in the room a wide variety of toys and other stimuli that would encourage a number of different conversational possibilities and expressions of need or declarations. If there are other children or adults in the situation, the clinician must remember that the functions expressed by the child are inextricably related to the behavior and utterances of other conversational participants.

Also, functions are only interpretable in light of the nonverbal context of communication. For instance, if a child points at a cow beside the highway and says "cow," we might assume the child is "labeling" or "commenting" about the animal. This would be suspected more strongly if the child's attention then went to something else. Another variable to bear in mind is the notion of sampling functions of communication in multiple settings. Our earlier example of how a child's use of language was dramatically different in the preschool setting as opposed to the clinic should illustrate the importance of multiple sampling. It would be a shame to target the regulatory function for training in the clinic, when the child frequently regulates the behavior of people in other situations. It is not necessarily a communication disorder when a child does not regulate in the clinic.

Some authors have suggested using standard eliciting tasks for basic communication functions. This has been done for imperatives and declaratives (Snyder, 1978, 1981; Dale, 1980; Staab, 1983) but not as widely for more specific functions of communication. Generally, declaratives seem to be elicited most effectively by presenting discrepant events and objects in the sampling situation. The child may then comment on the novel stimulus. Imperatives are more reliably obtained than declaratives because the clinician can maintain control over the stimuli and activities in the sampling situation. The child will ask for access to toys, or ask the clinician to assist in certain operations (winding of toys or the like). Chapman (1981) recommends that we assess functions in terms of how often they are verbally realized. Regulation, comment, greeting, and other functions may be expressed gesturally or behaviorally, and it would be important to determine if a child can use oral language to express these communications. Presently, there are no formal tests for all of the functions in early communication, and it is unlikely that there could be a standard valid method of assessing functional communication. It depends too much on child-initiated communications, which are not too easily contrived.

So far, in this portion of the chapter we have not mentioned form/structure of language. Earlier, we indicated that the process of language should not be fractionalized. The implication of this is that structure and function should be analyzed interactively. In cases where the child is nonverbal or at the single-word level, it is feasible to target communication functions in treatment. The clinician may want to increase the number of regulatory attempts in a particular child, or increase the verbal realizations of regulation in a client. When a child reaches the point of late single words and early multiword utterances, however, we recommend analysis of structure and function interactively.

### Assessment of Structure and Function in Early Utterances

Children in the single-word period can be examined for both the types of words they use and the apparent reasons they use them. The form of single-word utterances has been viewed in different ways by various authorities. Nelson (1974) categorized single words as members of specific classes (for example, general nominal, specific nominal, personal-social, action words, function words). Bloom and Lahey (1978: 484) separate single words "into nouns and relational words and then most of the relational words are categorized according to the content categories. . . ." These authors provide a lengthy discussion and examples of their system for early utterance analysis. Single words should be paired with functions such as those discussed by Chapman (1981).

As mentioned previously, there are existing methods of viewing and analyzing early semantic relations in children's utterances (Bloom, 1973; Brown, 1973; Leonard, 1976; Braine, 1976). There are also, as discussed above, a number of systems for examining communication functions in children (Halliday, 1975; Dore, 1975). Few systems, however, exist that interactively analyze structure and function in early utterances.

Bloom and Lahey (1978) have described an analysis system that takes into account structure and function. The system suggests that the clinician transcribe the child's utterances, the adult's utterances, and the nonverbal communication contextual events that are relevant to the communication. They prefer videotaping samples for use in their analysis because all linguistic and contextual information can be preserved and reviewed. If videotape equipment is unavailable, they recommend using audiotape and transcribing the nonlinguistic context. Finally, Bloom and Lahey recommend the use of hand transcription if it is not feasible to use instrumentation. They indicate that hand transcription is the least accurate of the three methods of recording because it must be done "on-line." Using notes is helpful in noisy situations where taping is not feasible. It is also possible to transcribe each third or fourth utterance instead of every one. Bloom and Lahey recommend that the beginning clinician start by gaining practice with a particular coding taxonomy in carefully scoring videotaped sessions. When speed and reliability are increased, then hand transcriptions may be easier and more accurate.

At the very least, we recommend that the clinician observe the child in an interaction with caretakers, teachers, or children so that utterances can be transcribed and the context of communication noted. We feel that the following assumptions are important in early multiword assessment:

1. It is important to determine if a child has a "basic" set of semantic relations or only limited usage of just a few (McClean and Snyder-McClean, 1978).
2. A child should be able to code verbally many relationships and aspects of the environment.
3. The clinician should obtain an inventory of communication functions used by a child to determine if there is a "basic set" of language uses.
4. Structure and function should be viewed interactively (Bloom and Lahey, 1978).
5. The clinician may find it valuable to get a feeling for the percentage of time a child initiates language versus adult-initiated utterances (Bloom and Lahey, 1978).
6. The clinician must be able to analyze utterances one to four words in length.
7. Early multiwords are typically analyzed using semantic grammar, which is different from the analyses done for later syntax (Brown, 1973; Bloom and Lahey, 1978; Bowerman, 1973).
8. The clinician should be sensitive to later developing forms present with the early multiwords (word endings, function words, and so on) to project development into later stages.

A number of taxonomies could be used in assigning semantic cases to early multiword utterances. Because neither function nor semantic relations can be assigned without taking into account the context in which they occur, the clinician must become very familiar with the cases and functions in the coding system so that functions and cases can be assigned immediately to utterances as they occur. If the clinician is present in the context, this could save much time, as nonverbal and verbal contributions of others need not be transcribed. The clinician can simply make an immediate judgment about structure and function based on a limited set of cases and uses. If a clinician is viewing a videotape or listening to an audiotape, notation about the nonlinguistic context should be made.

Appendix B contains a suggested transcription sheet for use with the analysis. The clinician should first write down the child's utterance either phonetically or orthographically and then follow this with the immediate interpretation of a semantic relation and function. Thus, the first three columns can be filled out at the time of each utterance. This procedure could be used as a preliminary part of an assessment to find out basic semantic relations and functions in a child's communication. It can also be carried forward as a means for monitoring treatment progress. From the data, later analysis can. determine the percentage of child-initiated versus adult-initiated utterances, as well as the percentage of use of each function and semantic relation in the sample. A summary sheet is presented in Appendix C. The remaining two columns of the transcription sheet can be filled out by the clinician after the evaluation session and used to complete the summary sheet.

As Bloom and Lahey (1978) state, an immediate note-taking system is not necessarily the ideal way to analyze early multiword utterances for the busy clinician. Its disadvantages are as follows:

1. The clinician must make an immediate decision about the form and function based on knowledge of the context. This is difficult at first, but becomes easier as the clinician becomes familiar with the coding system. Many of the child utterances will be quite clear in terms of form and function, but a core of them will be more problematic. It should also be pointed out that most of these children do not exhibit long utterances and typically do not speak frequently or rapidly; this reduced length and frequency of utterances make the transcription task more manageable.

2. The categories the clinician selects for form and use are a priori and may bias the view of the child's system (Leonard, Steckol, and Panther, 1983). This is true of any system approach. It is, however, better to use a system that looks at structure and function interactively rather than one that does not. Most often, the child enrolled in treatment for noninitiation of language (a problem with function) will also have structural problems. Rarely do we target for function alone in these early cases, and it is not often that we concentrate only on structure to the exclusion of use.

### Use of Formal Tests in Assessment

As we have indicated in the section on theoretical considerations, formal tests are best suited for comparing a child's performance on some measure to that of other youngsters who took the test. Formal tests, as Muma (1973a) stated, address the issue of whether or not a problem exists. These measures are not particularly good at determining the nature of the problem or selecting treatment targets. Table 4.1 lists commonly mentioned instruments. We make no attempt to critically analyze or detail these tests, because other sources provide substantial reviews and descriptions (*Ninth Mental Measurements Yearbook*, in press; Darley, 1979; Aram and Nation, 1982; Peterson and Marquardt, 1981). The reader will note, however, that the tests are calculated to tap a variety of language skills (expression, vocabulary, comprehension, imitation, cognitive), are targeted for use with a wide spectrum of age ranges, and represent a number of different theoretical points of view. The older tests obviously do not take into account current advances in thinking about language acquisition or assessment.

Clinicians who elect to use a formal test should consider the following: (1) the assumptions the test is based on; (2) the age, culture, and socioeconomic status of the population it was normed on; (3) the validity and reliability data provided; (4) the quality of information the test will provide as it relates to treatment; and (5) the aspects of language that are tested. Owens et al. (1983) provide a summary of specific grammatical forms examined by a wide variety of tests. Further

TABLE 4.1   Selected Language Assessment Instruments

| INSTRUMENT | AGE RANGE |
| --- | --- |
| Assessment of Children's Language Comprehension (Foster, Giddan, and Stark, 1973) | 3–0 to 6–11 |
| Bankson Language Screening Test (Bankson, 1977) | 4–1 to 8–0 |
| Basic Concept Inventory (Englemann, 1967) | 3–0 to 10–0 |
| Berry-Talbott Tests of Language: I—Comprehension of Grammar (Berry, 1966) | 5–0 to 8–0 |
| Boehm Test of Basic Concepts (Boehm, 1971) | Kindergarten to second grade |
| Carrow Elicited Language Inventory (Carrow, 1974) | 3–0 to 7–11 |
| Clinical Evaluation of Language Function (Semel and Wiig, 1980) | Kindergarten to tenth grade |
| Del Rio Language Screening Test: English/Spanish (Toronto et al., 1975) | 3–0 to 6–11 |
| Denver Developmental Screening Test (Frankenburg, Dodds, and Fandal, 1970) | 0–0 to 6–0 |
| Environmental Language Inventory (MacDonald, 1978) | None |
| Full Range Picture Vocabulary Test (Ammons and Ammons, 1948) | 2–0 to adult |
| Houston Test for Language Development (Crabtree, 1963) | 0–6 to 3–0 |
| Illinois Test of Psycholinguistic Abilities (Kirk, McCarthy, and Kirk, 1968) | 2–0 to 10–11 |

**TABLE 4.1**   (cont.)

| INSTRUMENT | AGE RANGE |
| --- | --- |
| Language Facility Test (Dailey, 1977) | 3–0 to 20–0 |
| Michigan Picture Language Inventory (Wolski and Lerea, 1962) | 4–0 to 6–0 |
| Miller-Yoder Language Comprehension Test (Miller and Yoder, 1984) | 3–0 to 8–0 |
| Northwestern Syntax Screening Test (Lee, 1969) | 3–0 to 7–11 |
| Oral Language Sentence Imitation Diagnostic Inventory (Zachman et al., 1978) | None |
| Peabody Picture Vocabulary Test—Revised (Dunn, 1980) | 2–6 to 18–0 |
| Picture Articulation and Language Screening Test (Rodgers, 1976) | Preschool |
| Porch Index of Communicative Ability in Children (Porch, 1974) | Preschool to 12–0 |
| Preschool Language Assessment Instrument (Blank, Rose, and Berlin, 1978) | 3–0 to 6–0 |
| Preschool Language Scale (Zimmerman, Steiner, and Evatt, 1969) | 1–6 to 7–0 |
| Receptive-Expressive Emergent Language Scale (Bzoch and League, 1971) | 0–0 to 3–0 |
| Reynell Developmental Scales (Reynell, 1969) | 0–6 to 6–0 |
| Riley Articulation and Language Test (Riley, 1971) | Kindergarten to second grade |
| Sequenced Inventory of Communication Development (Hedrick, Prather, and Tobin, 1975) | 0–4 to 4–0 |
| Test of Adolescent Language (Hammill et al., 1980) | Adolescent |
| Test of Auditory Comprehension of Language (Carrow, 1973) | 3–0 to 6–11 |
| Test of Language Development (Newcomer and Hammill, 1977) | 4–0 to 8–11 |
| Tina Bangs Language Scale (Bangs, 1961) | 2–0 to 6–0 |
| Token Test for Children (Disimoni, 1978) | 3–0 to 12–5 |
| Toronto Tests of Receptive Vocabulary: English/Spanish (Toronto, 1977) | 4–0 to 10–0 |
| Utah Test of Language Development (Mecham, Jex, and Jones, 1967) | 1–6 to 14–5 |
| Vane Evaluation of Language Scale (Vane, 1975) | 2–6 to 6–6 |
| Verbal Language Development Scale (Mecham, 1971) | 0–0 to 16–0 |
| Vocabulary Comprehension Scale (Bangs, 1975) | 2–0 to 6–0 |

portions of this chapter will address in more detail specific areas related to formal testing (such as comprehension and elicited imitation).

### Assessment of Children's Language Comprehension

Perhaps the area of children's linguistic assessment that has been the subject of the most test development has been language comprehension. A major reason behind the extensive development of language comprehension tests is the long-standing belief that in language acquisition reception precedes expression. The implication, then, is that one must understand language in order to express it adequately. Historically, programs for language training have been organized first in terms of receptive or comprehension modules, followed by expressive language training. Bloom (1974) discussed some basic differences between expression and reception of language. She brings up the important point that children's responses to language are multidetermined. That is, a child's correct response could be primarily in reaction to nonverbal contextual aspects of the situation. Following is a typical scenario:

> The mother says, "He can understand everything that we tell him. He just doesn't talk." The clinician leans forward and says, "Can you show me how you know he understands what you tell him?" The mother shifts uncomfortably in her chair and tells the child to "go turn off the light," as she points alternately between the light switch and the ceiling fixture. The child turns the light off and on several times. Later when the mother is told to provide only verbal stimuli, the child is not able to perform many one- and two-level commands when they were unaccompanied by gestures.

Thus, children and adults rely on the context in which language is used to aid in interpretation of what was said. Young children between and the ages of two and six are especially dominated by perception and tend to understand things in terms of how they appear rather than by the language or logic that is used to explain events (Ginsburg and Opper, 1969).

Chapman has discussed the notion of "comprehension strategies" exhibited by children. According to Chapman (1978: 310), a comprehension strategy is "a short cut, heuristic or algorithm for arriving at sentence meaning without full marshalling of the information in the sentence and one's linguistic knowledge. Thus, it sometimes yields the correct answer, although it may more usually give the appearance of understanding." Clinicians who attempt to assess early language comprehension should be wary of correct responses by children that could have been generated by attention to contextual stimuli or comprehension strategies. For example, many children process the name of an object and then they act on the object in a habitual manner. This gives the appearance of knowing an entire sentence ("Throw the ball") when, in actuality, the child may understand only the word "ball" and simply throws it as he usually does. Chapman gives many other comprehension strategies, and we encourage clinicians to become familiar with these patterns.

Bransford and Nitsch (1978) point out that comprehension involves a situation plus an input. A human organism is not a static system but has a history and background knowledge. A given input of language is placed in this "situation" along with the nonverbal context of communication. Many variables come to bear on the "understanding" of an input, not the least of which are the person's background as well as the linguistic and nonlinguistic contexts. Rees and Schulman (1978) have written an article in which they indicate that most tests of language comprehension measure only the literal meaning of things. Most comprehension tests are quite artificial when compared to the richness of language comprehension in a natural situation. The typical comprehension assessment situation involves presenting a child with test plates containing pictures. The child is asked to point to the picture that best represents some verbal stimulus uttered by the examiner. The pictures are often line drawings and the verbal stimuli are not discursively related to one another (in one case the child is asked to point to a "monkey" and in the next plate the topic is "shopping"). In these tests there is no temporal sequence of events that would allow a child to be able to predict what will be said, as in real language comprehension. Naturalistic situations also give the child the opportunity to ask for clarification or repetition in the face of information loss. We do not afford children this chance in comprehension testing. The above statements are meant only to reinforce the notion that real language comprehension is a highly complex phenomenon and cannot be assessed easily.

Millen and Prutting (1979) studied three language comprehension tests for consistency of response on specific grammatical features. They found that on the *Northwestern Syntax Screening Tests (NSST), Assessment of Children's Language Comprehension (ACLC),* and *Bellugi Comprehension Tests* there was general agreement in the overall scores generated by the measures. There were, however, significant differences among the tests for more than half of the specific grammatical features evaluated. The investigators logically suggest that the tests are not equivalent and not clinically sound for generating specific remediation targets. Other stimulus, task, and subject variables have been studied in comprehension tests. Haynes and McCallion (1981) found that children with a reflective cognitive tempo (long decision time) performed significantly better than impulsive (short decision time) children on the *Test of Auditory Comprehension of Language (TACL)*. Further, these researchers reported that scores on the *TACL* improved significantly over standard administration when the subjects were given two stimulus presentations or if the test was administered imitatively.

Thus, it appears that variables other than language comprehension enter into test performance, and failure to do well on a comprehension test could be explained by other factors. Attentional set, hearing impairment, ambiguous pictures, test administration procedures (Shorr, 1983), cognitive style, and unrelated stimuli—all could account for poor performance on a standardized test of language comprehension. Additionally, Gowie and Powers showed that a child's expectations about what a sentence was going to say significantly influenced their performance on a comprehension task. They say that ". . . knowing a word involves a set of expectations about the referents and about the types of messages in which the word is likely to occur" (1979: 40).

We have suggested that comprehension is difficult to test without contaminating influences from the context and comprehension strategies. Further, failure to perform well on a test of comprehension does not necessarily indicate the presence of a comprehension disorder. Based on the current literature, about all we can say with some conviction is that adequate performance on a standardized test of language comprehension probably means that the child is capable of comprehending some language in a highly artificial situation. This does not necessarily represent her comprehension in natural situations. Failure of a comprehension test, on the other hand, does not necessarily mean that the child is incapable of comprehending language either in the contrived testing situation or the natural environment.

Understanding of single words in young children appears to us to be testable. If they direct their attention to the appropriate object when uttered by an examiner (with appropriate controls for contextual cues) they probably recognize the lexical item. We begin to run into trouble when we try to test two-word utterances and larger sentences. Some attempts have been made to remove the effects of context by using anomalous commands in testing children (Kramer, 1977; Duchan and Siegel, 1979). This involves giving commands to children that are not likely to be expected from their past experience. A child may be told to "sit on the ball" or "kiss the phone." If the child performs, he is said to have comprehended both elements in the command. If the child does not perform (and this is where we run into the problem again), is it that he has not understood? Perhaps anomalous commands are silly to children and are disregarded. There may be a cognitive mismatch between the command and what the object is supposed to be used for. At any rate, failure to perform an anomalous command may not really mean lack of comprehension.

Currently, language comprehension is tested in four ways by speech pathologists. First, there are a number of standardized tests of comprehension (see Table 4.1). Second, some researchers have tested comprehension by having children act out certain commands (Leonard et al., 1978). Third, several investigators have used a decision task where the child makes judgments such as "good or bad" or he engages in a preference task to say which of two sentences was the better. Finally, similar to the standardized tests, clinicians have used pictures and/or objects and engaged children in an informal pointing task. Perhaps the "best" method of comprehension testing is to use several methods, both formal and informal. The clinician should also employ more naturalistic assessment methods, such as engaging the child in play or conversation, and evaluating the appropriateness of verbal and nonverbal responses. The clinician should also note if the child uses requests for clarification or repetition in conversation.

## LANGUAGE SAMPLING:
## A GENERAL LOOK AT THE PROCESS

A common thread throughout this chapter thus far has been the notion of ecological validity. When done appropriately, language sampling of a child's spontaneous conversation is perhaps the closest we come to evaluating a youngster's real communication. As Miller (1981) says, we must broaden our definition of what sampling is to include the very young child who may be a year old and not much of a conversationalist. We do, however, sample his communication. Perhaps a better name for this process would be "communication sampling." Sampling is the only way to hold content, form, and use intact; thus, it is one of our most powerful tools.

Most speech pathologists have sat in a small room with a young child and attempted to fill a cassette with a "representative" sample of language. Most of us also have experienced the despair and humiliation (if observed) of harvesting a string of one-word utterances and elliptical responses. Faced with this, we begin to put the pressure on the child for longer utterances and ask questions about the obvious. "What is in this picture?" we ask, when both the child and the clinician know the answer. "Tell me about what you did at school today," we cajole, and the child shrugs his shoulders, saying, "Nuthin."

A very wise observation was made by Hubbell (1981) after he studied spontaneous talking in young children. When children feel they are being interrogated and there is a great deal of pressure for them to talk, they tend to clam up. One of the worst liabilities the clinician can have is a mother who says to her child in the waiting room, "Now this lady wants you to talk to her, so be sure you do." This is, in many cases, the kiss of death for a decent language sample. Children need to feel at ease and not pressured to talk. Clinicians also should try to resist the very strong urge to "interrogate" children and, worst of all, to question them about the obvious. As we mentioned earlier, all communication is affected by the context in which it occurs, and language sampling is no different. Because each sampling session is a product of an individual child, clinician, and communication environment, it is impossible to provide guidelines that will work with all cases. All we can do is "play the probabilities" and provide some suggestions that may facilitate spontaneous talking with most cases.

For detailed treatments of language-sampling procedures the reader is referred to the ample sources dealing with the topic (Barrie-Blackley, Musselwhite, and Rogister, 1978; Miller, 1981). Some general watchwords are as follows:

1. Always tape-record the sample. We tend to subjectively "fill in" utterances that are incomplete, and it is distracting to a child if you are attempting to carry on a legitimate conversation and are scribbling on a yellow pad. Either we are engaging in a real conversation or we are not.

2. Try to use a good quality tape recorder and position it in such a way to promote optimal recording. This is one of the most often overlooked aspects of sampling language. It is a real disappointment when a clinician has done a masterful job of eliciting natural conversation from a child only to have it rendered unintelligible by a poor recording.

3. Try to minimize the use of yes/no questions. Remember, as soon as you ask these, you know the answer will be yes, no, or I don't know. Beginning clinicians typically bombard the child with yes/no questions and the sample may be so loaded with single-word utterances that the child's MLU is severely underestimated due to sampling error (see Miller, 1981, regarding sampling error).

4. Attempt to minimize questions that can be answered with one word, for example, "What color is your dog?" Although you have to ask some of these in the normal course of conversation, they do elicit single-word responses.

5. Try to ask broad-based questions, such as "What happened?" "What happened next?" "Tell me about. . . ." "Why?"

6. Don't be afraid to make contributions to the conversation. One of the most common errors of beginning clinicians is that they want the child to do all the talking. This is not a natural conversation situation. Also, the child's utterances are typically in the role of "responder." Think back to the last language sample you took and ask yourself if the child had opportunities to initiate conversation instead of merely responding to your interrogations. Also, ask yourself if you were a semitruthful conversational participant. Did you tell the child some of your feelings and experiences? Did you talk mostly about things that were obvious or trivial? As Hubbell (1981) states, a facilitator of conversation is a good conversational model. It has been our experience, that as soon as we stop the barrage of questions and begin to make some observations about what is going on in the session and what we think about things, the child begins to make some contributions to the conversation.

7. As Miller (1981) says, try not to "play the fool" during a language sample, especially with an older child. Give the child credit for the intelligence to know that you could easily describe the pictures and that you know how to do simple operations such as "washing clothes," etc.

8. Learn to tolerate periods of silence or pauses. Beginning clinicians seem to feel that they have to fill up pauses in communication with verbalizations. Give the child an opportunity to initiate conversation.

9. Stay on a topic long enough to converse about it. Do not change topics after the child says one utterance on the issue. This encourages a series of "one liners" from children, and the clinician is again placed in the position of having to interrogate.

10. Finally, be aware of children's cognitive levels when you ask questions. The clinician should be aware that children have differing conceptual frameworks from adults and altered perspectives of time and space. We have heard clinicians ask three-year-olds such questions as "Why do you think the truck goes so fast?"

There are variables that appear to affect the length and complexity of language samples obtained by researchers and examiners. First, the racial background of the participant could have a potential influence on a child's conversation. Several studies have suggested that young black children are especially prone to "style shifting" or "code switching" when confronted with a white adult examiner (Labov, 1970; Cazden, 1970). Cazden (1970) has stated that black children speak in a school register (for teachers and administrators) and a street register (for peers and family). Interestingly, the school register is different in content, has a shorter mean length of utterance, is less complex, and is more disfluent than the street register. This certainly has implications for language sampling. Clinicians should realize that the samples they obtain from young minority children may underestimate their linguistic abilities.

Verbalizations of the examiner may also affect language sampling. Lee (1974) suggests that the clinician attempt to speak with a variety of syntactic structures during sampling a child's language. The modeling literature has shown that children, in as little as a single session, can use language that is roughly similar in complexity to an adult model, whether the model uses extremely simple sentences or complex sentences involving embedding and conjoining (Haynes and Hood, 1978). Children are also sensitive to pragmatic aspects of a communication situation. If they are placed in a play situation with younger children, their language will be simpler than when they talk to adults.

Presupposition may also play a role in the length and complexity of samples obtained from children. Like adults, children will elaborate linguistically about objects and events that are not present in the current communication context (Strandberg and Griffith, 1969). If a child does not share visual access to the stimuli with the clinician, she will tend to elaborate linguistically to a greater degree (Haynes, Purcell, and Haynes, 1979).

Several studies have shown that children provide longer and more complex language samples if they are engaged in conversation as opposed to picture description tasks (Longhurst and Grubb, 1974; Longhurst and File, 1977; Haynes, Purcell, and Haynes, 1979). Picture description tends to lend itself to description and naming of elements in a picture rather than linguistic elaboration about a topic unknown to the clinician. These are typically single-word responses or elliptical answers. Especially, if the clinician views the picture with the child, the task becomes not one of conversation but of naming aspects of pictures. In the studies mentioned above, the children evidenced longer and more complex language samples when engaged in conversation than when they were describing pictures or objects. Conversation, of course, carries with it an element of presupposition because the clinician does not know what the child will talk about. Thus, the child is forced to elaborate linguistically because the clinician is not aware of the conversational aspects the child is attempting to convey. Picture description, however, is a viable method of sampling language for some children. Certainly some children will not readily engage in conversation, and picture description is needed to elicit some language for analysis (Atkins and Cartwright, 1982).

Several investigations have dealt with the difference between samples obtained at home and those in a clinical setting, as well as between samples gathered by mothers and those by speech pathologists. Kramer, James, and Saxman (1979) compared home and clinic samples and found that longer utterances were obtained in the home environment as compared to the clinical setting. They suggest that, if possible, samples obtained in the home environment may be obtained occasionally prior to the evaluation in order not to underestimate a child's language ability. Olswang and Carpenter (1978) studied language samples taken by experienced speech clinicians and by mothers of language-impaired children. They found that the mothers elicited more language from their children in a given time period. However, the quality of the language elicited by both groups was similar. That is, there was no significant difference in the lexical, semantic, or syntactic character of the child's language. This study suggests that speech pathologists should feel fairly confident that the samples they elicit from children are at least similar in quality to the samples elicited by mothers in a clinical setting.

Sometimes speech clinicians are interested in eliciting particular syntactic structures from a child as opposed to a general language sample. This occasion would arise if the clinician wanted to probe the child's use of certain constructions such as question forms in spontaneous speech. Mulac, Prutting, and Tomlinson (1978) suggest that a variety of tasks could be used to elicit a particular construction. They found that the most effective tasks for eliciting the "is interrogative" were those that required intent and had contextual referents and some inherent structure to the activity. One example was a guessing game in which children had to guess what was in a bag—"Is it a ——?" The notion of using several different informal elicitation tasks to evaluate certain syntactic structures has been supported by others as well (Leonard et al., 1978; Lund and Duchan, 1983; Musselwhite and Barrie-Blackley, 1980).

We have seen that obtaining a language sample is a critical part of language evaluation. There are a host of variables that can affect the size and quality of the sample obtained by the examiner. These variables, and their effect on sample size, may play a major role in the clinician's interpretation of the child's language sample and must be considered when analyzing the client's communication ability.

### Assessment of Utterances Using Length Measures

One of the most common measures recommended for use in a basic language evaluation is the mean length of utterance (MLU) (Miller, 1981). Length measures are not new in speech pathology, having been used historically as a mainstay of our clinical armamentarium (Johnson, Darley, and Spriestersbach, 1963). There are several reasons why authorities have continued to recommend computing a length measure of utterances obtained in a language sample. One is that there is a general correlation between MLU and chronological age in many groups of children up to age four (Miller, 1981). Thus, MLU may be used as a very gross indicator of language development in this age group; but the clinician cannot simply rely on length measures alone in an analysis. Another important reason for computing MLU is that Brown (1973) has used this length measure to demarcate his five stages of language development. Allegedly, MLU is a much better predictor of language development than chronological age. Brown (1973) has postulated that if two children are matched on MLU a clinician may predict that the constructional complexity of their language will be similar.

Brown (1973) and Miller (1981) provide suggestions for the computation of MLU. Miller recommends a distributional analysis to ensure that MLU has a relatively normal distribution around an average length. The analysis is simply a listing of the number of utterances at each morpheme level—1, 2, 3, 4, and so on. If the distributional analysis reveals an MLU with a small variation, perhaps an organic condition or a sampling error has played a role in the length of utterance. Miller and Chapman (1981) report normative data for MLU, and more recently, research on temporal reliability in older children has been published (Chabon, Udolf, and Egolf, 1982). The latter investigators report that MLU has weak temporal reliability in older children and its use for prediction of language level may be less sensitive than previously thought. There may be some difficulties with MLU as it is presently computed (Muma, 1983), and some investigators report stronger relationships between MLU and language ability if the measure is computed with single-word utterances removed (Klee and Fitzgerald, 1983).

The norms for MLU are presently reported for a rather narrow population, and further data gathering is necessary. The use of MLU seems to be in a state of transition, but until more conclusive data and viable alternatives are provided, we feel that MLU should be routinely calculated in a language evaluation of children younger than age five.

### Assessment of Syntax Using Elicited Imitation

Elicited imitation has been used in psycholinguistic research on language development for decades (Slobin and Welsh, 1971). There is a correlation between age and the ability to imitate sentences of increasing length and complexity (Brown, 1973). Elicited imitation, as an assessment procedure, carries with it certain assumptions that its user must believe to be true about language and linguistic processing. A basic assumption of imitative techniques is that children will repeat only those structures for which they have linguistic competence. If a child omits or misuses a syntactic element in a sentence imitation task, the examiner must suspect that the child does not "have" that element in his repertoire. Conversely, if the child does imitate an item, it is assumed that the youngster has that structure. This basic assumption of elicited imitation has been challenged during the last decade, and investigators have explored variables that affect the elicited imitation response other than linguistic competence.

One variable that has been recently explored is the use of a nonlinguistic context in conjunction with elicited imitation. Nelson and Weber-Olsen (1980) found greater mean length of imitative utterance and fewer errors when contextual support in the form of object manipulations was provided as compared to a no-context condition. Similarly, Haniff and Siegel (1981) found significantly fewer errors in an imitation task that was accompanied by picture stimuli as compared to a no-picture condition. These two studies suggest that imitation is improved when the clinician provides a context. Because the major subject-verb-object elements are depicted for them, a context may assist children in remembering elements presented in a model sentence or allow them to focus on more obscure aspects of a sentence. One study, however, does not support the finding that context improves imitative performance (Connell and Myles-Zitzer, 1982).

Elicited imitation is also affected by stress patterns in the model sentence (Slobin and Welsh, 1971; Blasdell and Jensen, 1970). If a child misses a syntactic element and the examiner stresses the element on the second trial, the probability of correct performance is increased. Clinicians must be aware of this when they use elicited imitation for pretest-posttest measures to evaluate treatment effects, as they may inadvertently stress elements that were the targets of training.

Two studies have suggested a trial or practice effect in elicited imitation (Lang and Moore, 1977; Haynes and Haynes, 1979). Haynes and Haynes (1979) gave children a sentence imitation task two times separated by two days. They found that more than 52 percent of the children's errors on the first trial had been corrected on the second trial even though only two days separated the performances. Interestingly, 22 percent of the children's errors remained the same, and 25 percent of the errors on the second day were new ones that had not occurred on the first trial. Fujiki and Brinton (1983) reported that sampling reliability for elicited imitation may not stabilize until a syntactic structure is repeated over three trials. This certainly gives one pause when contemplating the administration of an elicited imitation test in a single trial and makes one wonder about what the clinician learns from the imitative task.

Elicited imitation tests are typically composed of a series of unrelated sentences. Imitation, because of its nature, violates a host of pragmatic conventions, and one of these is discursiveness. If sentences are unrelated to each other, many of the linguistic forms (pronouns, questions, demonstratives, and so on) are used inappropriately. Haynes and Haynes (1979) explored the use of discursively related sentences that made up a story versus imitation of the same sentences that were randomly arranged. No significant difference was found in the imitative performance of normal language children in the related and unrelated sentence tasks. Thus, for normal children, the relatedness made little difference in performance. However, we do not know about this variable as it relates to language-impaired youngsters. On a subjective level, though, the experimenters noted that the normal children appeared to "enjoy" the task to a greater degree when the sentences were in a story format, and there were fewer lapses in attention.

Bonvillian, Raeburn, and Horan (1979) studied the effects of rate, intonation, and length of children's elicited imitation. They found that there were significantly more errors on longer sentences than in shorter ones. They also found a significant trend indicating that the children made fewer errors when the stimuli they imitated were presented at a rate of about two words per second (wps), a rate similar to the children's own speech rate (1.8 wps). Finally, there was significant interaction between length and intonation pattern. The children made fewer errors on the longer sentences when normal intonation patterns were used as compared to a monotone presentation. Perhaps intonation is a valuable cue used by children in decoding complex sentences.

Several investigators have expressed concern about the validity of elicited imitation as being representative of spontaneous grammatical performance (Prutting, Gallagher, and Mulac, 1975; Daily and Boxx, 1979; McDade, Simpson, and Larnt, 1982; Connell and Myles-Zitzer, 1982; Werner and Kreseck, 1980). Bloom (1974) has reported a case of a child who was incapable of effectively imitating his own spontaneous utterances that had been recorded and transcribed from a previous session. She attributed this performance decrement to a lack of context during the imitative task.

From this general review of the literature it can be seen that performance on an elicited imitation task is affected by many variables; thus, we cannot be certain what elicited imitation is measuring. Further, many studies have shown that elicited imitation performance can agree with or differ from spontaneous speech performance. As Prutting and Connolly (1976: 420) so aptly state: "Elicited imitations alone may underestimate, overestimate or accurately describe the child's language performance." On a theoretical plane, elicited imitation violates the integrative model of language because it separates structure from function and uses unrelated utterances with no communicative intent.

There are several advantages to the use of elicited imitation, however, First, an imitative task can be administered in a short time, usually in less than fifteen minutes. Second, with imitation, the clinician can assess specific structures instead of waiting for them to appear spontaneously in a language sample. Third, some tests (Carrow, 1974) include normative data for comparing children's performance in order to solve the problem/no problem issue. Finally, some authorities suggest that elicited imitation may be a most effective procedure when operating under severe time constraints. There are several tests that have been constructed in an elicited imitation format (Carrow, 1974; Zachman et al., 1978).

The present authors feel that elicited imitation is a useful procedure, but clinicians should never rely solely on an imitative assessment. Treatment targets should only be selected from spontaneous language samples, and if imitative techniques are used they should always be supplemented by spontaneous performance.

### Assessment of Syntax Using Analysis Packages

After the speech pathologist has obtained a language sample, judgments must be made regarding the syntactic development of the child. Analysis of syntax can be conceptualized on a continuum. On the left end of the continuum is the administration of formal tests. These measures can give the clinician some insight into general syntactic development. In the middle of the continuum the clinician can analyze a language sample in accordance with specific "packaged" assessment procedures (Lee, 1974) and obtain more precise information than is available from standardized tests. Finally, on the right end, the clinician can analyze the sample using his knowledge of linguistics and language development and not relying on a step-by-step package analysis procedure. The left end of the continuum requires less expertise than the right end in terms of clinician experience and training. Also, the left end of the continuum takes less time for the analysis than the right, but it provides less clinically relevant information. Thus, the clinician must make a decision as to the time available for the analysis, her expertise in linguistics, and the depth of information desired.

It is beyond the scope of this chapter to instruct clinicians in performing an analysis of a child's syntax. The best way to learn an analysis system is to obtain a sample and follow the guidelines provided by authors of complexity analysis packages. Typically, the authors provide explicit instructions for obtaining a sample, segmentation, and analysis. Beginning clinicians should realize that any syntactic analysis method requires practice in order to be used effectively. The most widely known analysis procedures are listed in Figure 4.6.

Muma (1978) points out that descriptive procedures have greater "power" than normative ones because they help the clinician to describe individual differences. Descriptive procedures, because they are based on spontaneous language samples, also provide the clinician with more relevant intervention targets, as they do not fracture the integrity of the content-form-use model as imitative and standardized tests do. Thus, there are advantages to performing a descriptive analysis, and package systems provide the clinician with guidelines for completing such an analysis. We should, however, remember that each analysis procedure reflects its author's bias regarding language and that most systems look at a language sample in only limited ways.

Consumers who intend to use an analysis package should be aware that the procedures differ importantly. These differences may determine whether or not a clinician finds it appropriate to use a particular package. We will use the *Developmental Sentence Scoring (DSS)* procedure in our examples because this methodology is widely known. Use of this procedure in our discussion is not meant to be a criticism of this particular approach.

1. Some package systems recommend obtaining a specific sample size before subjecting the language to analysis (Lee, 1974). For instance, Lee (1974) recommends using 50 subject-verb utterances for computation of the *DSS*. A later study, however, stated that a sample of 150 utterances may be more appropriate for reliable scoring. If the clinician does not have a large enough sample, perhaps a different procedure would be more appropriate.

2. Analysis packages vary considerably in the time required for completion. This may be due to several influences: Some procedures are quite detailed and lengthy (Bloom and Lahey, 1978; Crystal, Fletcher, and Garman, 1976); and other procedures use very specific terminologies and vocabulary or have complicated scoring systems that require much time and practice in order for the clinician to use the procedure economically.

FIGURE 4.6    Selected language sample analysis procedures.

- Assessing Children's Language in Naturalistic Contexts (Lund and Duchan, 1983)
- Assigning Structural Stage (Miller, 1981)
- Co-occurring and Restricted Structures Analysis (Muma, 1973b)
- Developmental Sentence Analysis (Lee, 1974)
- Indiana Scale of Clausal Development (Dever and Bauman, 1974)
- Language Assessment, Remediation and Screening Procedure (Crystal, Fletcher, and Garman, 1976)
- Language Sampling, Analysis and Training (Tyack and Gottsleben, 1974)
- Length Complexity Index (Miner, 1969)
- Length of T-Unit or Communication Unit (Loban, 1976)
- Linguistic Analysis of Speech Samples (Engler, Hannah, and Longhurst, 1973)
- Mean Length of Utterance and Distributional Analysis (Miller, 1981)
- A Method for Assessing Use of Grammatical Structures (Kahn and James, 1980)
- Structural Complexity Score (McCarthy, 1930)

3. The procedures differ in terms of how they segment or separate utterances obtained in the sample. The *DSS*, for instance, analyzes subject-verb utterances and does not score sentence fragments. Some clinicians, however, feel that there is much useful information in sentence fragments (for example, elliptical responses) that may be important to analyze.

4. Some systems are recommended by their authors as ideal for use with particular treatment approaches. Lee, Koenigsknecht, and Mulhern (1975) used the *DSS* as an input to their interactive language teaching strategy and continued to monitor progress using the system.

5. Another way that evaluation systems differ is in terms of the structures they do or do not analyze. For example, the *DSS* does not specifically analyze certain forms (prepositions, articles, and so forth), accounting for their presence or absence by assigning a "sentence point" to an utterance if it is grammatical. Other systems specifically analyze most structural elements of English, even structures that may not be of interest to the clinician.

6. Analysis packages differ in their provision of normative data. The *DSS* has normative data, whereas other packages are purely descriptive and make no attempt to cull numerical scores on normal and disordered children.

7. Finally, the analysis procedures are not uniform in applying the results to a normal language development progression. That is, some are designed to examine linguistic elements without locating the child on a language development continuum. Lee (1974), Bloom and Lahey (1978), and Crystal, Fletcher, and Garman (1976) apply their results to developmental progressions.

Several investigations have shown that some of the package analysis procedures appear to be capable of documenting language changes in children, at least in a general way (Longhurst and Schrandt, 1973; Sharf, 1972). Further, any method that a clinician selects will require specific training and practice in order to use it effectively. It should be remembered that any method used depends to a significant degree on the quality of the sample obtained and typically analyzes only the structural elements of language independent of pragmatics. Thus, any analysis package procedure will take the clinician time and practice to learn and in the end will look at language only from a specific point of view (Miller, 1981).

It is the preference of the present authors that if clinicians are going to spend time learning about analysis of the structural aspects of language, their time would be better spent learning linguistics and language acquisition instead of one specific analysis package that probably would not be appropriate for all clients anyway. An analysis package could always be learned later to supplement the clinician's linguistic knowledge and would probably be learned more easily due to the experience with linguistics. A knowledge of linguistics would allow the clinician to generally analyze samples for structures that are present, absent, or inconsistent and still choose treatment targets that are relevant instead of trying to find a package analysis procedure that is a "best fit" for the child. We feel that, ultimately, the clinician must determine (1) which structures the child appears to have acquired, (2) which structures are absent in obligatory contexts, (3) which structures are inconsistently used, and (4) which contexts seem to be associated with use and nonuse of the inconsistent structures.

Muma (1973b) and Kahn and James (1980) have advocated descriptive procedures that focus on determining present, absent, and inconsistent syntactic elements, and we view this as a commonsense approach to analysis that has direct clinical application. It also does not involve the clinician's commitment of time to learning one or two package procedures and their unique scoring systems.

Recently, computer analysis of language samples has come to the fore.[1] Software programs are available that provide detailed information about a language sample. However, the clinician must remember that typically much time is invested in coding the transcript into the computer. Often this may take more time than a paper and pencil analysis, if the clinician merely wants to define treatment targets. Also, the computer analysis may provide the clinician with more information than is really needed. The advantage of the computer would appear to lie in the multiple analyses that could be performed once the sample is inputted.

No doubt we will learn much in the next decade from these procedures about patterns of error and subtypes of language disorder. No single procedure can tell a clinician all she needs to know about a child's language. Again, ultimately , it is the clinician's judgment that must be applied to a particular case, whether it is a decision to choose among several package analysis systems or simply to focus on a more broad-based linguistic analysis.

### Assessment of Conversational Pragmatics

As mentioned earlier, the most productive aspect of assessing the pragmatics of children using semantic relations is to analyze their functions of communication or the reasons why they talk. In children whose MLUs are long, however, utterances serve multiple functions, and it is not necessarily as productive to analyze their communicative intent. Unfortunately, there are no tests for conversational pragmatics that have received widespread support, and it is quite unlikely that an effective one could be developed due to the nature of language use in context. One measure of "interpersonal language skills" has appeared that analyzes children's conversations surrounding a board game such as "Sorry" (Blagden and McConnell, 1983); however, this is a specialized type of context and not necessarily reflective of normal conversational processes. When the clinician focuses on conversation and discourse it is necessary to obtain a sample of the child's conversational performance and to transcribe the utterances of both the child and the interlocutor—a time-consuming task. However, if the clinician is to obtain data on the child's conversational performance, the contributions of both participants cannot be ignored.

There are several measures that the clinician might elect to use to analyze conversation, depending on which aspects of the discourse are of interest. These measures overlap to a certain degree and are really different methods of examining the same behavior.

---

[1] Referential Semantic Analysis, Teaching Texts, Box 303, Broadway, Va. 22815; and Lingquest Software, Inc., 3349 Beard Road, Napa, Calif. 94558.

Bloom, Rocissano, and Hood (1976) provide us with guidelines regarding the assessment of "contingency," which is also recommended by Gallagher (1982). Contingency is the extent to which a speaker's contribution to a conversation reflects the effect of a previous utterance. They define three types of adjacent utterances: (1) contingent speech, which shares the same topic with the preceding statement and adds new information; (2) imitative speech, which shares the same topic but does not add new information; and (3) noncontingent utterances, which do not share the same topic as prior utterances.

Bloom, Rocissano, and Hood have shown that contingent speech increases between Brown's (1973) language development stages I and V and imitative and noncontingent speech decreases. Early in stage I children are not particularly contingent, and they become progressively more able to stay on a topic and make additional contributions. Obviously, a person cannot be contingent all of the time due to topic shifts. Children in stage V are about 50 percent contingent in their utterances.

> Lamar, a twelve-year-old boy, was referred for a language evaluation and was billed as "autisticlike." His clinician, teachers, and parent were interviewed and they reported that he did not have much functional language, although he would frequently chant commercials and other routines he had memorized from television and radio. The clinician who accompanied Lamar "triggered" him on a commercial about a wrestling match to be held in a nearby city. He went on and on: "Big time championship wrestling at the memorial auditorium at 8:00, etc." We videotaped the evaluation in which we tried to engage Lamar in a variety of interactions, and toward the end of the session we tried to extinguish some of his commercials. We decided to analyze the tape for the percentage of Lamar's utterances that were contingent or related to another speaker's statement. We found that less than 10 percent of his utterances related to what someone else had said. At the subsequent staffing, we recommended that increasing contingent utterances and contextually relevant speech could be the treatment targets. The people from Lamar's school admitted that the commercials were a source of amusement and interest. Some school personnel mistakenly believed that these routines were "practice" in using language. Further discussion revealed that Lamar was frequently encouraged to say commercials for both entertainment and practice. They had not realized that so little of his communication was relevant and that they were playing a role in perpetuating his communication disorder.

Thus, one method of analyzing a child's conversational participation is to obtain an overall view of the contingency of the utterances. A child who is not capable of a reasonable degree of contingency will have trouble maintaining topics and perpetuating interactions with others.

Topic is another area that overlaps with contingency, but an analysis of topic may give the clinician slightly different information (Keenan and Schiefflin, 1976). Topics may use general knowledge shared by interactants, information physically present in the context or previous discourse. According to Keenan and Schiefflin (1976) much "conversational space" is taken up by communicators to establish a

topic. Once the topic is established, an interactant can use his turn to either maintain the topic (continuous discourse) or change the topic (discontinuous discourse).
When speakers continue a discourse topic by collaborating a previous utterance
with a related statement or incorporating information in a prior utterance into their
statement, the topic is maintained. When a speaker discontinues a discourse topic, it
is either by introducing a topic that is unrelated to previous utterances or reintro-
ducing a prior topic ("getting back to what we said about . . ."). Thus, topic-
maintaining utterances collaborate a prior statement or incorporate it into a new
statement that is still on the topic.

Developmentally, the length of continuous discourse increases with age. In
assessment, we need to determine how a child is able to secure the attention of a
listener in order to initiate a topic—crying, yelling, gesturing, tugging, loudness,
prosody, or an introduction such as "know what?" We can measure the length of
the topic unit in terms of number of turns taken per topic. We can also measure the
topic-maintaining and -shifting utterances used by a child. It is important in assessment to examine not only a child's ability to continue topics but also to initiate
them. In sampling, as mentioned previously, we do not often do this. Some studies
report a high percentage of adult interrogatives in conversations with children,
which is perhaps related to social control because it places constraints on the
listener (Hubbell, 1981). Mishler (1975) found this typical of the interaction
pattern between teachers and first-graders.

Another major category of measurement of conversational competence is the
contingent query. A number of studies (Garvey, 1977a, 1977b) show that contingent queries are used by adults and children to achieve cohesion in conversation.
Children as young as three years use contingent queries. Basically, the queries serve
multiple functions in conversation, many of which have to do with repair procedures that allow the conversation to continue. For instance, a contingent query can
be used to request a general repetition ("huh?"), a specific repetition ("a what?"),
a request for confirmation ("a tape recorder?"), and elaboration ("we have to go
where?"). There are more complex aspects of contingent queries that are explained
in the cited references. One can see, however, that these queries are important
mechanisms of conversational competence, and a child who does not know how to
ask for clarification, for instance, will have difficulty continuing a particular topic
with an interactant.

"Back channel responding" is another measure that has been used to describe
the performance of language-impaired children (Watson, 1977; Sheppard, 1980;
Stein, 1976; Fey and Leonard, 1983). Back channel responses are sentence com-
pletions, requests for clarification, and affirmations (such as "yeah," "uh, huh").
It is typically associated with communicative nonassertiveness because the response
is a way to keep the conversation going without adding much content. The child
can take a turn without making more detailed conversational contributions. An
analysis of this behavior could be an important part of evaluating a child's conversational competence.

Many reports in the literature attest to pragmatic differences in language-
impaired children. Some investigations report that language-impaired children have

difficulty organizing narratives and staying on a topic (Johnston, 1982; Lucas, 1980). Fey and Leonard (1983) have recently hypothesized that there may be subgroups of language-impaired children exhibiting a variety of pragmatic problems. There have been reports of the language-disordered child having difficulty taking listener perspective into account (Lucas, 1980; Muma, 1975). The problems described here may or may not be significant for the speech pathologist to evaluate and/or treat. The research on the pragmatic performance of language-impaired children has just begun, and there are methodological considerations that we must take into account when interpreting the investigations (Fey and Leonard, 1983).

There have been differences among pragmatic studies in the composition of the research dyad (child-child, child-adult, normal child–language-impaired child, language-impaired child–language-impaired child). There have also been differences in the measures used in the studies, as well as age differences in the children investigated. Some of the studies have used very small numbers of subjects (three dyads). Other reports are anecdotal and present no empirical data (Lucas, 1980). Finally, because almost all of the studies used language-disordered children whose linguistic structures were abnormal, it is altogether possible that their pragmatics were abnormal partly due to structural differences. There is some evidence, however, that structure and use are partly separate (Fey and Leonard, 1983).

Whatever the extent of a child's pragmatic differences, the speech pathologist can evaluate conversational competence from a variety of perspectives, as suggested above. It is in these kinds of analyses that the clinician can plumb communication competence (Hymes, 1971) and go beyond the basic evaluation of language structures. We will be called on more frequently to examine communication and not merely language. Recent interest has emerged in the older language-disordered child and adolescent (Boyce and Larson, 1983). In these children the syntax and phonology may be relatively normal, and the major difficulty may be in how to use language as a tool in school work, conversations, and survival skills. The area of pragmatics and the measures discussed will take on even more importance for the speech pathologist in the coming decade.

Damico (1980) has taken a different approach and advocated the analysis of specific discourse errors in children's language. He provides a listing of nine discourse errors that can be detected in conversation and computed into a percentage of utterances containing pragmatic difficulties. He recommends obtaining 180 utterances over two sessions in conversational interaction about home and school activities. The goal of the analysis is to describe specific discourse errors that exist in the interaction. Damico has gathered data on more than 150 normal and 300 language-disordered children and proposes some ranges for determining very generally the existence of a pragmatic problem and its severity.

### Assessment of Special Populations

Because the nature of language and the model that we subscribe to do not change with the client, the assessment of special populations should not be dramatically different from developmentally language-disordered children. That is, our business is still to assess the integrity of the communication system (cognitive, linguistic, social, pragmatic), and this process should be in operation regardless of the etiology. We feel, as Bloom and Lahey (1978) have indicated, that the diagnostic group of which a child is a member contributes very little insight into his language impairment. Certainly, however, there are some characteristics that are important to consider in evaluating specific populations. It is our view that the basic assessment of the communication of any client should focus on the process from an integrative vantage point. Thus, whether the clinician is confronted with a mentally retarded, an autistic, a hearing-impaired, or a learning-disabled child, the major task remains to determine the child's linguistic structural capability and the presence of cognitive/social/biological prerequisites to language, as well as to explore the child's use of language in the environment.

Dealing with special populations increases the probability of having to assess biological, social, and cognitive prerequisites to language. Clearly, a mentally retarded child is, by definition, cognitively impaired (Rogers, 1977; Weiss and Zigler, 1979; Cosby and Ruder, 1983; Kamhi and Johnston, 1982). The clinician must be certain that the child possesses the cognitive holdings necessary for learning a particular symbol system (objects, pictures, words, gestures). Autistic children also have been reported to have cognitive difficulties, and the clinician should attempt to gain insight into this area in the evaluation (Curcio, 1978; Rutter, 1978; Clune, Paolella, and Foley, 1979). This is a difficult enterprise, at best. Autistic children are frequently reported to be socially withdrawn, and their general nonverbal social interaction may have to be modified in treatment before they can be expected to use functional communication (Opitz, 1982; Baltaxe and Simmons, 1975). Thus, one implication of special populations is that they may involve the clinician in more broad-based analysis of both precommunicative as well as communicative behaviors presented by the child.

Another aspect involved in dealing with a special population is that the clinician has an increased probability prescribing a nonverbal/nonvocal response mode or prosthetic communication device. Recent research has shown that both mentally retarded and autistic children may benefit from training in gestural communication modes (Silverman, 1980). Thus, it may be incumbent on the diagnostician to determine the potential that a given client may have for learning a nonvocal system. Shane and Bashir (1980) provide some guidelines for considering a nonvocal communication system with severely involved clients.

Special populations, as a whole, generally have a poorer prognosis than language-impaired children without complicating difficulties. The prognosis decreases in proportion to the number of ancillary problems that the child exhibits (hearing impairment, neuromotor involvement, mental retardation, absent caretakers). Also, the existence of ancillary problems increases the likelihood that a multidisciplinary team will be involved in the evaluation. The assistance of special educators, audiologists, psychologists, and medical personnel are invaluable to the clinician in making treatment recommendations for children from special populations. Recently, due to changes in the public law, the speech pathologist has the opportunity to collaborate in staffings with other professionals to discuss assessment and treatment of language-disordered children. In most cases, we have found this to be stimulating and in the best interest of all concerned (especially in early language cases).

With certain types of children, the diagnostician should make an inventory of characteristic behaviors that may need to be modified in the treatment program. For instance, both autistic and mentally retarded children have been reported to engage in self-stimulatory behaviors (arm flapping, masturbation, rocking). Some authorities believe that new learning cannot effectively take place while the child is in a self-stimulatory state. Thus, one goal of treatment might be to reduce the occurrence of self-stimulation and to catalog these behaviors. With autistic and other behavior-disordered children, self-abusive behaviors have been reported. These should also be noted by the clinician as potential treatment targets.

## CONSOLIDATING DATA
## AND ARRIVING AT TREATMENT RECOMMENDATIONS

To a certain degree, even if the diagnostician adheres to an integrative model of language, the assessment process tends to fragment the child and the information obtained in the evaluation. Before arriving at treatment recommendations, suggestions for further testing, and/or referral decisions, the clinician should pause and take stock of what has been done in the assessment process. We have found it useful and insightful to summarize the following areas:

*Data obtained in the evaluation.* This section refers to the actual behaviors observed and the procedures administered to a child in the evalution. It does not include the different analyses of the data. For instance, a spontaneous language sample can be subjected to a variety of analyses (MLU, *DSS*, pragmatics). Often, at the end of an evaluation, a clinician will be struck by the need for additional data that could have been obtained in the initial phase of treatment. We sometimes wonder why we cannot make clinical judgments about certain aspects of a child's language, and then we find that we did not gather all of the data necessary to make these decisions. Appendix D provides a checklist for clinicians to use in summarizing the data collected. Where blanks are provided, specific measures should be filled in if applicable.

*Analyses performed in the evaluation.* This section allows the clinician to summarize the analysis procedures performed on the data collected. Each analysis procedure should be specified by name. On the surface this procedure may appear to be simplistic. However, because language has so many aspects that may be important to assess, it is easy to forget to gather certain data or perform certain analyses.

*Remarks on the data.*   This section is intended for the clinician to comment on any remarkable findings or difficulties in the data gathering. If the parents were hostile or the formal testing was considered unreliable due to fatigue, it can be reported here.

*Synthesis of findings.*   In this section the clinician makes brief summary statements about each aspect of the assessment model. Any remarkable or normal aspects of the prerequisites to communication should be noted. By making a summary statement about portions of the language assessment model and the various stages of language development, the clinician is confronted with any omissions in the data gathering or analysis. If the clinician cannot make an adequate summary statement about a child's social abilities, then she must make further observations. By being forced to respond with a summation of each relevant area in the assessment model, a clinician can see areas of strength and weakness in a child's communication system and be better prepared to make treatment recommendations and prognostic statements.

*Areas of concern and strength.*   By examining the summary statements about each area in the communication process and language development stages, the clinician will be impressed with areas of normality, strength, and concern. The clinician should look for hierarchical patterns in the data that are revealed when a judgment must be made about the overall effectiveness of each area in the language model. For instance, a child may evidence summary statements in the biological prerequisite area that indicate concern over poor motor coordination, remarkable birth, and developmental history. The same child may have performed poorly on cognitive tasks, and the clinician questions the child's conceptual prerequisites for language development. Similarly, in social areas of the model, the child is not operating according to age level and is not exhibiting optimal social prerequisites for communication. In the language development area, the child turns out to be nonverbal. When the clinician checks the areas of concern and strength, based on the summary statements, the child will get a minus for biological prerequisites and minuses for social and cognitive prerequisites as well. The child will also receive a minus for delayed language. By examining the summary statements, the clinician can develop a profile of areas of strength and concern for each case. If no clear-cut statement for concern or strength can be made, then the clinician should examine the data gathered and the analyses performed to determine if enough information has been accumulated. In most cases, an inability to make a general statement about areas of the model is due to insufficient information, poor quality information, or insufficient analysis.

*Recommendations.*   The areas that are covered in the recommendation section revolve around four topics. First, the child may require referral to other professionals to obtain further information. For instance, referral to a psychologist may be warranted to determine the child's mental ability and potential for learning. Audiometric referral may be another common need. Second, the clinician may have been unable to perform certain tests or analyses due to time constraints or lack of cooperation by the child. Before specific treatment recommendations can be made, more data may be required. By examining the sections on data obtained and analyses performed, the clinician can determine this need. Third, if enough data were obtained and analyses performed, the clinician is in a position to make treatment recommendations. By examining the child's areas of strength and weakness, the clinician can consider intervention avenues that are the most appropriate. For instance, if a child is biologically, cognitively, and socially ready for communication development and the clinician has located the child in the language development process, an appropriate goal might be to begin concentrating on the language forms that develop next according to the acquisition literature and the child's need to communicate. If the child is normal in most respects and the major concern is intelligibility, then this carries with it a treatment priority. If the child has cognitive and social problems in addition to language delay, then some of the treatment goals might revolve around these prerequisite areas (facilitating cognitive development, improving social nonverbal skills, and the like).

The areas of concern and strength also carry with them prognostic implications. To date, we have no certain method of computing a given child's prognosis for success in language treatment. So many variables deal with the child's capacities, skills, motivation, environment, caretaker participation, time in treatment. One approach to prognosis that will probably reflect reality is to regard the child with fewer concerns in the major areas of the model as having a more favorable prognosis than one who has many deficiencies. A fourth area in the recommendation section might involve further parent counseling and/or training.

## CONCLUDING REMARKS

We have attempted to show that language assessment in children is no simple matter. It requires the clinician to learn a multitude of skills and read a wide range of literature in order to perform it competently. The diagnosis of language disorder requires more than just a single test or procedure. It demands that the clinician examine the communication process differently for each type of child. There are high probability areas of investigation for certain types of cases, as we have tried to demonstrate. Finally, no chapter in a textbook can teach a clinician how to do a language assessment. The most we can do is to show the clinician some of the tools and procedures that authorities have indicated might be important in language diagnosis. The clinician must then read the cited primary sources, administer the measures to clients, and judge whether or not the information obtained is clinically useful. (See Appendixes A, B, C, and D on pp. 334–343.)

HIGHLIGHT   *Assessment Implications of Dialectical Syntactic Variations of Black English*

It is widely accepted that many black Americans speak a dialect of English that has its linguistic roots in Africa (Dillard, 1972) and is not simply an impoverished form of Standard English. Much has been written about the differences between Black English and Standard English that permeate pragmatic, phonological, semantic, and syntactic domains. Perhaps the most dramatic differences between Standard English and Black English are in the area of syntax. The speech clinician assessing language in young black children should be aware of possible syntactic alterations that are due to dialectical variation. It is important to be able to distinguish clinically significant problems from dialectical differences.

Interestingly, most formal language assessment procedures were designed for Standard English speakers and their norms do not take into account dialectical variations. Thus, a Black English speaker may appear to have a communication disorder on these measures when, in fact, he does not have a clinicially significant problem. Although there are a few tests available that take dialect into account, the bulk of these procedures do not. The clinician should always examine test materials to determine if the measure was normed on subjects from various ethnic groups or if there is some provision for scoring the instrument that takes into account dialectical variation.

Presently, the most effective way of accounting for dialectical variation in language assessment is increasing clinical awareness and knowledge in this area. Every time a black child is evaluated, the clinician must consider that she could be speaking Black English, and areas of dialectical difference should be noted as such. We will mention only a few syntactic differences here to demonstrate how a test or language sample could be altered by black dialect.

The following could be omitted by a Black English speaker:

| | |
|---|---|
| Regular past tense | -ed |
| Plural | -s |
| Contractible auxiliary "be" | "He goin to town" |
| Contractible copula "be" | "He in the garage" |
| Possessive | -s |
| Third-person singular present tense -s | "He walk" |
| Forms of "have" | "I been here" |

The following changes are also possible:

| | |
|---|---|
| Double negatives | |
| Invariant "be" forms | "He be here" |

The reader can see that a dialect speaker would be severely penalized on many language measures that emphasize grammatical morphemes of Standard English. There are some other important points for the clinician to bear in mind:

1. Not all blacks are black dialect speakers; many speak Standard English.

2. The recent position paper of the American Speech-Language and Hearing Association (Battle et al., 1983) has stated that Black English is a legitimate dialect and not a communication disorder.

3. The speech clinician may be in the position of having to explain the nature of dialectical variation to teachers who refer black children for language treatment. Each speech clinician will have to take a position on whether or not to work with dialect cases and justify the criteria used in these decisions.

4. Most data on Black English have been gathered from adolescents living in the inner cities of the United States. Dialectical differences, however, have been shown to vary from county to county in many areas of the rural South. The clinician should attempt to get in tune with local norms.

5. Several studies have shown that most black parents want their children to have some facility in Standard English, presumably because this makes school easier and job opportunities greater.

6. We presently have very little data on how Black English develops. Thus, we are placed in the unfortunate position of comparing black children to norms generated from Standard English, mostly white speakers. More data are needed in this area.

7. The clinician should remember that the phonological and functional differences referred to earlier must be taken into account in an assessment of a black child.

We recommend that beginning clinicians read some of the sources listed in our references to become acquainted with all significant dialectical variations in addition to Black English. Dialect is an extremely important variable for the clinician to consider in assessment and to include in deciding whether or not to enroll a child in language treatment.

## BIBLIOGRAPHY

ALLEN, D., L. BLISS, and J. TIMMONS (1981). "Language Evaluation: Science or Art?" *Journal of Speech and Hearing Disorders,* 46: 66–68.

AMMONS, R., and H. AMMONS (1948). *Full Range Picture Vocabulary Test.* Missoula, Mont.: Psychological Test Specialists.

ARAM, D., and J. NATION (1975). "Patterns of Language Behavior in Children with Developmental Language Disorders." *Journal of Speech and Hearing Research,* 18: 229–241.

—— (1982). *Child Language Disorders.* St. Louis, Mo.: C. V. Mosby.

ARWOOD, E. (1983). *Pragmaticism.* Rockville, Md.: Aspen Systems Corp.

ATKINS, C., and L. CARTWRIGHT (1982). "An Investigation of the Effectiveness of Three Language Elicitation Procedures on Headstart Children." *Language, Speech and Hearing Services in Schools,* 13: 33–36.

BALTAXE, C., and J. SIMMONS (1975). "Language in Childhood Psychosis: A Review." *Journal of Speech and Hearing Disorders,* 40: 439–458.

BALTHAZAR, E. (1973). *Balthazar Scales of Adaptive Behavior. II. Scales of Social Adaptation.* Palo Alto, Calif.: Consulting Psychologists Press.

BANGS, T. (1961). "Evaluating Children with Language Delay." *Journal of Speech and Hearing Disorders,* 26: 6–18.

—— (1975). *Vocabulary Comprehension Scale.* Boston: Teaching Resources Corp.

BANKSON, N. (1977). *Bankson Language Screening Test.* Baltimore: University Park Press.

BARRIE-BLACKLEY, S., C. MUSSELWHITE, and S. ROGISTER (1978). *Clinical Oral Language Sampling.* Danville, Ill.: Interstate Printers and Publishers.

BASHIR, A., et al. (1983). "Issues in Language Disorders: Considerations of Cause, Maintenance and Change," in *Contemporary Issues in Language Intervention,* ASHA Report 12, ed. J. Miller, D. Yoder, and R. Schiefelbusch. Rockville, Md.: ASHA.

BATES, E. (1976). *Language in Context.* New York: Academic Press.

BATES, E., et al. (1979). *The Emergence of Symbols: Cognition and Communication in Infancy.* New York: Academic Press.

BATTLE, D., et al. (1983). "Position Paper on Social Dialects." *Journal of the American Speech Language Hearing Association,* 25: 23–24.

BEARD, R. (1969). *An Outline of Piaget's Developmental Psychology for Students and Teachers.* New York: Basic Books.

BERRY, M. (1966). *Berry-Talbott Tests of Language. I. Comprehension of Grammar.* 4322 Pinecrest Rd., Rockford, Ill.

BLAGDEN, C., and N. McCONNELL (1983). *Interpersonal Language Skills Assessment.* Moline, Ill.: Linguisystems.

BLANK, M., S. ROSE, and L. BERLIN (1978). *Preschool Language Assessment Instrument.* New York: Grune & Stratton.

BLASDELL, R., and P. JENSEN (1970). "Stress and Word Position Determinants of Imitation in First Language Learners." *Journal of Speech and Hearing Research,* 13: 193–202.

BLOOM, L. (1970). *Language Development: Form and Function in Emerging Grammars.* Cambridge, Mass.: MIT Press,

—— (1973). *One Word at a Time: The Use of Single Word Utterances Before Syntax.* The Hague: Mouton.

BLOOM, L. (1974). "Talking, Understanding and Thinking," in *Language Perspectives—Acquisition, Retardation and Intervention,* ed. R. Schiefelbusch and L. Lloyd. Baltimore: University Park Press.

BLOOM, L., and M. LAHEY (1978). *Language Development and Language Disorders.* New York: John Wiley.

BLOOM, L., P. LIGHTBROWN, and L. HOOD (1975). "Structure and Variation in Child Language." *Monographs of the Society for Research in Child Development,* 40: 1–41.

BLOOM, L., L. ROCISSANO, and L. HOOD (1976). "Adult-Child Discourse: Developmental Interaction Between Information Processing and Linguistic Knowledge." *Cognitive Psychology,* 8: 521–552.

BOEHM, A. (1971). *Boehm Test of Basic Concepts.* New York: Psychological Corp.

BONVILLIAN, J., V. RAEBURN, and E. HORAN (1979). "Talking to Children: The Effects of Rate, Intonation and Length on Children's Sentence Imitation." *Journal of Child Language,* 3:459–467.

BOWERMAN, M. (1973). "Structural Relationships in Children's Utterances: Syntactic or Semantic?" in *Cognitive Development and the Acquisition of Language,* ed. T. E. Moore. New York: Academic Press.

BOYCE, N., and V. LARSON (1983). *Adolescents' Communication: Development and Disorders.* Eau Claire, Wis.: Thinking Ink Publications.

BRAINE, M. (1963). "The Ontogeny of English Phrase Structure: The First Phrase." *Language,* 39: 1–14.

—— (1976). "Childrens' First Word Combinations." *Monographs of the Society for Research in Child Development,* 41: 1–104.

BRANSFORD, J., and K. NITSCH (1978). "Coming to Understand Things We Could Not Previously Understand," in *Speech and Language in the Laboratory, School and Clinic,* ed. J. Kavanagh and W. Strange. Cambridge, Mass.: MIT Press.

BROWN, R. (1973). *A First Language: The Early Stages.* Cambridge, Mass.: Harvard University Press.

BROWN, R., and C. FRASER (1963). "The Acquisition of Syntax," in *Verbal Behavior and Learning: Problems and Processes,* ed. C. Cofer and B. Musgrave. New York: McGraw-Hill.

BZOCH, K., and R. LEAGUE (1971). *Receptive-Expressive Emergent Language Scale.* Gaines-ville, Fla.: Tree of Life Press.

CARROW, E. (1973). *Test of Auditory Comprehension of Language.* Austin, Tex.: Learning Concepts.

—— (1974). *Carrow Elicited Language Inventory.* Austin, Tex.: Learning Concepts.

CARROW-WOOLFOLK, E., and J. LYNCH (1982). *An Integrative Approach to Language Disorders in Children.* New York: Grune & Stratton.

CAZDEN, C. (1970). "The Neglected Situation of Child Language Research and Education," in *Language and Poverty: Perspectives on a Theme,* ed. F. Williams. Chicago: Rand McNally.

CHABON, S., L. UDOLF, and D. EGOLF (1982). "The Temporal Reliability of Brown's Mean Length of Utterance Measure with Post Stage V Children." *Journal of Speech and Hearing Research,* 25: 124-128.

CHAPMAN, D., and J. NATION (1981). "Patterns of Language Performance in Educable Mentally Retarded Children." *Journal of Communication Disorders,* 14: 245-254.

CHAPMAN, R. (1978). "Comprehension Strategies in Children," in *Speech and Language in the Laboratory, School and Clinic,* ed. J. Kavanagh and W. Strange. Cambridge, Mass.: MIT Press.

—— (1981). "Exploring Children's Communicative Intents," in *Assessing Language Production in Children: Experimental Procedures,* ed. J. Miller. Baltimore: University Park Press.

CHAPPEL, G., and G. JOHNSON (1976). "Evaluation of Cognitive Behavior in Young Nonverbal Children." *Language, Speech and Hearing Services in Schools,* 7: 17-27.

CHOMSKY, N. (1957). *Syntactic Structures.* The Hague: Mouton.

CLUNE, C., J. PAOLELLA, and J. FOLEY (1979). "Free Play Behavior of Atypical Children: An Approach to Assessment." *Journal of Autism and Developmental Disorders,* 9: 61-72.

COGGINS, T., and R. CARPENTER (1978). "Categories for Coding Prespeech Intentional Communication." Unpublished manuscript. Seattle: University of Washington.

CONNELL, P., and C. MYLES-ZITZER (1982). "An Analysis of Elicited Imitation as a Language Evaluation Procedure." *Journal of Speech and Hearing Disorders,* 47: 390-396.

CORMAN, H., and S. ESCALONA (1969). "Stages of Sensorimotor Development: A Replication Study." *Merrill Palmer Quarterly,* 15: 351-361.

COSBY, M., and K. RUDER (1983). "Symbolic Play and Early Language Development in Normal and Mentally Retarded Children." *Journal of Speech and Hearing Research,* 25: 404-411.

CRABTREE, M. (1963). *Houston Test for Language Development.* Houston: Houston Test Co.

CRYSTAL, D., P. FLETCHER, and M. GARMAN (1976). *The Grammatical Analysis of Language Disability: A Procedure for Assessment and Remediation.* London: Edward Arnold.

CURCIO, F. (1978). "Sensorimotor Functioning and Communication in Mute Autistic Children." *Journal of Autism and Childhood Schizophrenia,* 8: 281-292.

DAILEY, J. (1977). *The Language Facility Test.* Alexandria, Va.: Allington Corp.

DAILY, K., and J. BOXX (1979). "A Comparison of Three Imitative Tests of Expressive Language and a Spontaneous Language Sample." *Language, Speech and Hearing Services in Schools,* 10: 6-13.

DALE, P. (1976). *Language Development: Structure and Function.* New York: Holt, Rinehart & Winston.

—— (1980). "Is Early Pragmatic Development Measurable?" *Journal of Child Language,* 7: 1-12.

DAMICO, J. (1980). "Clinical Discourse Analysis." Miniseminar presented at the convention of the American Speech and Hearing Association, Detroit.

DARLEY, F. (1979). *Evaluation of Appraisal Techniques in Speech and Language Pathology.* Reading, Mass.: Addison-Wesley.

DEVER, R., and P. BAUMAN (1974). "Scale of Children's Clausal Development," in *Linguistic Analysis of Children's Speech,* ed. T. Longhurst. New York: MSS Information Corp.

DEVILLIERS, J., and P. DEVILLIERS (1973). "A Cross-Sectional Study of the Acquisition of Grammatical Morphemes in Child Speech." *Journal of Psycholinguistic Research,* 3: 267-278.

—— (1978). *Language Acquisition.* Cambridge, Mass.: Harvard University Press.

DILLARD, J. (1972). *Black English: Its History and Usage in the United States.* New York: Random House.

DISIMONI, F. (1978). *Token Test for Children.* Boston: Teaching Resources Corp.

DORE, J. (1975). "Holophrases, Speech Acts and Language Universals." *Journal of Child Language,* 2: 21–40.

—— (1978). "Requestive Systems in Nursery School Conversations: Analysis of Talk in Its Social Context," in *Recent Advances in the Psychology of Language,* ed. R. Campbell and P. Smith. New York: Plenum.

DORE, J., et al. (1976). "Transitional Phenomena in Early Language Acquisition." *Journal of Child Language,* 3: 13–28.

DOWNS, M. (1981). "Contribution of Mild Hearing Loss to Auditory Language Learning Problems," in *Auditory Disorders in School Children,* ed. R. Roeser and M. Downs. New York: Thieme-Stratton.

DUCHAN, J., and L. SIEGEL (1979). "Incorrect Responses to Locative Commands: A Case Study." *Language, Speech and Hearing Services in Schools,* 10: 99–103.

DUNN, L. (1980). *The Peabody Picture Vocabulary Test–Revised.* Circle Pines, Minn.: American Guidance Service.

DUNST, C. (1980). *A Clinical and Educational Manual for Use with the Uzigiris and Hunt Scales of Infant Psychological Development.* Baltimore: University Park Press.

ELDER, J., and D. PEDERSON (1978). "Preschool Children's Use of Objects in Symbolic Play." *Child Development,* 49: 500–504.

ENGLEMANN, S. (1967). *The Basic Concept Inventory.* Chicago: Follett.

ENGLER, L., E. HANNAH, and T. LONGHURST (1973). "Linguistic Analysis of Speech Samples: A Practical Guide for Clinicians." *Journal of Speech and Hearing Disorders,* 38: 192–204.

FEY, M., and L. LEONARD (1983). "Pragmatic Skills of Children with Specific Language Impairment," in *Pragmatic Assessment and Intervention Issues in Language,* ed. T. Gallagher and C. Prutting. San Diego, Calif.: College-Hill Press.

FILLMORE, C. (1968). "The Case for Case," in *Universals in Linguistic Theory,* ed. E. Bach and R. Harms. New York: Holt, Rinehart & Winston.

FOLGER, J., and R. CHAPMAN (1978). "A Pragmatic Analysis of Spontaneous Imitations." *Journal of Child Language,* 5: 25–38.

FOSTER, R., J. GIDDAN, and J. STARK (1973). *Manual for the Assessment of Children's Language Comprehension.* Palo Alto, Calif.: Consulting Psychologists Press.

FRANKENBURG, W., W. DODDS, and A. FANDAL (1970). *Denver Developmental Screening Test.* Denver: University of Colorado Medical Center.

FUJIKI, M., and B. BRINTON (1983). "Sampling Reliability in Elicited Imitation." *Journal of Speech and Hearing Disorders,* 48: 85–89.

GALLAGHER, T. (1982). "Pragmatics." Workshop presented at Auburn University, Auburn, Ala.

GARNICA, O. (1974). "Some Characteristics of Prosodic Input to Young Children." Paper presented at the SSRC Conference on Language Input and Acquisition, Boston.

GARVEY, C. (1977a). "Play with Language and Speech," in *Child Discourse,* ed. S. Ervin-Tripp and C. Mitchell-Kernan. New York: Academic Press.

—— (1977b). "The Contingent Query: A Dependent Act in Conversation," in *Interaction, Conversation, and the Development of Language,* vol. 5, ed. M. Lewis and L. Rosenblum. New York: John Wiley.

GINSBURG, H., and S. OPPER (1969). *Piaget's Theory of Intellectual Development: An Introduction.* Englewood Cliffs, N.J.: Prentice-Hall, Inc.

GOWIE, C., and J. POWERS (1979). "Relations Among Cognitive, Semantic and Syntactic Variables in Children's Comprehension of the Minimal Distance Principle: A Two Year Developmental Study." *Journal of Psycholinguistic Research,* 8: 29–41.

GRICE, H. (1975). "Logic and Conversation," in *Studies in Syntax, Semantics and Speech Acts,* vol. 3, ed. P. Cole and J. Morgan. New York: Academic Press.

HALLIDAY, M. (1975). *Learning How to Mean: Explorations in the Development of Language.* New York: Elsevier.

HAMMILL, D., et al. (1980). *Test of Adolescent Language: A Multidimensional Approach to Assessment.* East Aurora, N.Y.: Slosson Educational Publications.

HANIFF, M., and G. SIEGEL (1981). "The Effect of Context on Verbal Elicited Imitation." *Journal of Speech and Hearing Disorders,* 46: 27–30.

HAYNES, W., and M. HAYNES (1979). "Pragmatics and Elicited Imitation: Children's Performance on Discursively Related and Discursively Unrelated Sentences." *Journal of Communication Disorders,* 12: 471–479.

HAYNES, W., and S. HOOD (1978). "Disfluency Changes in Children as a Function of the Systematic Modification of Linguistic Complexity." *Journal of Communication Disorders,* 11: 79–93.

HAYNES, W., and M. McCALLION (1981). "Language Comprehension Testing: The Influence of Cognitive Tempo and Three Modes of Test Administration." *Language, Speech and Hearing Services in Schools,* 12: 74–81.

HAYNES, W., E. PURCELL, and M. HAYNES (1979). "A Pragmatic Aspect of Language Sampling." *Language, Speech and Hearing Services in Schools,* 10: 104–110.

HEDRICK, D., E. PRATHER, and A. TOBIN (1975). *Sequenced Inventory of Communication Development.* Seattle: University of Washington Press.

HOLLAND, A. (1975). "Language Therapy for Children: Some Thoughts on Context and Content." *Journal of Speech and Hearing Disorders,* 40: 514–523.

HOWE, C. (1976). "The Meanings of Two Word Utterances in the Speech of Young Children." *Journal of Child Language,* 3: 29–47.

HUBBELL, R. (1981). *Children's Language Disorders: An Integrated Approach.* Englewood Cliffs, N.J.: Prentice-Hall, Inc.

HYMES, D. (1971). "Competence and Performance in Linguistic Theory," in *Language Acquisition: Models and Methods,* ed. R. Huxley and E. Ingram. New York: Academic Press.

JOHNSON, W., F. DARLEY, and D. SPRIESTERSBACH (1963). *Diagnostic Methods in Speech Pathology.* New York: Harper & Row.

JOHNSTON, J. (1982). "Narrative: A New Look at Communication Problems in Older Language Disordered Children." *Language, Speech and Hearing Services in Schools,* 13: 144–155.

KAHN, L., and S. JAMES (1980). "A Method for Assessing the Use of Grammatical Structures in Language Disordered Children." *Language, Speech and Hearing Services in Schools,* 11: 188–197.

KAMHI, A., and J. JOHNSTON (1982). "Towards an Understanding of Retarded Children's Linguistic Deficiencies." *Journal of Speech and Hearing Research,* 25: 435–445.

KEENAN, E., and B. SCHIEFFLIN (1976). "Topic as a Discourse Notion: A Study of Topic in the Conversations of Children and Adults," in *Subject and Topic,* ed. C. Li. New York: Academic Press.

KIRK, S., and W. KIRK (1971). *Psycholinguistic Learning Disabilities.* Urbana: University of Illinois Press.

KIRK, S., J. McCARTHY, and W. KIRK (1968). *Illinois Test of Psycholinguistic Abilities.* Rev. ed. Urbana: University of Illinois Press.

KLEE, T., and M. FITZGERALD (1983). "The Relation Between Grammatical Development and Mean Length of Utterance in Morphemes." Paper presented at the Convention of the American Speech and Hearing Association, Cincinnati, Ohio.

KRAMER, C., S. JAMES, and J. SAXMAN (1979). "A Comparison of Language Samples Elicited at Home and in the Clinic." *Journal of Speech and Hearing Disorders,* 44: 321–330.

KRAMER, P. (1977). "Young Children's Free Responses to Anomalous Commands." *Journal of Experimental Child Psychology,* 24: 219–234.

LABOV, W. (1970). "The Logic of Nonstandard English," in *Language and Poverty: Perspectives on a Theme,* ed. F. Williams. Chicago: Rand McNally.

LAMBERT, N., M. WINDMILLER, D. THARINGER, and L. COLE (1981). *AAMD Adaptive Behavior Scale.* Monterey, Calif.: Publishers Test Service.

LANG, M., and W. MOORE (1977). "Some Variables Affecting Sentence Imitation of Normal Children." Unpublished research. Auburn University, Auburn, Ala.

LEE, L. (1969). *Northwestern Syntax Screening Test.* Evanston, Ill: Northwestern University Press.

—— (1974.) *Developmental Sentence Analysis.* Evanston, Ill.: Northwestern University Press.

LEE, L., R. KOENIGSKNECHT, and S. MULHERN (1975). *Interactive Language Development Teaching.* Evanston, Ill.: Northwestern University Press.

LEONARD, L. (1972). "What Is Deviant Language?" *Journal of Speech and Hearing Disorders,* 37: 427–446.

—— (1975). "On Differentiating Syntactic and Semantic Features in Emerging Grammars: Evidence from Empty Form Usage." *Journal of Psycholinguistic Research,* 4: 357–364.

—— (1976). *Meaning in Child Language: Issues in the Study of Early Semantic Development.* New York: Grune & Stratton.

—— (1978). "Cognitive Factors in Early Linguistic Development," in *Bases of Language Intervention,* ed. R. Schiefelbusch. Baltimore: University Park Press.

—— (1979). "Language Impairment in Children." *Merrill Palmer Quarterly,* 25: 205–232.

—— (1983). "Defining the Boundaries of Language Disorders in Children," in *Contemporary Issues in Language Intervention. ASHA Report 12,* ed. J. Miller, D. Yoder, and R. Schiefelbusch. Rockville, Md.: ASHA.

LEONARD, L., C. PRUTTING, C. PEROZZI, and R. BERKLEY (1978). "Nonstandardized Approaches to the Assessment of Language Behaviors." *Journal of the American Speech and Hearing Association,* May: 371–379.

LEONARD, L., K. STECKOL, and K. PANTHER (1983). "Returning Meaning to Semantic Relations: Some Clinical Applications." *Journal of Speech and Hearing Disorders,* 48: 25–35.

LOBAN, W. (1976). *Language Development.* Champaign, Ill.: National Council of Teachers of English.

LONGHURST, T., and J. FILE (1977). "A Comparison of Developmental Sentence Scores for Headstart Children in Four Conditions." *Language, Speech and Hearing Services in Schools,* 8: 54–64.

LONGHURST, T., and S. GRUBB (1974). "A Comparison of Language Samples Collected in Four Situations." *Language, Speech and Hearing Services in Schools,* 5: 71–78.

LONGHURST, T., and T. SCHRANDT (1973). "Linguistic Analysis of Children's Speech: A Comparison of Four Procedures." *Journal of Speech and Hearing Disorders,* 38: 240–249.

LOWE, M., and A. COSTELLO (1976). *The Symbolic Play Test.* London: National Foundation for Educational Research Publishing.

LUCAS, E. (1980). *Semantic and Pragmatic Language Disorders.* Rockville, Md.: Aspen Systems Corp.

LUND, N., and J. DUCHAN (1983). *Assessing Children's Language in Naturalistic Contexts.* Englewood Cliffs, N.J.: Prentice-Hall, Inc.

McCARTHY, D. (1930). "The Language Development of the Preschool Child," *Child Welfare Monographs,* No. 4, Minneapolis: University of Minnesota Press.

—— (1935). "The Language Development of the Preschool Child." *University of Minnesota Institute of Child Welfare Monograph Series IV.* Minneapolis: University of Minnesota Press.

McCLEAN, J., and L. SNYDER-McCLEAN (1978). *A Transactional Approach to Early Language Training.* Columbus, Ohio: Chas. E. Merrill.

McDADE, H., M. SIMPSON, and D. LARNT (1982). "The Use of Elicited Imitation as a Measure of Expressive Grammar: A Question of Validity." *Journal of Speech and Hearing Disorders,* 47: 19–24.

MacDONALD, J. (1978). *Environmental Language Inventory.* Columbus, Ohio: Chas. E. Merrill.

McNEILL, D. (1970). *The Acquisition of Language: The Study of Developmental Psycholinguistics.* New York: Harper & Row.

MECHAM, M. (1971). *Verbal Language Development Scale.* Circle Pines, Minn.: American Guidance Service.

MECHAM, M., J. JEX, and J. JONES (1967). *Utah Test of Language Development.* Salt Lake City: Communication Research Associates.

MENYUK, P. (1964). "Comparison of Grammar of Children with Functionally Deviant and Normal Speech." *Journal of Speech and Hearing Research,* 7: 199–121.

MERHABIAN, A., and M. WILLIAMS (1971). "Piagetian Measures of Cognitive Development for Children up to Age Two." *Journal of Psycholinguistic Research,* 1: 113–125.

MILLEN, K., and C. PRUTTING (1979). "Consistencies Across Three Language Comprehension Tests for Specific Grammatical Features." *Language, Speech and Hearing Services in Schools,* 10: 162–170.

MILLER, J. (1981). *Assessing Language Production in Children: Experimental Procedures.* Baltimore: University Park Press.

MILLER, J., and R. CHAPMAN (1981). "The Relation Between Age and Mean Length of Utterance in Morphemes." *Journal of Speech and Hearing Research,* 24: 154–161.

MILLER, J., and D. YODER (1984). *The Miller-Yoder Language Comprehension Test.* Baltimore: University Park Press.

MINER, L. (1969). "Scoring Procedures for the Length-Complexity Index: A Preliminary Report." *Journal of Communication Disorders,* 2: 224–240.

MISHLER, E. (1975). "Studies in Dialogue and Discourse. II. Types of Discourse Initiated by and Sustained Through Questioning." *Journal of Psycholinguistic Research,* 4: 99–121.

MOREHEAD, D., and A. MOREHEAD (1974). "From Signal to Sign," in *Language Perspectives—Acquisition, Retardation, and Intervention,* ed. R. Schiefelbusch and L. Lloyd. Baltimore: University Park Press.

MULAC, A., C. PRUTTING, and C. TOMLINSON (1978). "Testing for a Specific Syntactic Structure." *Journal of Communication Disorders,* 11: 335–347.

MUMA, J. (1973a). "Language Assessment: Some Underlying Assumptions." *Journal of the American Speech and Hearing Association,* 15: 331–338.

—— (1973b). "Language Assessment: The Co-Occurring and Restricted Structure Procedure." *Acta Symbolica,* 4: 12–29.

—— (1975). "The Communication Game: Dump and Play." *Journal of Speech and Hearing Disorders,* 40: 296–309.

—— (1978). *Language Handbook: Concepts, Assessment, Intervention.* Englewood Cliffs, N.J.: Prentice-Hall, Inc.

—— (1983). "Speech Language Pathology: Emerging Clinical Expertise in Language," in *Pragmatic Assessment and Intervention Issues in Language,* ed. T. Gallagher and C. Prutting. San Diego, Calif.: College-Hill Press.

MUSSELWHITE, C., and S. BARRIE-BLACKLEY (1980). "Three Variations of the Imperative Format of Language Sample Elicitation." *Language, Speech and Hearing Services in Schools,* 11: 56–67.

NATION, J., and D. ARAM (1977). *Diagnosis of Speech and Language Disorders.* St. Louis: C. V. Mosby.

NELSON, K. (1973). "Structure and Strategy in Learning to Talk." *Monographs of the Society for Research in Child Development,* 38: 11–56.

—— (1974). "Concept, Word and Sentence: Interrelations in Acquisition and Development." *Psychological Review,* 81: 267–285.

NELSON, L., and M. WEBER-OLSEN (1980). "The Elicited Language Inventory and the Influence of Contextual Cues." *Journal of Speech and Hearing Disorders,* 45: 549–563.

NEWCOMER, P., and D. HAMMILL (1977). *Test of Language Development.* Austin, Tex.: Empiric Press.

NEWHOFF, M., and L. LEONARD (1983). In *Diagnosis in Speech-Language Pathology,* ed. I. Meitus and B. Weinberg. Baltimore: University Park Press.

NICOLICH, L. (1977). "Beyond Sensorimotor Intelligence: Assessment of Symbolic Maturity Through Analysis of Pretend Play." *Merrill Palmer Quarterly,* 23: 89–101.

NINTH MENTAL MEASUREMENTS YEARBOOK (in press). Lincoln, Neb.: Buros Institute of Mental Measurements, University of Nebraska.

OLSWANG, L., and R. CARPENTER (1978). "Elicitor Effects on the Language Obtained from Young Language-Impaired Children." *Journal of Speech and Hearing Disorders,* 43: 76–86.

OPITZ, V. (1982). "Pragmatic Analysis of the Communicative Behavior of an Autistic Child." *Journal of Speech and Hearing Disorders,* 47: 99–108.

OWENS, R., et al. (1983). "Language Test Content: A Comparative Study." *Language, Speech and Hearing Services in Schools,* 14: 7–21.

PETERSON, H., and T. MARQUARDT (1981). *Appraisal and Diagnosis of Speech and Language Disorders.* Englewood Cliffs, N.J., Prentice-Hall, Inc.

PORCH, B. (1974). *Porch Index of Communicative Ability in Children.* Palo Alto, Calif.: Consulting Psychologists Press.

PROJECT RHISE (1979). *Manual for Administration of the Rockford Infant Developmental Evaluation Scales.* Bensenville, Ill.: Scholastic Testing Service.

PRUTTING, C., and J. CONNOLLY (1976). "Imitation: A Closer Look." *Journal of Speech and Hearing Disorders,* 41: 412–422.

PRUTTING, C., T. GALLAGHER, and A. MULAC (1975). "The Expressive Portion of the NSST Compared to a Spontaneous Language Sample." *Journal of Speech and Hearing Disorders,* 40: 40–48.

REES, N., and M. SHULMAN (1978). "I Don't Understand What You Mean by Comprehension." *Journal of Speech and Hearing Disorders,* 43: 208–219.

REYNELL, J. (1969). *Reynell Developmental Language Scales.* Buckinghamshire, England: National Foundation for Educational Research in England and Wales.

RILEY, G. (1971). *The Riley Articulation and Language Test.* Beverly Hills, Calif.: Western Psychological Services.

RODGERS, W. (1976). *Picture Articulation and Language Screening Test.* Salt Lake: Word Making Productions.

ROGERS, S. (1977). "Characteristics of the Cognitive Development of Profoundly Retarded Children." *Child Development,* 48: 837–843.

RUDER, K., and M. SMITH (1974). "Issues in Language Training," in *Language Perspectives— Acquisition, Retardation and Intervention,* ed. R. Schiefelbusch and L. Lloyd. Baltimore: University Park Press.

RUTTER, M. (1978). "Diagnosis and Definition of Childhood Autism." *Journal of Autism and Childhood Schizophrenia,* 8: 139–169.

SCHLESINGER, I. (1974). "Relational Concepts Underlying Language," in *Language Perspectives—Acquisition, Retardation and Intervention,* ed. R. Schiefelbusch and L. Lloyd. Baltimore: University Park Press.

SEMEL, E., and E. WIIG (1980). *Clinical Evaluation of Language Function.* Columbus, Ohio: Chas. E. Merrill.

SHANE, H., and A. BASHIR (1980). "Election Criteria for the Adoption of an Augmentative Communication System: Preliminary Considerations." *Journal of Speech and Hearing Disorders,* 45: 408–444.

SHARF, D. (1972). "Some Relationships Between Measures of Early Language Development." *Journal of Speech and Hearing Disorders,* 37: 64–74.

SHEPPARD, A. (1980). "Monologue and Dialogue Speech and Language Impaired Children in Clinic and Home Settings: Semantic, Conversational and Syntactic Characteristics." Master's thesis, University of Western Ontario.

SHORR, D. (1983). "Grammatical Comprehension Assessment: The Picture Avoidance Strategy." *Journal of Speech and Hearing Disorders,* 48: 89–92.

SIEGEL, G. (1975). "The Use of Language Tests." *Language, Speech and Hearing Services in Schools,* 6: 211–217.

SILVERMAN, F. (1980). *Communication for the Speechless.* Englewood Cliffs, N.J.: Prentice-Hall, Inc.

SLOBIN, D., and C. WELSH (1971). "Elicited Imitation as a Research Tool in Developmental Psycholinguistics," in *Language Training in Early Childhood Education,* ed. C. Lavatelli. Urbana: University of Illinois Press.

SNOW, C. (1972). "Mother's Speech to Children Learning Language." *Child Development,* 43: 549–565.

—— (1977). "The Development of Conversation Between Mothers and Babies." *Journal of Child Language,* 4: 1–22.

SNYDER, L. (1978). "Communicative and Cognitive Disabilities in the Sensorimotor Period." *Merrill Palmer Quarterly,* 24: 161–180.

—— (1981). "Assessing Communicative Abilities in the Sensorimotor Period: Content and Context." *Topics in Language Disorders,* 1: 31–46.

STAAB, C. (1983). "Language Functions Elicited by Meaningful Activities: A New Dimension in Language Programs." *Language, Speech and Hearing Services in Schools*, 14: 164–170.

STECKOL, K., and L. LEONARD (1981). "Sensorimotor Development and the Use of Prelinguistic Performatives." *Journal of Speech and Hearing Research*, 24: 262–268.

STEIN, A. (1976). "A Comparison of Mothers' and Fathers' Language to Normal and Language Deficient Children." Doctoral dissertation, Boston University.

STRANDBERG, T., and J. GRIFFITH (1969). "A Study of the Effects of Training in Visual Literacy on Verbal Language Behavior." *Journal of Communication Disorders*, 2: 252–263.

TOFFLER, A. (1981). *The Third Wave*. New York: Bantam.

TORONTO, A. (1977). *Toronto Tests of Receptive Vocabulary: English/Spanish*. Austin, Tex.: Academic Tests.

TORONTO, A., et al. (1975). *Del Rio Language Screening Test English/Spanish*. Austin, Tex.: National Education Laboratory Publications.

TOUGH, J. (1977). *The Development of Meaning*. New York: Halsted Press.

TRANTHAM, C., and J. PEDERSEN (1976). *Normal Language Development*. Baltimore: Williams & Wilkins.

TYACK, D., and R. GOTTSLEBEN (1974). *Language Sampling, Analysis and Training: A Handbook for Teachers and Clinicians*. Palo Alto, Calif.: Consulting Psychologists Press.

UZIGIRIS, I., and J. HUNT (1975). *Assessment in Infancy*. Urbana: University of Illinois Press.

VANE, L. (1975). *Vane Evaluation of Language Scale*. Brandon, Vt.: Clinical Psychology Publishing Co.

WATSON, L. (1977). "Conversational Participation by Language Deficient and Normal Children." Paper presented at the Convention of the American Speech and Hearing Association, Chicago.

WEISS, A., L. LEONARD, L. ROWAN, and K. CHAPMAN (1983). "Linguistic and Nonlinguistic Features of Style in Normal and Language-Impaired Children." *Journal of Speech and Hearing Disorders*, 48: 154–163.

WEISZ, J., and E. ZIGLER (1979). "Cognitive Development in Retarded and Nonretarded Persons: Piagetian Tests of the Similar Sequence Hypothesis." *Psychological Bulletin*, 86: 831–851.

WERNER, E., and J. KRESECK (1981). "Variability in Scores, Structures and Errors on Three Measures of Expressive Language." *Language, Speech and Hearing Services in Schools*, 12: 82–89.

WESTBY, C. (1980). "Assessment of Cognitive and Language Abilities Through Play." *Language, Speech and Hearing Services in Schools*, 11: 154–168.

WOLFUS, B., M. MOSCOVITCH, and M. KINSBOURNE (1980). "Subgroups of Developmental Language Impairment." *Brain and Language*, 10: 152–171.

WOLSKI, W., and L. LEREA (1962). *The Michigan Picture Language Inventory*. Ann Arbor: University of Michigan Press.

WOOD, B. (1981). *Children and Communication: Verbal and Nonverbal Language Development*. Englewood Cliffs, N.J.: Prentice-Hall, Inc.

ZACHMAN, L., R. HULSINGH, C. JORGENSEN, and M. BARRETT (1978). *Oral Language Sentence Imitation Test*. Moline, Ill.: Linguisystems.

ZIMMERMAN, I., V. STEINER, and R. EVATT (1969). *Preschool Language Scale*. Columbus, Ohio: Chas. E. Merrill.

# CHAPTER FIVE
# ASSESSMENT OF ARTICULATION DISORDERS

Many speech pathologists and laypeople tend to view disorders of articulation as relatively minor, even trivial. Perhaps one reason for this perception is the ubiquity of misarticulations in all children as they progress through communication development. There are also many famous personalities with articulation disorders who have proved successful in their fields and appear frequently in the media. Because all children exhibit misarticulations during development, they are viewed as natural phenomena by many parents and professionals. Frequently, physicians will tell parents that articulation problems are likely to be "outgrown" by children, and in many cases they are correct. Sometimes, however, physicians and parents wait too long to refer to the speech pathologist, and severe articulation disorders are difficult to remediate in the short time between age four and school entrance.

The early research literature in speech pathology is replete with studies attempting to determine the nature and etiology of articulation disorders. As a result, speech pathologists feel that if there is an area they "know," it is articulation. Most clinicians would probably indicate that the disorder area that they feel most competent in assessing and treating is articulation. We even hear such phrases as "simple articulation disorder" or "just an articulation problem." The disorder appears to be so fathomable that many laypeople are quite adept at diagnosing some gross aspects of childhood misarticulations. They come to the clinic saying, "He has trouble with his /r/ sounds" or "He doesn't say his words right" or "We can't understand him when he talks."

All of the above-mentioned illustrations probably contribute to the conception of an articulation disorder as being a relatively simple problem to diagnose, an easy problem to treat, and a difficulty that really is not significantly penalizing to the client. It is true that of all the disorders the speech pathologist deals with, articulation problems probably are the ones with which they have the most clinical success. We do have some effective basic procedures, many of which have not changed significantly since the 1940s, and this fact should give us some confidence in the articulation area. There is no doubt that we can effectively assess and treat the vast majority of articulation disorders, and we do not question this. The challenge of the 1980s, however, is not to learn how to assess and treat articulation disorders on a basic level. Rather, it is to learn how to assess and treat them more efficiently. How can we dismiss our clients in less time?

Although it is possible to trivialize the articulation disorders of some adults, the impact of an intelligibility problem on young children should not be minimized. Most parents are extremely anxious when their child cannot be understood, especially when the youngster's peers in the neighborhood or preschool setting are readily intelligible. If the child reaches the age of school entrance with a significant intelligibility problem, although treatment can be requested, the potential for negative effects on social and educational areas is great. Articulation-disordered children may be at high risk for language problems, reading difficulties, and, as a result, general educational difficulties (Winitz, 1969; Powers, 1971; Bernthal and Bankson, 1981).

At any rate, an articulation disorder severe enough to interfere significantly with intelligibility is certainly as debilitating a communication problem as many other disorders. A child's social development might be adversely affected if he is unintelligible to others. Even in cases of adult misarticulations, some research has indicated that individuals with certain phonemic problems are perceived as handicapped and rated less favorably by other adults (Mowrer, Wahl, and Doolan, 1978; Silverman, 1976). Thus, the commonality of misarticulations should not diminish their importance, nor should our ability to assess and treat these difficulties lead us to a feeling of complacency. As we will point out, articulation disorders are not simple at all, and they are not necessarily easy to diagnose effectively.

## THE ARTICULATORY PROCESS

In the early part of this century articulation was conceptualized by most clinicians as primarily a motor act. The sensorimotor aspect of articulation was studied and trained in therapy. It was not uncommon for articulation treatment to emphasize almost exclusively the movements of the oral musculature through an emphasis on diagrams, models, and motoric drills (Scripture and Jackson, 1927). With the advent of greater attention to language in the 1950s, however, it was noted that articulation had more components than simply motor activity. Several authors suggest that linguistic activity contributes to the articulatory process (Shriberg and Kwiatkowski, 1982a; Schwartz, 1983; Shelton and McReynolds, 1979).

Many events occur before the actual motor act of articulating. First, there is a biological component to articulation. The speaker must have a vocal tract and intact sensory and motor systems. Second, there is a cognitive-linguistic component in which the speaker conceives of "something to say." The thought then undergoes linguistic processing in which semantic elements are selected, words are arranged in proper syntactic order, and the utterance is appropriately tailored to the communication situation by the speaker, taking pragmatics into consideration. Finally, the selection of phonemic elements and their order is accomplished by applying phonological rules of our language.

The details of linguistic processing of an utterance are not fully understood. It is enough to say, however, that linguistic processing involving semantic, syntactic, pragmatic, and phonological areas must be necessary at some point in expressing an utterance. Subsequent to language processing, motor commands of some sort must be sent to the articulators in order to make them produce the sequence of sounds dictated by phonological programming. (Much research has been directed toward determining the basic unit of articulatory motor programming; we do not know its size or identity.) The motor production in the vocal tract then gives rise to acoustic vibrations that travel through a medium of air and arrive at the ears of our listeners.

This brief sketch of the processes that occur in articulatory production is highly simplified. It is possible to categorize the articulatory process into at least three major areas. First, the biological component provides the basic structures for articulation, such as the vocal tract, the articulators, and the intact nervous system, that allow us to perform the sensory (auditory, tactile, kinesthetic, proprioceptive) and motor functions necessary for controlled movement. Second, there is a cognitive-linguistic component that includes the thought, semantic-syntactic-pragmatic processing, and the application of phonological rules. Third, there is a sensorimotor-acoustic component, which includes motor programming and motor learning of actual sequences of physical movement in a wide variety of phonetic contexts.

It is the view of the present authors that this gross separation of the articulatory process into biological, cognitive-linguistic, and sensorimotor components carries with it several important implications. The diagnostician must be prepared to assess and treat any or all aspects of the process in a given client. Bernthal and Bankson (1981:3) indicate, for instance, that articulation disorders can be "motorically based errors (the ability to produce a target sound is not within the person's repertoire of motor skills) . . . or linguistically based (the client can produce a sound but does not use the sound in appropriate contexts)." They further state that differentiating a motoric from a linguistically based disorder is not always an easy task. If the client exhibits primarily a linguistically based problem (a phonological simplification such as deletion of certain final consonants, for instance), we should be able to examine a sample of speech for patterns of error that represent these phonological reductions. Oral-peripheral, audiological, and ultimately medical evaluation procedures can pinpoint difficulties with the biological foundations of articulation. Examination of a client's ability to sequence rapidly phonetic strings can give the clinician insight into articulatory motor learning and programming. The implication, then, is that a client can have difficulties with one or several parts of the process, and the diagnostician should be equipped to assess these.

Another implication of a multicomponent conception of articulation is that no single measure is capable of adequately examining all parts of this complex process. It is naive to believe that administration of a traditional articulation test, stimulability, and an oral-peripheral examination are all that is necessary to perform a complete assessment of articulatory behavior. The articulatory process is too complex and the disordered population too heterogeneous to rely on a "standard battery" for all clients. This is not to say that the clinician should not have a standard way of conducting the initial phases of an articulation evaluation. We are emphasizing the importance of knowing where to go and what to do to gain insight into aspects of articulation that are revealed to be problematic by the initial testing. As with any disorder area, no single chapter can possibly tell a student how to do everything well. Our goal is simply to make clinicians aware of the possibilities in articulatory assessment and refer the reader to the appropriate literature.

## TYPES OF ARTICULATORY DISORDERS

There are several ways of categorizing misarticulations. Historically, speech pathologists have used the traditional classifications of (1) substitution of one sound for another ("thoup" for "soup"), (2) omission of a sound ("kool" for "school"), (3) distortion of a sound (nonstandard production of a sound), and (4) addition of a sound ("puhlease" for "please"). These historical classifications have persisted because they do describe most articulatory deviations. If there is any fault with the categories, it is that they are not specific enough. The diagnostician must say more than "the child has substitutions and omissions in his speech." We need to know which sounds are substituted for others, how often, and in what contexts. The same could be said for distortions, omissions, and additions. Another superficiality of the historical categories is that they do not imply what part of the articulatory process is affected. That is, we cannot discern from the category of "substitution" whether the error is related to deficiencies in the client's sensorimotor, biological, or linguistic-phonological system.

The traditional classifications, however, are a good place to begin the articulatory assessment. We can then assess further and attempt to determine variability of performance in specific phonetic contexts, as well as how the misarticulation varies in utterances of different linguistic complexities. Articulatory errors can also be divided into categories of organic (some physical cause for the misarticulation) and functional (no demonstrable organic cause). The latter term has come under criticism for quite some time (Powers, 1971). Powers (1971) calls the term "functional" a "diagnosis by default." This is because the diagnosis of organic requires some positive proof of organicity, whereas the diagnosis of functional requires no positive evidence. The classification of functional is made only when a lack of evidence of organicity exists. The words most frequently associated with the functional classification are "learned" and "habit."

Thus, although the classification of functional has been justifiably criticized, it is still widely held that the vast majority of articulation disorders have no significant, maintaining organic basis, and the treatment is behavioral in nature. Future research may yet uncover subtle organic or behavioral differences in these individuals (Bernthal and Bankson, 1981). Assessment of organically based articulation disorders such as dysarthria and apraxia will be dealt with in Chapter 7. The present chapter focuses on misarticulations that have no obvious organic component.

### Seven Important Factors in Articulation Disorders and Evaluation

Before we discuss assessment of articulation disorders, there are several areas that the clinician should be familiar with. Actually, there are more areas that could be considered, but these seven seem to be the critical prerequisites to performing a diagnostic evaluation.

*Knowledge of the anatomy and physiology of the speech mechanism.*   Before attempting to deal with an articulatory evaluation, the clinician should be fully familiar with the normal oral mechanism. Most students obtain this knowledge in their undergraduate training. There are many textbooks that provide this information (Daniloff, Schuckers, and Feth, 1980; Dickson and Maue-Dickson, 1982; Kahane and Folkins, 1984; Palmer, 1984; Zemlin, 1981).

*Knowledge of phonetics.*   It is one thing to know about the anatomy and physiology of the vocal mechanism, but it is quite another to be aware of how that apparatus actually produces the variety of consonant and vowel sounds in English. References have described sound productions and articulatory movements associated with them (Shriberg and Kent, 1982; Van Riper and Smith, 1979; Carrell and Tiffany, 1960). Aside from knowing articulatory phonetics, the clinician must have well-developed skills in phonetic transcription. This is important in order to record a client's productions accurately for later analysis. Phonetic transcription abilities are especially important in order to accomplish phonological analyses (Shriberg and Kwiatkowski, 1980).

*Knowledge of articulatory development.*   A major goal in diagnosis is to compare a child's articulatory performance to the behavior of other children in the same age range. In this way we can tell if a child's misarticulations are developmental or clinically significant. There are at least three interpretations of articulatory development the clinician should be familiar with before doing an assessment.

The most abundant normative data available are traditionally oriented studies of children's phoneme production of words with the target sound in the initial, medial, and final positions (Templin, 1957; Wellman et al., 1931; Poole, 1934).

Although their criteria for "acquisition" differ slightly, they provide ages at which children master phonemes. More recent data (Sander, 1972; Irwin and Wong, 1983; Prather, Hendrick, and Kern, 1975) suggest earlier development of speech sounds and provide age ranges of development of "customary production" (two of three word positions) and mastery. The data provided by Irwin and Wong (1983) deal with sound production in connected spontaneous speech as opposed to the typical single-word responses reported in other traditional studies. Figure 5.1 is an example of normative sound development data.

**FIGURE 5.1**   Average age estimates and upper age limits of customary consonant production. The solid bar corresponding to each sound starts at the median age of customary articulation; it stops at the age level at which 90 percent of all children are customarily producing the sound. (Sander, 1972: 62;  © 1972, the American Speech-Language-Hearing Association, Rockville, Maryland.)

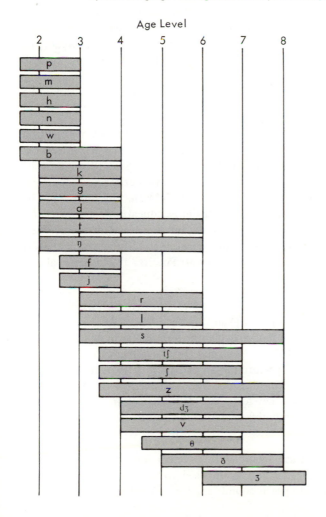

Another type of developmental data involves distinctive feature acquisition. Several sources report a developmental order in distinctive feature acquisition (Singh, 1976; Blache, 1978). These data could be used when analyzing a child's distinctive feature system as opposed to more traditional norms.

Finally, data are beginning to emerge regarding the occurrence of phonological reduction processes in normally developing children (Shriberg and Kwiatkowski, 1980; Ingram, 1976). Shriberg and Kwiatkowski (1980) indicate that several large-scale investigations are underway dealing with children's phonological development and we await these data. Ingram (1976) has provided some general age cutoffs for certain phonological processes. If a clinician sees a child who is deleting final consonants, for instance, she cannot use traditional norms to determine when this tendency diminishes in normal children. Data must be gathered on the occurrence of phonological processes beyond the preliminary information we presently have access to.

Bernthal and Bankson (1981) point out that there are very little longitudinal developmental data and most of our information has been gleaned from cross-sectional investigations. No doubt, as in other aspects of development, a variety of articulatory acquisition strategies will eventually be found. A major point we wish to make here is that the clinician can look at an articulatory sample from a variety of perspectives. Traditional, distinctive feature and phonological norms should be useful, depending on which framework the clinician is using.

*Knowledge of factors related to articulation disorders.*   Whenever a clinician undertakes an articulatory evaluation, he can expect that parents will often ask questions regarding the etiology of the problem. The clinician, then, must be familiar with the pertinent literature dealing with research on etiological factors, as well as skills and abilities of articulation-disordered children. Questions may be asked about language development, reading, spelling, educational performance, dentition, oral structures, gross and fine motor skills, intelligence, auditory abilities, and much more. Several sources summarize this research handily and should assist clinicians in answering any questions (Winitz, 1969; Powers, 1971; Bernthal and Bankson, 1981).

*Knowledge of dialectical variation.*   Many sources have reported articulatory differences as a product of regional dialect (Van Riper and Smith, 1979; Carrell and Tiffany, 1960). Other authorities report articulatory differences in minority populations (Stoller, 1975; Dillard, 1972). According to the American Speech and Hearing Association, the clinician performing an articulatory evaluation must be able to differentiate a communication disorder from a dialectical variation (Battle et al., 1983). Since there are so few tests that take dialect into account, the clinician must become familiar with this material and routinely consider it when evaluating misarticulations.

*Coarticulation.*   For at least twenty years, researchers have known that speech is produced in a parallel fashion as opposed to a serial, discrete manner (Winitz, 1975). This means that speech sounds are not isolated entities but overlap motorically and acoustically in time. Put simply, sounds are influenced by other phonemes that surround them. This influence of one sound on another is called coarticulation and is one of the most basic facts about the articulatory process. The phonetic environment or phonetic context a sound is produced in influences the production of the phoneme.

There are two major types of coarticulation that can be described in terms of the direction of the influence of one sound on another. Left to right coarticulation refers to a preceding sound having an effect on a following sound (the *t* in "boots" is produced with some lip rounding because of the rounding /u/ vowel that precedes it). This type of coarticulation is perceived by some to be a type of "overflow" of movement from the first sound to the second. Thus, the left to right coarticulation is thought to be primarily the result of mechanical-inertial factors. The other type of coarticulation is right to left. This means that a sound later in the speech sequence affects a sound earlier in the stream of speech. For example, the *t* sound in the word "tea" is produced differently than the *t* in the word "too." The difference in the two situations is that in the word "tea" the sound is followed by a vowel that is not produced with rounded lips. Thus, the *t* sound in "too" might be produced with lip rounding because the following vowel is rounded. Note that in both of these cases the sound that influences the *t* occurs after the *t* has been uttered. Researchers and theorists have suggested that the right to left influence is probably the result of articulatory preprogramming. That is, early sounds in a sequence are produced differently in anticipation of sounds that are yet to be said. This implies some sort of motor planning.

There are many studies of coarticulation that have used cinefluorography, electromyography, and spectrographic analyses. These investigations have shown conclusively that coarticulation does, in fact, occur in speech sequences. Because it is a fact that coarticulation will be present in any utterance, it is a phenomenon that the speech pathologist can choose to deal with in assessment and treatment. Whether or not we use coarticulatory influences in assessment and treatment to increase the efficiency of our clinical work, the effects will still occur. Most authorities feel that as long as coarticulation exists, we might as well use it to the best interest of our client.

The implications of the existence of coarticulation for articulatory assessment are significant. One implication is that testing sounds in isolation is an unrealistic and artificial enterprise. What a child can do with a sound in isolation may be totally different from his production in connected speech. A second implication has to do with testing in single words. When we speak, we typically do not put oral pauses or "spaces" between our words as in the ones you are reading right now. The speech stream has been called an "unsegmentable whole" (Kent and Minifie, 1977). Research on coarticulation has shown that the effects of one sound on another can cross both word and syllable boundaries (McClean, 1973; Moll and Daniloff, 1971; Daniloff and Moll, 1968; Amerman, Daniloff, and Moll, 1970). Thus sounds located in two adjacent words can have an effect on one another. This means that testing sound production on the single-word level may not be representative of sound production in spontaneous speech, because connected words may provide different coarticulatory effects as compared to single words alone (Faircloth and Faircloth, 1970).

Another implication has to do with possible facilitating and sabotaging effects of phonemes surrounding a particular target sound. For instance, a misarticulated /r/ sound may be produced correctly by a child if it is preceded by a /k/, perhaps because both sounds require grossly similar positioning of the tongue in the vocal tract (Hoffman, Schuckers, and Ratusnik, 1977). Conversely, an /r/ might be misarticulated as a /w/ if words surrounding the target sound contain a /w/ or some other lip-rounded phoneme (Winitz, 1975). Therefore, the effects of coarticulation can be either positive or negative, facilitating or sabotaging, and this is especially important for the clinician to consider in assessment and treatment. Perhaps the most important implication is in accounting for articulatory inconsistency. Most misarticulations are notoriously inconsistent and if the clinician analyzes these productions, she can find that this "inconsistency" may actually be quite consistent indeed. Phonetic context is often the common denominator among errors that appear inconsistent on the surface.

*The linguistic-articulatory connection.*    An important postulate in discussing articulatory assessment is the intimate relationship between language and articulation. This connection has been shown in several ways in the literature.

1.  Theoretically, phonology has been considered a classic component of language models. Chomsky, for instance, includes phonological rules in his model of transformational grammar (1957), along with semantics and syntax.
2.  Many bound morphemes (*-ed,* plural *-s,* possessive *-s,* and so on) are realized in speech as single phonemes. The *-ed* in the word "walked" is really pronounced as a /t/ sound in a consonant blend at the end of the word /wɔkt/. Thus, a single sound makes a difference in word meaning and that same single unit is a grammatical morpheme. A sound, therefore, is much more than merely a phonetic unit; it makes a difference in word meaning and carries linguistic value.
3.  Several studies have shown that misarticulations are affected by linguistic complexity (Panagos, Quine, and Klich, 1979; Schmuach, Panagos, and Klich, 1978; Haynes, Haynes, and Jackson, 1982). That is, more misarticulations will occur as syntactic complexity increases. This is a clear relationship between articulation and language.
4.  Shriberg and Kwiatkowski (1980) have suggested that even the type of word in terms of its syntactic class may affect sound productions. They found, for instance, that blends may be reduced differently in verbs as compared to the same blend in nouns.
5.  Pragmatics has also been implicated as affecting sound productions in several investigations (Weiner and Ostrowski, 1979; Leonard, 1971; Campbell and Shriberg, 1982). That is, children may produce sounds more correctly in conditions of increased information load and misarticulate more frequently when the communication value is lessened. This means that when there is a greater chance of being misunderstood, the child may articulate more correctly.
6.  A relationship between language and articulation can be inferred from the high co-occurrence of the two disorders in children. Generally, children who

have articulation problems are at high risk for language disorders and vice versa.

7. Another connection was shown in a study of treatment effects by Matheny and Panagos (1978). These investigators examined children with both articulation and language disorders and demonstrated that the subjects trained only on language tended to improve their articulation skills and others trained on articulation only improved their language abilities. This also shows a possible connection between the two domains.

The implications of these connections between articulation and language are significant for assessment. First, routine assessment of articulation with an exclusive sensorimotor orientation is not appropriate. Language and articulation are hopelessly intertwined when a person speaks spontaneously (Locke, 1983). Second, when the speech pathologist is looking for sources of inconsistency, he may find significant effects from semantic, syntactic, or pragmatic variables. Phonetic context, then, is not the only source of inconsistent productions. A final implication is that an articulatory deviation can be due more to linguistic influences of the child's phonological system rather than a product of sensorimotor difficulties. Thus, a more productive view would be to consider both sensorimotor and linguistic components in the assessment repertoire (Schwartz, 1983).

## TESTING FOR ARTICULATION DISORDERS

### Case Detection Screening

Commonly, public school speech clinicians conduct surveys to identify those children with communication disorders. The purpose of screening is to select children with significant communication problems by assessing a total population with a brief but discriminating testing procedure. The objective, then, is detection, not description, of persons with disordered speech.

A screening test must be swift, yet discerning. The examiner must be able to detect individuals with impaired speech while rapidly passing over all the normal speakers. Although brief, the detection process should provide a sufficient sample of each person's oral communication to permit critical judgment of articulation and voice, fluency, and language abilities. Because screening procedures and materials differ with various age groups, we shall describe methods for target populations: preschool and early elementary school children (age three through third grade), later elementary school children (fourth through eighth grade), and older groups. See also the work of Black (1964), Irwin (1965), and Van Hattum (1983) for descriptions of screening programs used in school settings.

*Preschool and early elementary school children.* There are essentially five ways to screen the speech of a young child. We must remember, however, that our goal in screening is to determine if enough of a difference exists in a child's communication to warrant recommending a full diagnostic evaluation. In cases of very young children it is quite possible that they will not talk to the clinician at all, especially if they are taken to a strange setting with an unfamiliar adult. We have a finite amount of time to spend with each child in a screening, and if a disproportionate amount of time is invested in a particular child the purpose of a rapid screening is defeated. Thus, with children who simply will not speak, it is prudent to recommend a rescreening or a diagnostic evaluation after all attempts at obtaining direct and indirect samples have failed. The clinician is operating at a disadvantage in a screening because there is little time to establish a relationship with each child, and some of these youngsters will not spontaneously communicate until they are comfortable with their listener.

One way to obtain information about the communication of a reluctant child is to interview the parents or teachers, if they are available. Much important information can be provided by people who interact with the child day after day. They can provide "ball park" data on the child's mean length of utterance, types of word combinations, fluency, vocal quality, and intelligibility and summarize the occasions when the child communicates most. This interview process is no substitute for observing the child's communication firsthand, but it certainly can pinpoint significant problems in any area and can be the basis for recommending a diagnostic evaluation.

A second way of obtaining information about a young child is to observe him during free play, perhaps with other children. This procedure is very effective but time consuming. One advantage of this process is that the child is not taken away from his environment and isolated with a strange adult. The clinician can also interact with the child as he performs his schoolroom tasks and involve other children to stimulate diverse interactions.

A third method of screening young children is to obtain a short sample of conversational speech. Recently it was found that screening judgments made by an experienced clinician from a two- to three-minute sample were as good or better than formal measures (Eveleigh and Warr-Leeper, 1983). This is similar to the high correspondence between formal and informal measures in language assessment (Allen, Bliss, and Timmons, 1981).

Another method of screening is to have the child repeat words or phrases. The examiner's model tends to influence the child's speech and thus may not provide a representative sample. If the clinician must screen large numbers of children rapidly, however, an imitative protocol may be the most expedient method of obtaining the information in the shortest amount of time.

A fifth technique to use in screening is to have the child name colors, count, and identify pictures or objects. This is a common method used, especially with low functioning children; it is easy and takes little time, and children seem to respond well to the task.

Many of the published diagnostic inventories cited later in this chapter include portions designed to serve as screening tests for children. For example, the first fifty items of the *Templin-Darley Tests of Articulation* (1969) are a useful screening device; the authors provide tables of norms that permit comparison of an individual child's score with that of others at the same age level. The *Triota Ten Word Test* devised by Irwin (1972) takes only one minute to administer and yields a composite error score by age. Several tests are designed specifically as screening instruments (Monsees and Berman, 1968; Riley, 1971; Rogers, 1972; Fluharty, 1974).

*Later elementary school children.*  Speech pathologists may use reading passages and conversation to screen children in grades four through eight who are typically referred by classroom teachers. The clinician may choose from among several published reading passages for later elementary children (Avant and Hutton, 1962; Eisenson and Ogilvie, 1977; Irvin, 1965).

To obtain a sample of spontaneous speech, questions about favorite hobbies and interests are useful. Actually, later elementary school children are often engaging conversationalists; they are sufficiently mature to enjoy relating to a new adult but not old enough to resent being scrutinized. Indeed, they are often intrigued with the screening test and want to know how they have done. It is usually wise to provide a brief explanation of any noted articulation errors.

*Older groups.*  Reading passages, sentences loaded with consonant sounds most frequently defective, and conversations are commonly used to obtain speech samples in screening programs for older individuals. The clinician can construct a reading passage or use any of the several published versions, which include "My Grandfather" (Van Riper, 1963), "Arthur the Young Rat" (Johnson, Darley, and Spriestersbach, 1963), "The Rainbow Passage" (Fairbanks, 1960), and "Directions" (Anderson and Newby, 1973).

Many universities require that students enrolled in teacher education be screened for speech disorders to prevent them from becoming poor models for children. In addition to an oral reading, some questions are asked to elicit a sample of spontaneous speech. Queries such as "What are you majoring in and how did you select that field?" or "If I were to come to your home area as a tourist, what are some things I might want to see?" are good examples of starters.

### Problems in Screening

Several problems may be encountered in conducting screening programs. Here are a few of the most salient challenges to the clinician:

*The routine nature of the task.*  Screening a large number of individuals makes it extremely difficult for the clinician to establish a genuine relationship with each person being evaluated. However, it takes little time or energy to personalize the procedure; you never know whether the individual being screened might be your next client. Personal comments about a particular item of clothing or the individual's place of residence, a smile, or some small bit of humor can be helpful. When the testing is completed, a child may want to know the results; it seems only common courtesy to discuss the information, if the child is mature enough to understand it. In our experience, if the clinician is enjoying the job and shows it, if she treats each individual not as a subject but as an interesting and unique person, then she not only makes the child or adult feel better but she also makes the redundant task more palatable (Siegel, 1967). Avoid stereotyped interactions with the individuals being screened; vary the wording of your questions to reduce monotony.

*The traffic problem.*   In order to screen large groups, it is necessary to make provisions for getting people in and out of the testing site as swiftly and quietly as possible. In public schools, older children have been used as guides and monitors; it is often helpful to have an extra room or space adjacent to the testing site as a waiting room. Screening tests should be done individually and privately, if possible; however, some clinicians prefer to screen children in small groups.

*Fear and resistance.*   Young children are sometimes threatened by the prospect of speech screening. We find it helpful to go into kindergarten and first-grade classrooms before the screening and tell the children exactly what we plan to do.

> Another ploy that frequently eases the anxiety surrounding screening is to begin the procedure with a positive experience. Nothing is worse than picking a child from a class roster who is resistant and shy and then comes back to the classroom in tears after the screening. In this case, the other children wonder what went on when their classmate was taken away. Visions of inoculations dance through their heads. It is helpful to ask the teacher for her most gregarious, friendliest child to begin with. This child returns to the classroom smiling and raving about the pictures and how "good a job" she did. Then the clinician can ask the class, "Who wants to be next?" and invariably several hands shoot up. After this, the anxiety of the entire class has been lessened and the screening has been shown to be painless and indeed a prized activity to participate in.

**Predictive Screening**

A significant number of children entering kindergarten and first grade will not have acquired the normal complement of consonant sounds (Pendergast et al., 1966). This places the clinician in a dilemma: At least half of these children will mature into normal articulation without therapeutic intervention—but which ones? Some of the children's speech differences are merely the result of late maturation and do not require treatment. But how do you separate the normal speakers from the potentially permanent misarticulators? If therapy is postponed for those who genuinely need assistance, their speech errors could become habituated and more resistant to treatment. In addition, the child may be educationally and socially penalized if his speech pattern draws undue attention. A few clinicians select certain children and not others, operating on an ad hoc basis. They then find it difficult to explain their selection process to teachers, parents, and administrators. The opposite extreme is to work with all first-grade children who present articulation errors.

In an effort to provide some "objective" means of determining which children should be enrolled in treatment, several test instruments have been developed that attempt to "predict" which children are at high risk for articulation disorders (Van Riper and Erickson, 1969; McDonald, 1968; Templin and Darley, 1969). These tests vary in terms of whether they are administered imitatively or spontaneously, and they differ in the distribution of phonemes tested. Recently, Ritterman et al. (1982: 432) compared the *McDonald Screening Deep Test,* the *Templin-Darley Screening Test* and the *Predictive Screening Test of Articulation (PSTA)* in terms of the pass/fail judgments indicated on ninety-one first-graders and found that there was a "poor correspondence among the tests as to the individuals failed. That is, only three subjects were failed by more than a single test." The three instruments evaluate either consistency of sound production (McDonald) or the total number of correctly produced spontaneous or imitative productions (Templin; *PSTA*).

Certainly, a child who is dramatically delayed in articulatory development would fail all three of these tests, but this type of child is not particularly problematic to the clinician. It is the borderline child who presents difficulties. Clinicians should not rely exclusively on such measures to determine if a child requires enrollment in treatment. Ultimately, it comes down to a clinical judgment that must be made for each case, based on normative data, and, although a formal screening test might be considered in concert with other variables, it cannot be the sole determiner of enrollment. Ritterman et al. (1982: 432) state that

> Research has indicated that each of the underlying variables on which the *Templin-Darley Screening Test of Articulation,* the *Predictive Screening Test of Articulation,* and the *Screening Deep Test of Articulation* are based have some degree of merit as pass/fail selection criteria. The results of the present study, however, would seem to indicate that these variables are not well correlated in that different children failed for different reasons on the three tests.

Other variables that might enter into decision making for a particular case might be (1) the child's perception of herself as communication-disordered, (2) parent and teacher perceptions and desires, (3) presence of concomitant disorders (such as language), and (4) existence of characteristically resistant articulatory deviations (such as lateral sibilants; vocalic /r/ distortions, omissions of consonants).

## TRADITIONAL ARTICULATORY ASSESSMENT

Subsequent to failure of an articulatory screening, a child may be scheduled for a complete assessment of articulatory ability with parental permission. There are a variety of types of articulatory assessments. They differ in their theoretical assumptions, method of sample elicitation, type of information obtained, and therapeutic implications. Perhaps the most common type of assessment is what we will call "traditional." The theoretical orientation of traditional testing is that each English phoneme must be evaluated in the initial, medial, and final positions of words. These words are typically elicited from the client by means of pictures, word lists, sentences, or conversational sampling. Even though the data for the analysis might range from words to connected speech, the orientation of the clinician is to determine omissions, substitutions, and distortions of phonemes in differing word positions.

Many tests are available for use in traditional assessment (Cypreansen, Wiley, and Laase, 1959; Bryngelson and Glaspey, 1962; Edmonson, 1969; Hejna, 1963; Pendergast et al., 1969; Goldman and Fristoe, 1969; Fudala, 1970; Templin and Darley, 1969; Mecham, Jex, and Jones, 1970; Ingram, 1971; Ham, 1971; Fisher and Logemann, 1971; Anderson and Newby, 1973; Bzoch, 1974; Haws, 1975). Most of these inventories include stimulus pictures for testing children and structured sentences for older clients to read; one also employs a filmstrip (Goldman and Fristoe, 1967). Several provide norms against which a child may be compared, and one (Fudala, 1970) features a method of scaling the degree of articulatory defectiveness.

Traditional diagnostic procedures have in common other basic operations. Most traditional assessments accrue a phonetic inventory from the client. This is a listing of all phonemes produced in the sample. One reason for obtaining a phonetic inventory is to compare the sounds produced correctly by a given client to normative data on articulatory development. Most normative studies are based on traditional notions and report phoneme productions of sounds in the three word positions (Templin, 1957; Wellman et al., 1931; Poole, 1934; Sander, 1972; Prather, Hedrick, and Kern, 1975).

Another traditional procedure is test a client's stimulability, or his response to stimulation. In other words, we evaluate the impact that the examiner's model has on the client's production. Is there some modification in the direction of normalcy, or is there no change in the articulatory behavior? Testing for stimulability (Milisen et al., 1954: 6-7) is an extremely useful diagnostic procedure. If a client can produce the error correctly by imitating a standard model, either in isolation, in nonsense syllables, or in words, then there may be no serious organic obstacles that would prevent the eventual acquisition of the sound (Darley, 1964: 65). Stimulability is also a useful prognostic sign; clients who can modify their articulation errors by imitating the examiner's standard production may improve more swiftly in treatment than those who cannot. Stimulability certainly has been implicated as a potential predictor of children who may develop normal speech through maturation (Farquhar, 1961).

> Stimulability is frequently given "short shrift" by practicing speech clinicians and students in training. Sometimes it is totally omitted. Often, we see students hurry through the stimulability testing, frequently giving inadequate instructions and rather imprecise models to the client. The spirit of stimula-

bility testing is to see how the client performs under maximal, multimodality stimulation. This is why most tests recommend that the model be presented two or three times after the client has been given a strong attentional set. Students sometimes indicate that the client was not stimulable for error phonemes after rather cursory testing. Subsequent stimulability trials, done more intensively, may reveal that the client, in fact, can produce the target sound. Prior to making negative stimulability statements in a clinical report, the clinician should be certain that the stimulation task was administered effectively.

It is our contention that traditional testing is a good starting point in an articulatory assessment. In many cases a traditional assessment may be all that is needed, especially when the client has only a few articulatory errors and is stimulable. In cases like this the clinician knows what the errors are and how often they occur in a test and in spontaneous speech if analyzed traditionally. Further, the clinician has a place to start production of the target sound, as the client can make it correctly with stimulation.

In the majority of cases, however, traditional testing does not go far enough. For instance, our discussion of coarticulation suggested that sound will be produced differently in different phonetic environments. Most traditional tests examine only a limited number of these phonetic contexts. If a child or adult is not stimulable, the clinician may want to rely on experimentation with different coarticulatory transitions to determine if there is a facilitating context. Traditional tests are just not equipped to do this. Also, traditional testing procedures are not directed toward detecting patterns of error in a client's speech. In order to define patterns of error, a phonological analysis is perhaps the most efficient method to use. Traditional analyses do not systematically examine the effects of syllable complexity (Panagos, Quine, and Klich, 1979) and linguistic complexity on misarticulation. Finally, traditional analyses do not focus on certain parameters that may be relevant to certain cases such as distinctive feature acquisition and use.

In short, no one method can do everything, and so it is with the traditional approach. The traditional test, however, is a viable instrument to use generically. If other analyses are required, they should be done as appropriate.

It is far easier to describe articulation testing than it is to administer an articulation test. A student's first attempt is generally a confusing situation that requires careful listening, attention to visual cues, recording the client's responses appropriately, and maintaining a positive client-clinician relationship. We recommend that the beginning clinician listen for only one sound at a time. When possible, have the child repeat the test words a number of times. Tape-record or, better yet, video-tape the child's responses to assist in later scoring of the test. Experienced speech pathologists are able to save time by testing more than one sound simultaneously (Fristoe and Goldman, 1968).

It is especially true with articulation assessment that the clinician is really the "test." Commercial articulation tests are nothing more than stacks of pictures bound together with metal or plastic. Because articulatory responses are so transient and fleeting, clinicians must listen carefully, practice frequently, and, above all, check their reliability. Studies have shown that speech pathologists are fairly reliable when the judgments they make are rather molar such as "correct" or "incorrect" (Winitz, 1969). When judgments become more "fine grained," as in determining the nature of specific substitutions in certain word positions, our reliability tends to deteriorate. One can easily see that very complex analysis procedures such as those used in distinctive features and phonology are even more susceptible to misjudgments on the part of the clinician. Clinicians must always strive to improve their reliability through practice and rechecking their results. Our evaluation results are only as good as our ability to perceive the reality of the client's responses. No one, as a professor said, has immaculate perception.

## TEST PROCEDURES THAT EVALUATE
## PHONETIC CONTEXT EFFECTS

After a traditional assessment a client may be judged not stimulable. Procedures then need to be initiated to determine if a facilitating phonetic context can be found. As we mentioned in the section on coarticulation, phonemes are significantly influenced by other sounds that surround them. This phenomenon results in the existence of facilitating contexts that can encourage the correct production of a target consonant. The concept that certain phonetic environments can facilitate correct production was suggested in the early writings of Van Riper and Irwin (1958) where they indicated there were "key words" in which a phoneme could be produced more effectively. If certain key words are discovered for a nonstimulable client, then treatment could commence in these contexts.

In 1964, McDonald devised the *Deep Test of Articulation (MDT)*, which, among other things, is based on the idea that phonemes will be produced differently, depending on the sounds that precede and follow them. Through systematically permuting a variety of consonants before and after a specific phoneme, the contexts in which correct production is observed can be noted by the clinician and serve as a starting point for treatment. In the *Deep Test*, each phoneme can be observed forty or more times as the initiating or terminating sound in a syllable. Because it is the basic unit of speech, it seems appropriate that the focus of testing should be the syllable (Priestly, 1977).

Here is a part of a session in which the examiner is administering the /s/ portion of the McDonald instrument to a second-grade boy with a lateralized /s/:

*Clinician*: Okay, Tony, we are ready to start with the numbered pages. You understand now that you are to make a funny "big word" from the names of the objects on the two pictures, like we did in the example "tubvase," without stopping between the words? Fine! Here is the first one:

1. Housepipe        No change
2. Housebell        No change

| | | |
|---|---|---|
| 3. | Housetie | Improvement-moderate |
| 4. | Housedog | Improvement-moderate |
| 5. | Housecow | No change |
| 6. | Housegun | No change |

Note that the word "house," with a final /s/, is tested as it precedes all other phonemes. The examiner listens carefully to identify any changes in the child's misarticulations. Then the examiner reverses the procedure so that /s/ follows all other phonemes (cupsun, tubsun, kitesun, and so on). For older clients, McDonald has prepared a series of sentences to be read aloud. The diagnostician will want to be familiar with this test.

The *McDonald Deep Test* has certain limitations. For instance, when we combine two lexical items into one nonsense word, we are no longer dealing with sound production in real linguistic units. Also, as the *MDT* progresses, some children find the big words neither "funny" nor interesting. We have found that it is too lengthy for initial assessment purposes and that some children experience considerable difficulty blending the two test items into one large word (Goda, 1970). If there is a pause between the two words, the purpose of the test is defeated (McDonald, 1964). Finally, depending on the child's pattern of misarticulation, many of the intended phonetic contexts are altered (for example, "housecow" becomes "house-tow"). This changes the ability of the instrument to evaluate all the contexts it is designed to elicit.

We prefer to use the test during the initial stages of treatment, exploring with the client for loci of improved, or at least altered, sound production. Additionally, researchers find the *Deep Test* invaluable for charting improvement during the course of treatment because it deals with many contexts.

The evaluation of a variety of phonetic contexts provides an interesting contrast to the limited number of environments evaluated by traditional measures. Schissell and James (1979) compared the evaluation of articulatory abilities in children using a more traditional test (*Arizona*) and the *McDonald Deep Test*. It was found that the traditional test missed some of the children who did not have consistent control of certain sounds, and it was also noted that the traditional test failed children on certain sounds when in actuality they performed the sound productions well in a significant number of contexts on the *MDT*. One interpretation of the disparity in results between these two measures is that the traditional test evaluated a limited number of phonetic contexts, and for some children the environment happened to be facilitative and for others it did not. The implication, of course, is that the more phonetic contexts examined, the more realistic picture obtained of the clients' articulatory performance. Also, we might find a place to begin our treatment.

Another way to examine phonetic context effects in children and adults is the use of sound-in-context sentences (Haynes, Haynes, and Jackson, 1982). These sentences can be read spontaneously by adults or imitated by children. Most work with these sentences has been done in research projects directed toward finding facilitating contexts for particular target consonants (mainly the /s/ and /r/ phonemes). The use of these sentence stimuli has shown that there are, in fact, facilitating contexts for /r/ and /s/ that occur for many clients. The essence of these sentences is that a clinician can have the client say any number of utterances that are constructed to determine phonetic context effects. For instance, if the clinician wants to evaluate the effects on /s/ production of a preceding /k/ sound and a following /p/ sound (for example, /KSP/) a sentence can be constructed such as "The dress had a black spot." Also, phrases may be used instead of sentences. The clinician, then, can use knowledge of coarticulation and devise stimuli to probe phonetic context effects on a given client's articulation.

Finally, Kent (1982: 75) urges continued experimentation with phonetic context effects in clinical and research settings because there is much we do not yet understand about this phenomenon:

> The selection of so-called facilitating contexts involves decisions regarding stress, word position, expected or permissible allophonic variation, frequency of occurrence and the influence of neighboring sounds. . . . The final selection of a facilitating context also should recognize as precisely as possible the nature of the articulation error. It should not be assumed, for example, that the same context will facilitate correct production of /s/ in children who distort the sound by dentalization, lateralization and palatalization.

With a knowledge of the effects of coarticulation, the clinician may construct a variety of utterance types for a particular client and need not rely solely on instruments devised by others. A thorough assessment could provide significant information that could be used at the outset of treatment if more attention were paid to ferreting out sources of error inconsistency attributable to phonetic context. The clinician should also be willing to experiment with a variety of segmental, suprasegmental, and linguistic complexity variables in the search for sources of inconsistency (Shriberg and Kwiatkowski, 1980).

### Distinctive Feature Analysis

As we mentioned previously, neither traditional analyses nor appraisals of phonetic context effects examine all pertinent aspects of a child's articulatory system. An evaluation of a child's distinctive feature system will provide yet another kind of information that the clinician may wish to consider in making treatment recommendations.

Researchers indicate that the most basic unit that speech can be distilled into is the distinctive feature, and the "reality" of features has been demonstrated both acoustically and physiologically (Singh, 1976). That is, as humans, we seem to pay attention to certain aspects of the speech signal both in perception and production. Phonemes are evidently made up of "bundles" of distinctive features that combine to produce a variety of different consonant and vowel sounds in a language. Singh (1976: 229) states: "Children do not acquire phonemes one by one; rather, they acquire a feature that provides them with a basis for manifesting a number of phonemes distinctively in speech production and discrimination tasks."

Features, then, are prerequisite to phonemes, because without the knowledge of and ability to produce a given feature of language, certain sounds containing that feature will not be produced. For instance, if a child does not learn that the feature of "voicelessness" is important in differentiating certain sounds from each other, the phonemes with the (−) voice feature—for example, /s, f, p, k/—will not be produced.

What are distinctive features? In this concept, speech sounds are not indivisible entities but, rather, are considered to be composed of intersecting subcomponents or attributes (voicing, nasality) that are termed "features" (Compton, 1970). Distinctive feature theory attempts to specify the characteristics of phonemes, according to the presence (+) or absence (−) of each feature that distinguishes or contrasts one speech sound from another. Let us illustrate with a distinctive feature comparison of /s/ and /θ/, two speech sounds that are often confused by children:

| /θ/ | Features | /s/ |
|-----|----------|-----|
| (−) | vocalic | (−) |
| (+) | consonantal | (+) |
| (−) | high | (−) |
| (−) | back | (−) |
| (−) | low | (−) |
| (+) | anterior | (+) |
| (+) | coronal | (+) |
| (−) | voice | (−) |
| (+) | continuant | (+) |
| (−) | nasal | (−) |
| (−) | strident | (+) |

To repeat, an analysis of phonemes (in this case /s/ and /θ/) yields a description of each speech sound with respect to the presence or absence of each feature (McReynolds and Engmann, 1975); definitions of the features can be found in Chomsky and Halle (1968). When particular features (in the example above the feature of stridency) serve to differentiate one phoneme from another, they are said to be distinct (Weston and Leonard, 1976).

One difficulty that is immediately apparent to a student studying distinctive features is the number of "systems" available (Singh, 1976). Further, these systems have been derived by different procedures and thus have disparate bases (acoustic, articulatory, perceptual). The feature systems also differ in the phonemes included in the scheme, the notation (binary, ternary, quarternary), and the number of features thought to be important. One source of solace to the clinician is the fact that most systems have some things in common. There are certain features that appear to be so significant and strong that they are included in the majority of systems. Specifically, the features of voice, nasality, duration, and place are the most common.

Several investigations have suggested that there are at least two different types of distinctive feature problems exhibited by children (McReynolds and Huston, 1971; Pollack and Rees, 1972; Ruder and Bunce, 1981). One type of distinctive feature difficulty is exemplified by a child who has not acquired the use of a feature at all. The child is not aware of the importance of the feature to differentiate English sounds and has difficulty producing the feature. The child might have one "aspect" or half of the feature (+ voicing) but does not have the other half (− voicing). Features are rather like light switches; they are only useful when you know about both turning them on and turning them off. Thus, a child has not really acquired the feature of voice until both voiced and voiceless sounds can be produced appropriately.

A second type of distinctive feature problem is shown in a child who has acquired the feature but does not use it appropriately. Control of features, like many things, is on a continuum. A child may be aware of the importance of a feature, and be capable of producing both aspects (+ and −) of it, yet there are specific contexts in which the feature is not used appropriately. On the other hand, a child may not be able to produce the feature aspects without great difficulty in any context. Several authorities have suggested that these two cases represent slightly different diagnostic groups: One child does not "have" the feature, and the other "has" it but is a feature misuser in certain contexts.

One can take several approaches to distinctive feature analysis. A distinctive feature analysis is useful primarily for children presenting four or more errors and reduces all of the client's articulation errors to a few underlying principles by which sound production is regulated. McReynolds and Engmann (1975) have prepared a manual featuring detailed clinical worksheets to guide the diagnostician in performing a distinctive feature analysis. The clinician first obtains a sample of the client's articulation—at least ten productions of each phoneme are recommended—and the responses are transcribed carefully according to number of correct productions, errors of omission, and substitutions (the actual sound substituted). Then, using a table of distinctive features, the clinician computes the percentage of the time a particular feature was used incorrectly by the client.

McReynolds and Engmann have provided some arbitrary percentages that indicate the severity of the feature problems of a client. The figure of 80 percent incorrect means that the feature has not been acquired by the client. Lower percentages of incorrect production of features are less well defined. The present authors, however, find the cutoff of 80 percent to be a reasonable indicator of a child who does not have control over a feature. A child who uses a feature correctly 50 to 60 percent of the time, however, probably has a different kind of problem than the one who has far less control over the feature.

The therapy program recommended by McReynolds and Engmann (1975) appears to be targeted toward introducing the feature into the child's system initially and not simply increasing the use of a feature that has been largely acquired. Thus, a major decision that must be made in a distinctive feature analysis is whether a child has not acquired a feature or whether he is a feature misuser. This decision is typically quite easy for a clinician to make after looking at the child's phonetic inventory to see if whole classes of sounds and features are missing. An experienced clinician can examine a child's speech sample and accurately predict which features are most in error without resorting to the lengthy procedure provided by McReynolds and Engmann. In many cases this may be enough to guide the clinician as to whether the treatment should be directed toward establishing a feature in a child's repertoire or altering the use of a feature that has already been acquired but is being used inconsistently.

What are the advantages of a distinctive feature analysis? We see four: (1) It provides a model for understanding articulation disorders in many children; an error on a given feature (for example, voicing) that is shared by more than one phoneme accounts for the misarticulation of many phonemes by reducing the seemingly random errors to a simpler pattern; (2) it provides one gauge of severity of sound substitution, in that the more feature differences between a target sound and its substitution, the more severe the problem may be; (3) it provides a basis for the selection of a target sound for therapy; the clinician can select the phoneme that shares features with many other misarticulated sounds; and (4) it may provide a basis for more efficient therapy (Ritterman and Freeman, 1974; Costello and Onstine, 1976) by facilitating generalization to sounds not being directly treated. Therapy directed toward one sound often improves others that are phonetically similar. Considered within the framework of distinctive features, it makes sense that training in features common to many sounds would result in greater improvement in misarticulation than specific training for each sound error.

Despite the many advantages, however, there are a number of factors that may limit the application of distinctive feature theory to clinical problems. First of all, the procedures for assessment as described by McReynolds and Engmann (1975) are quite time consuming; the clinician has to weigh this factor against the purported increase in efficiency. A second limiting factor is the obvious complexity of the system of analysis. Another drawback is that, on a phonetic level, the distinctive features advocated by Chomsky and Halle may have no conceptual reality (LaRiviere, 1974). By that we mean there may be no one-to-one relationship between distinctive features (an acoustic classification) and articulatory production (a physiological level) (Parker, 1976).

The physical act of articulation clearly is not a binary function that is either present (+) or absent (−) but is multivaried, a matter of varying degrees. According to Walsh (1974), the categories employed in distinctive feature analysis are overgeneralized and may encompass too great a phonetic space to be of clinical value. Leonard (1973: 141-142) points out that "articulation therapy involves giving phonetic instructions. Therefore, the features we deal with must have a specific physical interpretation." Where it is necessary to use a subphonemic system of analysis, we advocate, with others (Fisher and Logemann, 1971; Leonard, 1973; Walsh, 1974; McClean, 1976; Sommers and Kane, 1974; Eisenson and Ogilvie, 1977; Nation and Aram, 1977), the selection of one based on a model of speech production rather than on a system limited to an abstract classificatory function.

Sommers (1983) has suggested a less formal shortcut method of analyzing distinctive features from a sample of speech. He indicates that the briefer method yields similar results at a considerable savings of analysis time. We believe that whatever method the clinician uses to analyze distinctive features in a given client, the following are important:

1. The diagnostician should "think features" at some point in the analysis of a child with multiple articulation errors. In other words, one should at least be able to judge whether or not all features are present or if error patterns reflect consistent, repeated misuse of specific features in certain contexts.

2. The clinician should determine if a child (a) has not acquired a feature or (b) is a feature misuser. If the child does not evidence a particular feature in her system, then treatment may best be directed toward basic introduction of the feature into her repertoire (McReynolds and Engmann, 1975; McReynolds and Huston, 1971; Pollack and Rees, 1972). If the child is a feature misuser, then further phonological analysis (which implies feature use) is indicated, and the clinician must determine the extent and loci of feature misuse. Typical feature analysis techniques (McReynolds and Engmann, 1975) do not allow for determining specific contexts in which features are in error. Phonological analysis techniques are more equipped to do this.

3. Substitution errors especially should undergo a distinctive feature substitution analysis where the feature bundles of the target and substituted sounds are compared and misused features are noted by the examiner. Then percentages of incorrect occurrences of each feature across all relevant phonemes can be computed. Detailed distinctive feature analysis may not be appropriate for all clients. However, the clinician should at least be able to make a list of features most often misused and arrive at "ball park" estimates of feature error. This would enable the speech pathologist to decide whether to introduce an absent feature into a child's system or to do more contextually oriented treatment.

### Phonological Analysis

Another approach to analyzing a child's articulatory behavior is to perform a phonological analysis. In 1976, a landmark book by David Ingram, *Phonological Disability in Children,* sparked an interest in a more linguistic approach to misarticulation analysis. Ingram cited many sources that reported common patterns of articulatory simplification in children's speech (Stampe, 1969; Compton, 1970, 1976; Oller et al., 1972; Smith, 1973). That is, most children develop the ability to articulate gradually and before perfecting an adult production, they reduce the complexity of words in characteristic ways.

A phonological approach rests on certain assumptions. For instance, phonologists assume that there is a structure to every child's sound system and that even in the most unintelligible child, there is a pattern of phonemic production. Sounds do not occur in random combinations. Also, a phonological approach assumes an underlying system that gives rise to the observable sound combinations that we hear from children. The implication is that a phonological error may be a product of the underlying system that organizes the overt sound combinations.

Earlier in this chapter we indicated that there can be both linguistically based and sensorimotor-based misarticulations. The linguistically based errors could be construed as products of rules generated by the child's underlying phonological system. Rules, to a certain degree, imply patterns of performance, and phonological "rules" can be written simply to describe these patterns. Phonological rules, then, are descriptive of the way a child uses classes of phonemes. Many investigators have reported that, in development, it is commonly observed that children tend to simplify their word productions in comparison to the adult model. The simplifications are typically in the direction of producing physiologically easier sounds for more difficult ones. Studies in linguistics have shown that normally developing children naturally simplify adult productions by engaging in characteristic behaviors.

For reasons not known, some children appear to persist in using these simplification strategies, and if enough of them are retained, the child is likely to be quite unintelligible. Most authorities report that many of the patterns of error found in disordered children are those observed in normally developing youngsters at earlier ages (Ingram, 1976; Shriberg and Kwiatkowski, 1980). Ingram (1976), however, also points out that deviant rules not typically found in normally developing children may appear in phonologically disordered youngsters.

Phonological rules can describe these simplification techniques, and each rule implies a change in the use of distinctive features. That is, a child who substitutes stops for continuants is altering an important distinctive feature of the target phonemes.

| + Continuant | − Continuant |
|---|---|
| s | t |
| ʃ | t |
| f | p |
| θ | t |

The clinician wishing to gain insight into phonological processes has at least two levels of analysis to choose from. First, there are instruments available that are targeted toward discovering phonological processes in children. These measures provide picture or object stimuli and ask the child to give a single-word or phrase response. These responses are analyzed by the clinician for particular phonological simplifications. We will discuss these measures in a bit more detail. Figure 5.2 summarizes some of the specific phonological processes examined by the instruments discussed. The reader should consult these references for examples and guidelines in defining the processes.

The *Phonological Process Analysis (PPA)* (Weiner, 1979) is a descriptive procedure that is not sound-specific but focuses on patterns. The *PPA* uses delayed imitation and is directed toward children between the ages of two and five. It uses action pictures to sample single-words and sentence phrases. The stimulus items are organized by phonological process rather than by the traditional grouping by phoneme or age of development of sounds. Another measure is the *Compton-Hutton Phonological Assessment* (1978). The *Compton-Hutton* uses fifty picture stimuli to

**FIGURE 5.2   Summary of some phonological processes.**

*Hodson and Paden (1983)*
Cluster reduction
Stridency deletion
Stopping
Liquid deviations
Assimilation
Velar deviations
Backing
Final consonant deletion
Syllable reduction
Prevocalic voicing
Glottal replacement
Metathesis
Coalescence
Epenthesis
Diminutive

*Compton-Hutton Phonological Assessment
(1978)*
Gliding
Stopping
Affrication
Velar fronting
Consonant cluster reduction
Assimilation
Final consonant deletion
Vocalization
Final consonant devoicing
Fronting palatals

*Phonological Process Analysis
(Weiner, 1979)*
Final consonant deletion
Consonant cluster reduction
Weak syllable deletion
Glottal replacement
Labial assimilation
Alveolar assimilation
Velar assimilation
Prevocalic voicing
Final consonant devoicing
Stopping
Affrication
Fronting
Gliding of fricatives
Gliding liquids
Vocalization
Denasalization
Neutralization

*Assessment of Phonological Processes
(Hodson, 1980)*
Syllable reduction
Cluster reduction
Prevocalic obstruent omissions
Postvocalic obstruent omissions
Stridency deletion
Velar fronting
Prevocalic voicing
Postvocalic devoicing
Glottal replacement
Backing
Stopping
Affrication
Deaffrication
Palatalization
Depalatalization
Coalescence
Epenthesis
Metathesis
Gliding
Vocalization
Nasal assimilation
Velar assimilation
Labial assimilation
Alveolar assimilation
Reduplications
Diminutives
Nasalization
Denasalization

*Natural Process Analysis
(Shriberg and Kwiatkowski, 1980)*
Final consonant deletion
Velar fronting
Stopping
Palatal fronting
Liquid simplification
Assimilation
Cluster reduction
Unstressed syllable deletion

*Phonological Analysis of Children's Language
(Ingram, 1981)*
Final consonant deletion
Reduction of consonant clusters
Syllable deletion
Reduplication
Fronting palatals
Fronting velars
Stopping fricatives/affricates
Simplification of nasals
Simplification of liquids

elicit consonants in initial and final positions of words. The test is aimed at children between the ages of three and seven, and each word is elicited two times to evaluate consistency of productions. Two phonemes are examined in each word sampled. A third instrument is the *Assessment of Phonological Processes (APP)* (Hodson, 1980). The *APP* elicits and requires transcription of fifty-five utterances. Toys are used instead of pictures, and the child spontaneously names each object while the examiner transcribes the responses. All consonants are assessed a minimum of two times pre- and postvocalically. Thirty-one consonant clusters are assessed. The *APP* assesses forty-two phonological processes and "articulatory shifts."

The measures briefly reviewed above can be administered in a reasonable time (less than one hour), and the scoring time will vary with the clinician's experience using the test and the severity of the phonological disorder under evaluation. The measures, however, do not evaluate spontaneous connected speech, and therefore the phonological rules obtained may only approximate those typically used by the child in conversation.

The analysis of a spontaneous speech sample is a second level of analysis recommended by Shriberg and Kwiatkowski (1980) in the *Natural Process Analysis (NPA)*. This procedure specifically targets eight processes for analysis and provides a unique and useful phonetic inventory. The *NPA* can provide valuable information for the practitioner and represents a well-planned procedure. Ingram (1981) developed procedures for the *Phonological Analysis of Children's Language*, which includes phonetic analysis, homonym analysis, substitution analysis, and phonological process analysis. Although only 27 specific processes are targeted, Ingram states that the analysis is open-ended and can continue "until all the substitutions in a child's speech have been explained" (1981: 7). This procedure, because of its detail, should take as much and probably more time to complete than the *NPA*.

There appears to be some agreement that certain processes are at high risk in articulation-disordered children. Different authorities implicate specific phonological processes as being more important than others. Figure 5.2 includes the processes thought to be significant enough to test in formal assessment procesures. Although there is considerable variation in the length of the lists, there is also a high degree of agreement regarding processes that seem to be most at risk in unintelligible children. Studies aimed at uncovering a child's phonological processes range broadly in the number of processes tested. The actual number of processes targeted would seem to be related to the clinician's goals in the analysis (Ingram, 1981).

It should be noted that all of the evaluation techniques discussed allow for the assessment of other processes as discovered by the examiner, even though the process may not be specifically evaluated. If the clinician is attempting to account for all a child's misarticulations with a rule written for each, then a large number of potential processes must be targeted. If, on the other hand, only major processes are of interest due to their impact on intelligibility, then a smaller number of processes may be included. The probability is that if a child is exhibiting unstressed syllable deletion, final consonant deletion, and stopping, these will be initial treatment targets and "lesser" rules, such as epenthesis and vocalization, will not be objects of immediate concern.

Several cautions are in order regarding phonological analysis of a child's misarticulations. First a phonological approach requires that a clinician transcribe words and/or sentences of a spontaneous speech. Although most speech clinicians have completed courses in phonetics during their undergraduate education, many of these courses did not offer students the opportunity to transcribe disordered speech from a variety of male, female, adult, and child speakers. Some clinicians may not have adequate experience to transcribe connected speech reliably. One clinician of our acquaintance remarked that "the only thing I have used my phonetics for in the past ten years is to fill in the little blocks on the *Goldman-Fristoe* score sheet." It may be quite a leap, then, for some clinicians to transcribe words or connected speech in practice. Second, if our reliability is low in scoring phoneme errors, then we can only assume that reliability is even more of an issue in phonological transcription and analysis (Shriberg and Kwiatkowski, 1977).

A third concern is the compelling and captivating nature of phonological analysis. It makes an articulatory assessment rather like an interesting puzzle, and when the clinician reaches the "solution" and divines the phonological rules, it is tempting to view the child's problem only from a linguistic-phonological perspective and apply this type of treatment. Children of various etiological groups will demonstrate phonological regularities in their speech. Even if the disorder has a sensorimotor basis, phonological rules can be written and the child perceived as a phonological-linguistic case. Shriberg and Kwiatkowski (1982a) suggest that the clinician must examine linguistic, sensorimotor, and psychosocial aspects of a child's behavior and select appropriate treatment goals. Clinicians should not assume a linguistically oriented treatment simply because the child exhibits a systematic phonology. The treatment of choice for each child may require different emphases, and these could include focusing on sensorimotor aspects of articulation.

There is no doubt that phonological analyses are useful and a major innovation in articulatory assessment, but the clinician must be cautious to check reliability and not apply a phonological-linguistic interpretation to all cases without examining sensorimotor and social aspects as well.

If a clinician wishes to write phonological rules from a child's conversational sample, there are certain basic issues common to most procedures:

*Glossing and segmentation.* The clinician must interpret the child's utterances and provide adult interpretations or "glosses" of what the child was trying to say. One cannot arrive at a phonological rule system unless the intended utterance is known. Several methods of segmenting or arranging the data have been reported. One method is to arrange correct and incorrect child productions and glosses word by word in phonetic transcription:

| Child's Production | Adult Gloss |
|---|---|
| /ki/ | /ki/ |
| /b æ kI/ | /b æ skIt/ |
| /p æ / | /f æ n/ |
| /go/ | /go/ |

This allows the clinician the opportunity to compare productions with the adult model and hypothesize a phonological reduction pattern (for example, final consonant deletion in the words "basket" and "fan").

Another method of segmentation is to retain spontaneous connected speech intact and divide the sample into utterances:

Child's Production      Adult Gloss
/tidəgɔgi/              /siðədɔgi/

This method of segmentation can sometimes help the clinician account for certain phonological reductions in a word that are influenced by sounds in previous words. Different authors (Ingram, 1981; Shriberg and Kwiatkowski, 1980) recommend a variety of methods for organizing segments once they have been glossed (alphabetically, by syllable shape, by consonant). The purpose of these varied organizational schemes is to aid in the retrieval and comparison of individual words and sounds when attempting to prove the existence of a phonological rule.

*Hypothesizing a natural process.*    After arranging the data from a sample, the clinician attempts to account for errors by hypothesizing a phonological reduction pattern. For instance, when comparing a child's production of a word to the adult gloss, a deletion of the final consonant may be noted. The clinician may hypothesize the process of final consonant deletion. The high-risk processes listed in Figure 5.2 should be ruled out before any deviant processes are suspected.

*Finding support for hypothesized rules.*    It is not enough simply to postulate that final consonant deletion has occurred in a child's sample. Evidence must be obtained from the utterances to determine whether the process has, in fact, occurred. For instance, the child may have deleted the final consonant in a CVC word. The clinician should examine all other words in the sample that end in singleton consonants to determine the frequency of occurrence of the hypothesized phonological reduction. If there is widespread support for the occurrence of final consonant deletion, then the clinician may write the rule. If only certain final consonants are deleted consistently and others are produced normally, then the clinician must change the hypothesis to a rule that specifies particular kinds of final consonant deletion (stop and nasal deletion, for instance). This is where the use of distinctive features is helpful.

*Specification of frequency of occurrence.*    Authorities differ in their methods of specifying the frequency of occurrence of certain phonological rules. Some processes appear to be obligatory (occur virtually all the time) and others seem to be optional. In specifying optionality of a phonological rule, some authors recommend the three-stage system of "always," "sometimes," and "never" (Shriberg and Kwiatkowski, 1980). Other authorities (Ingram, 1981) recommend the use of percentage ranges such as 0–20, 21–40, 41–60, 61–80, and 81–100. Whatever method is used, the important variable is to indicate how often the process is occurring.

*Writing the rule.* After the clinician has gathered support for a rule from the transcript, the rule is written specifying the target phonemes, how they are changed, what context they are changed in and how often the rule occurs. A phonological rule for final stop consonant deletion may look like this:

$$
\begin{matrix} p \\ b \\ t \\ d \\ k \\ g \end{matrix} \longrightarrow \emptyset \quad / \ \ CV-\# \quad 80\text{--}100\%
$$

This rule says that the consonants *p, b, t, d, k,* and *g* are deleted in the context of the CVC word when the target sound is at the end. The slash stands for "in the context of," the blank represents the location of the target sound, and # refers to a word boundary. Note that the percentage of occurrence is indicated after the rule.

*Recycling of rules.* As each rule is written and proof is gathered for each phonological reduction, the clinician repeats the process of examining the errors, hypothesizing a phonological process, looking for data to support the rule, and writing the rule. Soon the clinician can account for the majority of the errors in the child's transcript with the exception of a small residue of words that the rules do not describe. At this point, the clinician may wish to hypothesize a phonological rule that is not normally seen in children's articulatory development. For instance, the child may delete initial consonants of certain types. The procedure, however, is still the same. The clinician must hypothesize the rule and find support for it before it can be written.

The detection of phonological simplification patterns can be a powerful tool in the hands of the clinician. A sample of speech that appears to have many unrelated misarticulations can be reduced to only a few phonological reduction patterns. The clinical implication of these processes is that the child does not need to work on a single sound but may need to focus on the pattern of error. The assumption is that the observable error pattern is generated by an underlying rule, and if the rule is to be altered, then many of the segments it affects should be targeted (Ingram, 1976; Hodson and Paden, 1983; Compton, 1976).

Again, the only way to discover these patterns of misarticulation is to search for them through a phonological analysis technique. Traditional tests are not constructed for this purpose, although they certainly could be suggestive for further analyses and provide hints for the clinician as to error patterns.

## OTHER TESTING

Four additional areas of examination relate significantly to a competent evaluation of an articulation-disordered client, depending on the type of case and its severity. The clinician should be prepared to assess these areas as appropriate.

*Language assessment.*   The clinician examining a child's articulatory system should expect the bulk of these cases to exhibit some language deviations as well. Many authorities report the high co-occurrence of articulation and language disorders. Paul and Shriberg (1982) report that 86 percent of articulation-disordered children are also likely to exhibit syntactic delays. The clinician should routinely gather a spontaneous language sample and administer standardized language tests for each articulation-disordered client.

*Audiometric screening.*   A second diagnostic procedure that should be routinely administered is an audiometric screening. It is critical that the possibility of hearing impairment be eliminated before treatment is begun. This becomes especially important if the parents report suspected auditory problems or if the child has a history of ear infections.

*The oral-peripheral examination.*   This is an integral part of the articulation examination (see Chapter 3 for guidelines in conducting this procedure). Oral-peripheral examination results may be important in distinguishing a sensorimotor from a linguistic disorder of articulation. Fletcher (1972) provides some normative data on diadochokinetic rates for children, and this should also be included as part of the examination for sensorimotor difficulties.

*Auditory discrimination.*   This area has been classically explored in articulation evaluation. Historically, many investigations have shown that articulation-disordered children do not perform as well as normal speakers on auditory discrimination tasks (Winitz, 1969; Powers, 1971; Bernthal and Bankson, 1981). Early treatment programs incorporated an obligatory module of auditory discrimination training (Van Riper and Irwin, 1958), and many authorities continue to believe that the assessment of auditory discrimination is an important part of an evaluation (Winitz, 1975).

Within the past ten years, however, criticisms have emerged regarding methods of auditory discrimination testing (Schwartz and Goldman, 1974; Beving and Eblen, 1973) and the efficacy of auditory discrimination training in treatment (Williams and McReynolds, 1975; Shelton et al., 1978). Recently, the most defensible position appears to be assessing the auditory discrimination of misarticulated sounds only (Locke, 1980; Bernthal and Bankson, 1981) rather than all phonemes and to evaluate it in a way that avoids the use of paired comparisons (mass-math). At present it is not clear if auditory discrimination testing needs to be a part of routine articulatory evaluations or if it should be embarked on only when some suspicion of a discrimination problem is evidenced in trial therapy. The present authors would favor the latter option.

## INTEGRATING DATA FROM THE ASSESSMENT

It is reasonable that after an articulation evaluation, the clinician should, at the very least, be able to make statements on the following areas:

1. Biological prerequisites (hearing, structure/function of the speech mechanism)
2. Linguistic ability
3. Phonetic inventory
4. Distinctive features acquired, used correctly, absent, or misused
5. Response to stimulation on sounds the child should have acquired according to normative data
6. Phonological processes evident in the sample
7. An indication of facilitating phonetic contexts, if any, in cases where stimulability is unproductive
8. A subjective rating of intelligibility
9. Severity/prognosis

There are a variety of ways to assess articulatory ability, and the broader the view taken by the clinician, the more realistic the picture obtained of the client. For instance, if only the results of a traditional articulation test are considered, the clinician may be able to summarize a phonetic inventory and make some preliminary judgments about distinctive feature acquisition, but perhaps an inventory of phonological processes may not be possible due to limited sampling. Further, the norms that might be used in comparing the child's phonetic inventory to that of other children (Sander, 1972; Templin, 1957) are not applicable to phonological processes. The nine areas mentioned above are simply different ways of looking at the child's articulatory system and should at least be considered in every case to the extent that the clinician can make a statement about each area. Then further exploration might be undertaken in areas of concern, such as writing a phonology from a spontaneous speech sample if problems are indicated on measures such as *PPA* or *APP*. If a child is noted to be missing entire classes of phonemes, then a more intensive distinctive feature analysis might be indicated. The point is that results from a variety of areas need to be considered and used as indicators for further analyses.

Recently, Shriberg and Kwiatkowski (1982a) have suggested that clinicians should consider possible causal correlates of articulation disorders. They recommend gathering data on each client in the areas of cognition/language, speech mechanism integrity, and psychological/social parameters. Consideration of these areas helps to keep the clinician from becoming too narrowly focused in the conception of articulation assessment and treatment. It also forces the clinician to at least consider the possibility of a variety of single or interactive maintaining factors in the articulation disorder. If a clinician is enamored with phonology and a linguistic interpretation of most articulation problems, such an approach forces him at least to gather some information on psychosocial and speech mechanism variables. Conversely, if a clinician has a sensorimotor orientation, the approach forces the evaluation of more linguistic aspects. The findings of such a broad-based analysis may provide the clinician with important information on prognosis and treatment goals that would otherwise have not been considered.

Several investigators have considered the problem of assigning a severity rating to children's misarticulation problems. We often hear clinicians rate a child's difficulty as "mild" or "moderate." When asked how this was determined, they sometimes have no empirical basis. Shriberg and Kwiatkowski (1982b) suggest the use of the percentage of consonants correct (PCC) in a spontaneous sample as being a most reliable predictor of severity ratings. Hodson and Paden (1983) offer the Composite Phonological Score as a measure of severity. The system considers age in the calculation, as well as other variables. Although both methods may be criticized by some, they are at least attempts to objectify severity in cases of articulation disorders and are available for use by practicing clinicians.

HIGHLIGHT *Intelligibility*

No matter how a child performs on an articulation test, a major concern of both the clinician and the parent is intelligibility in spontaneous speech. How understandable is the child in his daily interactions? Intelligibility is difficult to measure because it is affected by many variables. For instance, a child will be more intelligible to those who know him well because they have unconsciously decoded his system of substitutions and omissions. Another variable affecting intelligibility is the sound that the child misarticulates. Some sounds occur more frequently in the language than others, and if the child's error is on a sound that occurs frequently, intelligibility will be affected to a greater degree than when errors are on infrequently occurring phonemes.

An obvious factor that affects intelligibility is the number of phonemes a child misarticulates. The more sounds in error, the worse the intelligibility. Shriberg and Kwiatkowski (1982b) have gathered data on "severity of involvement" in articulation disorders. They had judges rank-order variables that were thought to contribute to severity, and intelligibility was ranked first as an influencing factor. They also had clinicians rate tape recordings of spontaneous speech on severity (mild, mild-moderate, moderate-severe, severe). Statistical analyses showed that the measure most predictive of severity rating was the percentage of consonants correct (PCC). Basically, the PCC is a calculation of the number of correct consonants divided by the number of correct plus incorrect consonants. The resulting number is multiplied by 100 to arrive at the PCC. Shriberg and Kwiatkowski (1982b) outline specific procedures and a worksheet for use in computation of the PCC. The point here is that the percentage of consonants correctly articulated relates to severity and severity relates to intelligibility. The number of errors a child has will obviously affect the PCC.

Another variable affecting intelligibility is the consistency of the error in the child's speech, which also affects the PCC calculation. A final factor that can affect intelligibility is the type of error the child exhibits. A child with many omissions of sounds and syllables is likely to be less understandable than one who substitutes one sound for another.

Fudala (1970) recommends using a continuum for rating intelligibility similar to the following:

1. Speech not intelligible
2. Speech usually not intelligible

3.  Speech difficult to understand
4.  Speech intelligible with careful listening
5.  Speech intelligible although noticeably in error
6.  Speech intelligible with occasional error
7.  Speech totally intelligible

There are few data relating intelligibility to age, although we know that children become more intelligible as they get older. The present authors have used the informal cutoff of age three for a child to be generally intelligible to strangers. If a three-year-old is not understandable it could affect social and language development. This also permits early intervention to begin.

Every assessment of articulatory ability should contain some judgment regarding intelligibility—this judgment is a factor that can be an important deciding variable in making treatment recommendations.

## BIBLIOGRAPHY

ALLEN, D., L. BLISS, and J. TIMMONS (1981). "Language Evaluation: Science or Art?" *Journal of Speech and Hearing Disorders,* 46: 66–68.

AMERMAN, J., R. DANILOFF, and K. MOLL (1970). "Lip and Jaw Coarticulation for the Phoneme /ae/." *Journal of Speech and Hearing Research,* 13: 148–161.

ANDERSON, V., and H. NEWBY (1973). *Improving the Child's Speech.* 2nd ed. New York: Oxford Univesity Press.

AVANT, V., and C. HUTTON (1962). "Passage for Speech Screening in Upper Elementary Grades." *Journal of Speech and Hearing Disorders,* 27: 40–46.

BATTLE, D., et al. (1983). "Position Paper—Social Dialects." *Journal of the American Speech Language Hearing Association,* 25: 23–24.

BERNTHAL, J., and N. BANKSON (1981). *Articulation Disorders.* Englewood Cliffs, N.J.: Prentice-Hall, Inc.

BEVING, B., and R. EBLEN (1973). "Same and Different Concepts and Children's Performance on Speech Sound Discrimination." *Journal of Speech and Hearing Research,* 16: 513–517.

BLACHE, S. (1978). *The Acquisition of Distinctive Features.* Baltimore: University Park Press.

BLACK, M. (1964). *Speech Correction in the Schools.* Englewood Cliffs, N.J.: Prentice-Hall, Inc.

BRYNGELSON, B., and E. GLASPEY (1962). *Speech in the Classroom (With Speech Improvement Cards).* 3rd ed. Chicago: Scott, Foresman.

BZOCH, K. (1974). *Bzoch Error Pattern Diagnostic Test.* Gainesville, Fla.: University of Florida Press.

CAMPBELL, J., and L. SHRIBERG (1982). "Associations Among Pragmatic Functions, Linguistic Stress and Natural Phonological Processes in Speech Delayed Children." *Journal of Speech and Hearing Research,* 25: 547–553.

CARRELL, J., and W. TIFFANY (1960). *Phonetics: Theory and Application to Speech Improvement.* New York: McGraw-Hill.

CHOMSKY, N. (1957). *Syntactic Structures.* The Hague: Mouton.

CHOMSKY, N., and M. HALLE (1968). *The Sound Pattern of English.* New York: Harper & Row.

COMPTON, A. (1970). "Generative Studies of Children's Phonological Disorders." *Journal of Speech and Hearing Disorders,* 35: 315–339.

———(1976). "Generative Studies of Children's Phonological Disorders," in *Normal and De-*

*ficient Child Language,* ed. D. Morehead and A. Morehead. Baltimore: University Park Press.

COMPTON, A., and S. HUTTON (1978). *Compton-Hutton Phonological Assessment.* San Francisco: Carousel House.

COSTELLO, J., and J. ONSTINE (1976). "The Modification of Multiple Articulation Errors Based on Distinctive Feature Theory." *Journal of Speech and Hearing Disorders,* 41: 199–215.

CYPREANSEN, L., J. WILEY, and L. LAASE (1959). *Speech Development, Improvement and Correction.* New York, Ronald Press.

DANILOFF, R., and K. MOLL (1968). "Coarticulation of Lip Rounding." *Journal of Speech and Hearing Research,* 11: 707–721.

DANILOFF, R., G. SCHUCKERS, and L. FETH (1980). *The Physiology of Speech and Hearing: An Introduction.* Englewood Cliffs, N.J.: Prentice-Hall, Inc.

DARLEY, F. (1974). *Diagnosis and Appraisal of Communication Disorders.* Englewood Cliffs, N.J.: Prentice-Hall, Inc.

DICKSON, D., and W. MAUE-DICKSON (1982). *Anatomical and Physiological Bases of Speech.* Boston: Little, Brown.

DILLARD, J. (1972). *Black English: Its History and Usage in the United States.* New York: Random House.

EDMONSON, W. (1969). *The Laradon Articulation Scale.* Denver, Colo.: Laradon Hall.

EISENSON, J., and M. OGILVIE (1977). *Speech Correction in the Schools.* 4th ed. New York: Macmillan.

EVELEIGH, K., and G. WARR-LEEPER (1983). "Improving Efficiency in Articulation Screening." *Language, Speech and Hearing Services in Schools,* 14: 223–232.

FAIRBANKS, G. (1960). *Voice and Articulation Drillbrook.* 2nd ed. New York: Harper & Row.

FAIRCLOTH, M., and S. FAIRCLOTH (1970). "An Analysis of the Articulatory Behavior of a Speech Defective Child in Connected Speech and Isolated Word Responses." *Journal of Speech and Hearing Disorders,* 35: 51–61.

FARQUHAR, M. (1961). "Prognostic Value of Imitative and Auditory Discrimination Tests." *Journal of Speech and Hearing Disorders,* 26: 342–347.

FISHER, H., and J. LOGEMANN (1971). *The Fisher-Logemann Test of Articulation Competence.* Boston: Houghton Mifflin.

FLETCHER, S. (1972). "Time-by-Count Measurement of Diadochokinetic Syllable Rate." *Journal of Speech and Hearing Research,* 15: 763–770.

FLUHARTY, N. (1974). "The Design and Standardization of a Speech and Language Screening Test for Use with Preschool Children." *Journal of Speech and Hearing Disorders,* 39: 75–88.

FRISTOE, M., and R. GOLDMAN (1968). "Comparisons of Traditional and Condensed Articulation Tests Examining the Same Number of Sounds." *Journal of Speech and Hearing Research,* 11: 583–589.

FUDALA, J. (1970). *The Arizona Articulation Proficiency Scale.* Beverly Hills, Calif.: Western Psychological Services.

GODA, S. (1970). *Articulation Therapy and Consonant Drillbook.* New York: Grune & Stratton.

GOLDMAN, R., and M. FRISTOE (1969). *Goldman-Fristoe Test of Articulation.* Circle Pines, Minn.: American Guidance Service.

HAM, D. (1971). *The Evaluation of Sounds: An Articulation Index for the Young Public School Child.* Springfield, Ill.: Chas. C Thomas.

HAWS, E. (1975). *The Haws Screening Test for Functional Articulation Disorders.* Salt Lake City: Educational Support Systems.

HAYNES, W., M. HAYNES, and J. JACKSON (1982). "The Effects of Phonetic Context and Linguistic Complexity on /s/ Misarticulation in Children." *Journal of Communication Disorders,* 15: 287–297.

HEJNA, R. (1963). *Developmental Articulation Test.* Ann Arbor, Mich.: Speech Materials.

HODSON, B. (1980). *The Assessment of Phonological Processes.* Danville, Ill.: Interstate Printers and Publishers.

HODSON, B., and E. PADEN (1983). *Targeting Intelligible Speech: A Phonological Approach to Remediation.* San Diego: College-Hill Press.
HOFFMAN, P., G. SCHUCKERS, and D. RATUSNIK (1977). "Contextual-Coarticulatory Inconsistencies of /r/ Misarticulation." *Journal of Speech and Hearing Research,* 20: 631–643.
INGRAM, D. (1971). *Edinburgh Articulation Test.* London: Edward Arnold.
—— (1976). *Phonological Disability in Children.* New York: Elsevier.
—— (1981). *Procedures for the Phonological Analysis of Children's Language.* Baltimore: University Park Press.
IRWIN, J. (1972). *Disorders of Articulation.* Indianapolis: Bobbs-Merrill.
IRWIN, J., and P. WONG (1983). *Phonological Development in Children 18 to 72 Months.* Carbondale: Southern Illinois University Press.
IRWIN, R. (1965). *Speech and Hearing Therapy.* Pittsburgh: Stanwix House.
JOHNSON, W., F. DARLEY, and D. SPRIESTERSBACH (1963). *Diagnostic Methods in Speech Pathology.* New York: Harper & Row.
KAHANE, J., and J. FOLKINS (1984). *Atlas of Speech and Hearing Anatomy.* Columbus, Ohio: Chas. E. Merrill.
KENT, R. (1982). "Contextual Facilitation of Correct Sound Production." *Language, Speech and Hearing Services in Schools,* 13: 66–76.
KENT, R., and F. MINIFIE (1977). "Coarticulation in Recent Speech Production Models." *Journal of Phonetics,* 5: 115–133.
LaRIVIERE, C., et al. (1974). "The Conceptual Reality of Selected Distinctive Features." *Journal of Speech and Hearing Research,* 17: 122–133.
LEONARD, L. (1971). "A Preliminary View of Information Theory and Articulatory Omissions." *Journal of Speech and Hearing Disorders,* 36: 511–517.
—— (1973). "Some Limitations in the Clinical Application of Distinctive Features." *Journal of Speech and Hearing Disorders,* 38: 141–143.
LOCKE, J. (1980). "The Inference of Speech Perception in the Phonologically Disordered Child. I. A Rationale, Some Criteria, the Conventional Tests." *Journal of Speech and Hearing Disorders,* 45: 431–444.
—— (1983). "Clinical Phonology: The Explanation and Treatment of Speech Sound Disorders." *Journal of Speech and Hearing Disorders,* 48: 339–341.
McCLEAN, J. (1976). "Articulation," in *Communication Assessment and Intervention Strategies,* ed. L. Lloyd. Baltimore: University Park Press.
McCLEAN, M. (1973). "Forward Coarticulation of Velar Movement at Marked Junctural Boundaries." *Journal of Speech and Hearing Research,* 16: 236–246.
McDONALD, E. (1964). *Articulation Testing and Treatment.* Pittsburgh: Stanwix House.
—— (1968). *A Screening Deep Test of Articulation.* Pittsburgh: Stanwix House.
McREYNOLDS, L., and K. HUSTON (1971). "A Distinctive Feature Analysis of Children's Misarticulation." *Journal of Speech and Hearing Disorders,* 36: 155–166.
McREYNOLDS, L., and D. ENGMANN (1975). *Distinctive Feature Analysis of Misarticulations.* Baltimore: University Park Press.
MATHENY, N., and J. PANAGOS (1978). "Comparing the Effects of Articulation and Syntax Programs on Syntax and Articulation Improvement." *Language, Speech and Hearing Services in Schools,* 9: 57–61.
MECHAM, M., J. JEX, and J. JONES (1970). *Screening Speech Articulation Test.* Salt Lake City: Communication Research Associates.
MILISEN, R., et al. (1954). "The Disorder of Articulation: A Systematic Clinical and Experimental Approach." *Journal of Speech and Hearing Disorders.* Monograph Supplement 4.
MOLL, K., and R. DANILOFF (1971). "Investigation of the Timing of Velar Movements During Speech." *Journal of the Acoustical Society of America,* 50: 678–684.
MONSEES, E., and C. BERMAN (1968). "Speech and Language Screening in a Summer Headstart Program." *Journal of Speech and Hearing Disorders,* 33: 121–126.
MOWRER, D., P. WAHL, and S. DOOLAN (1978). "Effect of Lisping on Audience Evaluation of Male Speakers." *Journal of Speech and Hearing Disorders,* 43: 140–148.
NATION, J., and D. ARAM (1977). *Diagnosis of Speech and Language Disorders.* St. Louis: C. V. Mosby.

OLLER, K. D., et al. (1972). "Five Studies in Abnormal Phonology." Unpublished. Seattle: University of Washington.

PALMER, J. (1984). *Anatomy for Speech and Hearing.* New York: Harper & Row.

PANAGOS, J., H. QUINE, and P. KLICH (1979). "Syntactic and Phonological Influences in Children's Articulations." *Journal of Speech and Hearing Research,* 22: 841-848.

PARKER, F. (1976). "Distinctive Features in Speech Pathology: Phonology or Phonemics." *Journal of Speech and Hearing Disorders,* 41: 23-39.

PAUL, R., and L. SHRIBERG (1982). "Association Between Phonology and Syntax in Speech Delayed Children." *Journal of Speech and Hearing Research,* 25: 536-546.

PENDERGAST, K., et al. (1966). "An Articulation Study of 15,255 Seattle 1st Grade Children with and without Kindergarten." *Exceptional Children,* 33: 541-547.

—— (1969). *Photo Articulation Test.* Danville, Ill.: Interstate Printers and Publishers.

POLLACK, E., and N. REES (1972). "Disorders of Articulation: Some Clinical Applications of Distinctive Feature Theory." *Journal of Speech and Hearing Disorders,* 37: 451-461.

POOLE, E. (1974). "Genetic Development of Articulation of Consonant Sounds in Speech." *Elementary English Review,* 11: 159-161.

POWERS, M. (1971). "Functional Disorders of Articulation: Symptomathology and Etiology," in *Handbook of Speech Pathology and Audiology,* ed. L. Travis. New York: Appleton-Century-Crofts.

PRATHER, E., D. HEDRICK, and C. KERN (1975). "Articulation Development in Children Aged 2 to 4 Years." *Journal of Speech and Hearing Disorders,* 40: 179-191.

PRIESTLY, T. (1977). "One Idiosyncratic Strategy in the Acquisition of Phonology." *Journal of Child Language,* 4: 45-65.

RILEY, G. (1971). *Riley Articulation and Language Test.* Los Angeles: Western Psychological Services.

RITTERMAN, S., and N. FREEMAN (1974). "Distinctive Phonetic Features as Relevant and Irrelevant Stimulus Dimensions in Speech Sound Discrimination Learning." *Journal of Speech and Hearing Research,* 17: 417-425.

RITTERMAN, S., et al. (1982). "The Pass/Fail Disparity Among Three Commonly Employed Articulatory Screening Tests." *Journal of Speech and Hearing Disorders,* 47: 429-432.

ROGERS, W. (1972). *Picture Articulation and Screening Test.* Salt Lake City: Word Making Productions.

RUDER, K., and B. BUNCE (1981). "Articulation Therapy Using Distinctive Feature Analysis to Structure the Training Program: Two Case Studies." *Journal of Speech and Hearing Disorders,* 46: 59-65.

SANDER, E. (1972). "When Are Speech Sounds Learned?" *Journal of Speech and Hearing Disorders,* 37: 55-63.

SCHISSEL, R., and L. JAMES (1979). "A Comparison of Children's Performance on Two Tests of Articulation." *Journal of Speech and Hearing Disorders,* 44: 363-372.

SCHMAUCH, V., J. PANAGOS, and P. KLICH (1978). "Syntax Influences and Accuracy of Consonant Production in Language Disordered Children." *Journal of Communication Disorders,* 11: 315-323.

SCHWARTZ, A., and R. GOLDMAN (1974). "Variables Influencing Performance on Speech Sound Discrimination Tests." *Journal of Speech and Hearing Research,* 17: 25-32.

SCHWARTZ, R. (1983). "Diagnosis of Speech Sound Disorders in Children," in *Diagnosis in Speech-Language Pathology,* ed. B. Weinberg and I. Meitus. Baltimore: University Park Press.

SCRIPTURE, M., and E. JACKSON (1927). *A Manual of Exercises for the Correction of Speech Disorders.* Philadelphia: F. A. Davis.

SHELTON, R., A. JOHNSON, D. RUSCELLO, and W. ARNDT (1978). "Assessment of Parent-Administered Listening Training for Preschool Children with Articulation Deficits." *Journal of Speech and Hearing Disorders,* 43: 242-254.

SHELTON, R., and L. McREYNOLDS (1979). "Functional Articulation Disorders: Preliminaries to Treatment," in *Speech and Language: Advances in Basic Research and Practice,* Vol. 2, ed. N. Lass. New York: Academic Press.

SHRIBERG, L., and R. KENT (1982). *Clinical Phonetics.* New York: John Wiley.

SHRIBERG, L., and J. KWIATKOWSKI (1977). "Phonological Programming for Unintelligible

Children in Early Childhood Projects." Paper presented to the Convention of the American Speech and Hearing Association, Chicago.
—— (1980). *Natural Process Analysis.* New York: John Wiley.
—— (1982a). "Phonological Disorders. I. A Diagnostic Classification System." *Journal of Speech and Hearing Disorders,* 47: 226–241.
—— (1982b). "Phonological Disorders. III. A Procedure for Assessing Severity of Involvement." *Journal of Speech and Hearing Disorders,* 47: 256–270.
SIEGEL, G. (1967). "Interpersonal Approach to the Study of Communication Disorders." *Journal of Speech and Hearing Disorders,* 32: 112–120.
SILVERMAN, E. (1976). "Listener's Impressions of Speakers with Lateral Lisps." *Journal of Speech and Hearing Disorders,* 41: 547–552.
SINGH, S. (1976). *Distinctive Features Theory and Validation.* Baltimore: University Park Press.
SMITH, N. (1973). *The Acquisition of Phonology.* Cambridge: Cambridge University Press.
SOMMERS, R. (1983). *Articulation Disorders.* Englewood Cliffs, N.J.: Prentice-Hall, Inc.
SOMMERS, R., and A. KANE (1974). "Nature and Remediation of Functional Articulation Disorders," in *Communication Disorders,* ed. S. Dickson. Glenview, Ill.: Scott, Foresman.
STAMPE, D. (1969). "A Dissertation on Natural Phonology." Ph.D. Dissertation. University of Chicago.
STOLLER, P. (1975). *Black American English.* New York: Delta.
TEMPLIN, M. (1957). "Certain Language Skills in Children: Their Development and Interrelationships." *Institute of Child Welfare Monograph 26.* Minneapolis: University of Minnesota Press.
TEMPLIN, M., and F. DARLEY (1969). *The Templin-Darley Tests of Articulation.* 2nd ed. Iowa City: University of Iowa Bureau of Educational Research and Service.
VAN HATTUM, R. (1983). *Speech-Language Programming in the Schools.* 2nd ed. Springfield, Ill.: Chas. C Thomas.
VAN RIPER, C. (1963). *Speech Correction: Principles and Methods.* 4th ed. Englewood Cliffs, N.J.: Prentice-Hall, Inc.
VAN RIPER, C., and R. ERICKSON (1969). "A Predictive Screening Test of Articulation." *Journal of Speech and Hearing Disorders,* 34: 214–219.
VAN RIPER, C., and J. IRWIN (1958). *Voice and Articulation.* Englewood Cliffs, N.J.: Prentice-Hall, Inc.
VAN RIPER, C., and D. SMITH (1979). *An Introduction to General American Phonetics.* 3rd ed. New York: Harper & Row.
WALSH, H. (1974). "On Certain Practical Inadequacies of Distinctive Feature Systems." *Journal of Speech and Hearing Disorders,* 39: 32–43.
WEINER, F. (1979). *Phonological Process Analysis.* Baltimore: University Park Press.
WEINER, F., and A. OSTROWSKI (1979). "Effects of Listener Uncertainty on Articulatory Inconsistency." *Journal of Speech and Hearing Disorders,* 44: 487–493.
WELLMAN, B., et al. (1931). *Speech Sounds of Young Children.* Studies in Child Welfare No. 5. Iowa City: University of Iowa.
WESTON, A., and L. LEONARD (1976). *Articulation Disorders: Methods of Evaluation and Therapy.* Lincoln, Nebr.: Cliffs Notes.
WILLIAMS, G., and L. McREYNOLDS (1975). "The Relationship Between Discrimination and Articulation Training in Children with Misarticulations." *Journal of Speech and Hearing Research,* 18: 401–412.
WINITZ, H. (1969). *Articulatory Acquisition and Behavior.* New York: Appleton-Century-Crofts.
—— (1975). *From Syllable to Conversation.* Baltimore: University Park Press.
ZEMLIN, W. (1981). *Speech and Hearing Science.* Englewood Cliffs, N.J.: Prentice-Hall, Inc.

# CHAPTER SIX
# STUTTERING

Stuttering is a curious, sometimes astonishing, and certainly a difficult way to talk. Why is the flow of speech, seemingly so easy and automatic for others, marred by tense interruptions? Unfortunately, the answer to that question still eludes clinicians and researchers—stuttering remains an enigma.

The puzzling nature of stuttering creates a dilemma for students. Confronted with a voluminous literature, a large number of treatment possibilities—each with its advocates—it is easy to give up in despair. Perhaps the negative attitude toward stutterers held by so many clinicians in part stems from overwhelming confusion about the disorder.[1] Yet, for some beginning clinicians, the dramatic nature of the disorder and even the confusion among experts have a fascinating appeal; they present a challenge.

This is a good place to review the fund of reliable truth we possess about stuttering, as filtered through our perceptual biases. We present below a list of "facts" about stuttering gleaned from the literature and an extensive clinical practice. For purposes of exposition we have eschewed lengthy lists of references. Each item can be documented, however, even though some might disagree with our particular selection or interpretation.

1. Stuttering as a disorder has existed throughout recorded history and is found among all peoples of the world.

[1]Current research (Turnbaugh, Guitar, and Hoffman, 1979, 1981; St. Louis and Lass, 1981; Ragsdale and Ashby, 1982) reveals that speech clinicians have strong unfavorable stereotypes about stuttering and stutterers.

2. The relative prevalence of stuttering and its forms may vary across cultures; the most commonly reported prevalence in the United States is slightly less than 1 percent.

3. Stuttering is a disorder of childhood, generally having its onset before the age of six; rarely does it begin in older persons, and when it does it may be a distinct subtype of the disorder (for example, neurotic stuttering).

4. Stuttering is found more frequently among males.

5. Stuttering tends to run in families.

6. Stuttering may be precipitated (and perpetuated) by certain environmental events, particularly the impact (in a critical, demanding way) of significant others, usually the parents.

7. Stuttering tends to appear more frequently in children described as "sensitive," who may be vulnerable or susceptible to stress. Stutterers may have a low threshold for autonomic arousal.

8. Stuttering tends to appear more frequently in children who were slow in acquiring speech or who manifest certain inadequacies of oral communication (articulation errors, language disturbances) other than fluency breakdowns.

9. Stuttering, in its developed state, has both overt and covert dimensions.

10. Stuttering is intermittent in occurrence. Many stutterers exhibit a decrease in blocking with repeated oral readings of the same material; moments of stuttering also tend to occur consistently on particular words.

11. Stuttering is eliminated or markedly reduced in a variety of conditions: speaking while alone, choral speaking, singing, prolonged or slow speaking, talking in time to rhythm or under masking conditions.

12. The basic speech characteristics of stuttering consist of relatively brief part-word repetitions (phonemic, syllabic) and prolongations. These oscillations and fixations may be audible or silent and tend to occur more frequently at the beginning of an utterance and on words and phrases motorically more complex—longer words, less frequently used words.

13. Stuttering tends to change in form and severity as the individual matures.

14. Stuttering tends to exhibit cycles of frequency and severity in a given individual.

15. Stuttering is apparently "outgrown" by a significant number of individuals.

16. Stuttering, in its developed form, consists largely of escape and avoidance behavior; that is, much of the overt abnormality results from the individual's attempt to cope with the emission of the basic speech characteristics described in item 12.

17. Stuttering is also characterized by speech and voice abnormalities other than disfluency—narrow pitch range, vocal tension, lack of vocal expression, muscular lags, and asynchronies—which can be detected in nonstuttered speech. These anomalies *may* reflect a basic impairment of phonation (difficulty in initiating phonation, making consonant-vowel transitions), respiration (abnormal reflex activity), neuromotor coordination, or cortical integration; they *may*, however, simply be effects of stuttering.

18. Stuttering, in its developed form, is often associated with an expectancy or anticipation of its occurrence.

19. Stuttering is a personal problem; individuals who stutter report fear, frustration, social penalties, dissatisfaction with themselves, lower level of aspiration, felt loss of social esteem. There is a tendency for problems common to

all human beings to become associated with the speech disturbance. However, there is no particular "stuttering personality" nor is the disorder a manifestation of psychoneurosis.

20. Stuttering is a social-psychological event. The acoustic and visual phenomena that occur during the motor act of stuttering are noxious stimuli in a communication context, and listeners tend to react in various explicit or implicit ways. The stutterer tends in turn to react to these listener responses.

For more detailed discussions of stuttering, the reader should consult the work of Van Riper (1982) and others (Bloodstein, 1981; Andrews et al., 1983; Fiedler and Standop, 1983). We trust that we have not discouraged the reader unduly by our somewhat somber presentation; for, even though the fluency disorder of stuttering remains a tantalizing mystery, there is much that we can do to help persons who seek our services. We hope to show by our case presentations and discussion that if we focus on the *client,* rather than the disorder, our mission becomes clearer.

## DIFFERENTIAL DIAGNOSIS

There are two important dimensions of differential diagnosis in regard to fluency disorders: identifying subtypes within the stuttering population and distinguishing the problem of stuttering from other conditions in which speech fluency is also disrupted.

Are there different kinds of stuttering? Does the label *stuttering* impart a linguistic unity to a generic disorder that may encompass several disparate types of fluency disturbances? We are not able to answer those questions, but we do know that, clinically, stuttering wears a variety of sad and confining disguises. Although the research is negligible in this area, we have seen several distinct subtypes—for example, interiorized and exteriorized stutterers (Douglass and Quarrington, 1952), predominantly clonic and predominantly tonic stutterers, clients who feature escape techniques, those who are addicted to avoidance, those who can predict an occurrence of stuttering, and those who cannot (Silverman and Williams, 1972). Perhaps there are even variations in stuttering that stem from cultural influence (Leith and Mims, 1975). We find these distinctions useful in planning therapy; persons with different behavioral histories require different management. Several observers have noted and attempted to classify subgroups of stutterers, but as yet no one system has been accorded widespread acceptance.

We are concerned not only with types of stutterers but also with varieties of fluency disturbance. There are several kinds of fluency breakdowns that can be confused with stuttering. In our clinical experience we have seen individuals with five rather distinct forms of abnormal disfluency:

*Episodic stress reaction.* It is well known that most speakers exhibit some degree of disfluency—revisions, interjections, word and phrase repetitions, and the like. Furthermore, everyone occasionally stutters (part-word repetitions and prolongations) at some point. In fact, speech fluency is a sensitive barometer of a person's psychological and physical integrity. Stress, particularly communicative stress, tends to increase a speaker's disfluency. Van Riper (1963) speculates that there is a positive relationship between communicative stress and progressive deterioration of speech:

> With minor stress, repetitions of sentences or phrases occur; with more stress, words are repeated, with even more pressure, the oscillating occurs on syllables. When complete disruption occurs but the urge to speak still remains, first prolongations of an audible sound ("mmmmmmother") are shown and finally even this breaks down to a silent posture. (Van Riper, 1963: 320)

Other situations of stress, such as battle conditions (Gavis, 1946; Grinker and Spiegal, 1945), intense excitement, emotional upheaval, and stage fright, can also precipitate a fluency breakdown.

Fluency breakdowns due to episodic stress show a number of consistent identifying features: an acknowledged source of intense or prolonged stimulation; tension overflow throughout the body (including the oral area), which may also produce a tremulous voice; an exacerbation of "normal" disfluency—broken words, incomplete phrases, interjections, repetitions of whole words; some part-word repetitions, usually syllabic but always with the correct vowel, never with the /ə/ vowel replacement; no avoidance, fear, rarely any penalty—perhaps some embarrassment after the incident is over. Finally, the most crucial characteristic is that the disfluency decreases markedly or stops when (or shortly after) the stress terminates. It is likely that all but the most stoic of persons have experienced an episodic fluency breakdown. It is interesting to note that nonprofessionals often react to stutterers with the same advice often tendered to persons under stress: "calm down," "take it easy," "slow down," and so on. The unfortunate consequence of such recommendations, for some stutterers, is an elaborate charade they play, attempting to simulate speakers under stress, often feigning confusion or bewilderment.

*Neurotic or hysterical stuttering.* Most stutterers, particularly confirmed adult cases, acquire a negative feeling tone about their problem. One of our clients summarized it succinctly when he said, "Stutterers are bugged because they are plugged." A few stutterers, however, show symptoms of a primary neurosis—they are "plugged because they are bugged." For these individuals, stuttering is a maladaptive solution to an acute psychological problem:

> Colleen, an eighth-grade parochial school pupil, began to stutter suddenly following the death of her parents in an automobile accident. She collapsed upon hearing the tragic news and remained mute, almost transfixed and catatonic, for several hours. During the planning for the funeral and the extended period of the wake, she started to stutter—a monotonous repetition of the initial syllable of words. She showed no struggle, no avoidance behavior. She looked directly at the auditor when she spoke and smiled bravely. We followed this case closely until the remission of stuttering two months later, and her disfluency was always the same—it never varied in form or severity from

situation to situation. When she read a passage several times, she did not show the typical reduction (adaptation) in stuttering. School documents, as well as interviews with several relatives, indicated that Colleen had had no prior speech difficulty. One maternal aunt whom we interviewed did recall, however, that the girl had several "spells" of uncontrolled weeping and laughing during her first menses a year before. The child had received an incredible amount of attention and solace after her parents' death—perhaps even more so because of her "stuttering"—from sympathetic adults.

Neurotic stuttering is characterized by a sudden onset (often in an older child), a monosymptomatic speech pattern, little situational variation, and seeming unconcern or indifference; the individual may be experiencing chronic stress or a sudden acute emotional upheaval; there may be a history of neurotic symptoms (Weiner, 1981; Deal, 1982).

*Fluency breakdowns following brain injury.* Speech fluency is a sensitive barometer of a person's physical (as well as psychological) health. We have observed disfluency in clients suffering from Parkinson's disease, some types of cerebral palsy, apraxia, and other neurological impairments (LeBrun, Retif, and Kaiser, 1983; Koller, 1983). There are also reports of fluency disruptions in alcoholics, drug addicts, and in patients afflicted with dialysis dementia (Madison et al., 1977). Although the acquired disfluency exhibited by persons suffering from these various impairments may sound like developmental stuttering, it is clearly a different type of disorder. Palilalia, a fluency disorder caused by bilateral subcortical brain damage, is a case in point. Palilalics repeat words and entire phrases—not sounds or syllables—with increasing speed and diminishing loudness (LaPointe and Horner, 1981; Kent and LaPointe, 1982).

Several aphasics with whom we have worked, particularly those clients who show good progress in word finding but have residual syntactic difficulty, exhibited fluency breakdowns superficially similar to stuttering:

> Miss Horn had suffered an aneurysm in the Circle of Willis leaving her hemiplegic, apraxic, and with mild expressive aphasia. When we examined her, almost a year after the cerebral vascular episode, her speech pattern resembled clonic stuttering. She would begin a word, repeat a phoneme or syllable several times, back up, and try again; if blocked once more, a repetition might reverberate almost endlessly. She frequently pounded on the table as if to time her utterances. We could discern no evidence of fear or avoidance, just severe frustration. Interestingly, when she spoke or read swiftly her fluency increased dramatically; she also talked quite freely when distracted from closely monitoring the act of speaking. Here is a sample of her speech taken from a tape recording during a group therapy session: "I can't—I can't (sigh) . . . I-I-I-I have tr-trouble with my, ah, with my speech . . . and, ah, my leg is, is, you know, stiff. . . ."

The disfluencies noted are rather typical—whole-word repetitions, revisions, interjections, broken words, gaps in the flow of speech. This client had difficulty formulating messages and then programming the proper motor sequences to utter the thought; unlike stutterers who have difficulty getting started, Miss Horn's fluency breakdowns occurred at any point in a sentence (Rosenbek et al., 1978; Donnan, 1979; Brown and Cullinan, 1981).

*Stuttering among the retarded.*  Some observers have reported a rather high prevalence of stuttering among mentally retarded, especially mongoloid, children (Van Riper, 1982: 38–41). We are frankly puzzled by these reports, as our experience agrees quite closely with the findings of Sheehan, Martyn, and Kilburn (1968) and Martyn, Sheehan, and Slutz (1969). We found only one stutterer in a population of 217 severely retarded children (ages four to twelve) in a residential hospital. It was our impression that the group of children evaluated, which included a large number with Down's syndrome, simply did not have a sufficient flow of speech on which to stutter; the majority were limited to one- or two-word utterances or an assortment of unintelligible grunts. Interestingly, we did observe stuttering emerge in two mongoloid children during a language-building program.

We have seen several stutterers among public school special education ("educable") pupils; it is our impression that the relative incidence of stuttering in this group is similar to that in most published surveys for normal school-aged populations. Their stuttering behavior exhibited the following characteristics: (1) an uncomplicated, typically clonic or repetitive, pattern; (2) little word or sound fear; (3) no anticipation of difficulty—most of these clients showed little awareness of their disfluency; and (4) almost no avoidance behavior (except sullen withdrawal). The frustration and struggle they did exhibit seemed to stem more from word-finding difficulty rather than expectation of fluency breakdown (Bonfanti and Culatta, 1977). Finally, the children we have examined seemed to clutter rather than stutter—they were trying to speak more rapidly than their system could tolerate (Farmer and Brayton, 1979).

*Cluttering.*  Cluttering is sometimes confused with stuttering:

Ralph was referred to us as a stutterer by his industrial education supervisor during his semester of student teaching. When we examined him, he revealed no fears or avoidances, exhibited only a few part-word repetitions, and had no fixations; he said that he enjoyed talking, did a lot of it, and that he was asked frequently to repeat himself, "especially when I talk fast." Ralph's difficulty seemed to take place on the phrase or sentence level; his interruptions broke the integrity of a *thought* rather than a *word*. In addition, he frequently omitted syllables and transposed words and phrases; he said "plobably," "posed," and "pacific" for "probably," "supposed," and "specific." Ralph's speech was sprinkled with spoonerisms (he said "beta dase" for "data base") and malapropisms (he described getting lost while hunting because the road he was following "dissipated" and told us he had a good "dialect" going with his roommate). His speech was swift and jumbled; it emerged in rapid torrents until he jammed up, and then he surged on again in another staccato outburst. In spontaneous talking, his message was characterized by disorganized sentences and poor phrasing. He gave the overall impression of being in great haste. When we asked him to slow down and speak carefully, there was a dramatic improvement, but he soon forgot our admonishment and reverted to his hurried, disorganized style. By and large, Ralph was unaware and indifferent to his fluency problem. He was an impatient, impulsive young man, always on the go. His course work was characteristically done in a great, almost compulsive, rush; he had difficulty reading, and his handwriting was a scrawl.

The major features of cluttering are, first, the excessive speed of speaking; second, the disorganized sentence structure; and third, the slurred or omitted syllables and sounds. Many clinicians suspect that cluttering may be one symptom of a central language disturbance or learning disability. They cite the difficulties their clients often have with reading, writing, spelling, and other language-dependent skills (DeFusco and Menken, 1979; Irvine and Reis, 1980).

The diagnostician should be aware that some stutterers may also exhibit features associated with cluttering; and it may be necessary to determine which fluency problem is primary (generally cluttering) or the most problematical.

Each of the fluency disorders described above requires distinctly different clinical management, even though the objective distortion of the speech signal may be somewhat similar. The diagnostician must keep in mind that a speech disorder involves more than a disturbance in the acoustic characteristics of an individual's oral output.

## EVALUATION AT THE ONSET OF STUTTERING

Experienced clinicians agree that the problem of stuttering is much easier to prevent in children than to treat in chronic adult clients. Indeed, the early detection and management of children beginning to stutter is one of the most significant contributions a speech clinician can make. The diagnostician must seek answers for a great many questions: Is the child stuttering? If he is stuttering, how far has the disorder progressed? When did it begin? What factors were associated with the onset of the problem? How aware is the child that his speech is blocked? How do listeners attempt to help him, and how does he respond to their efforts? How can we alter the child's environment to prevent the problem from getting worse?

Throughout this volume we have repeatedly suggested that diagnosis and therapy are not separate undertakings. The careful assessment of a client's problem is often therapeutic; only by working with an individual for a period of time do we truly come to know the dimensions of her problem. This is particularly true in the management of children beginning to stutter. In order to illustrate the activities of the diagnostician-clinician, we present below a case study of a three-and-one-half-year-old child brought to the clinic as an "incipient" stutterer. Our account is chronological and reports what was done from the initial contact to the termination of treatment. The family was seen for a total of six counseling sessions (not including brief follow-up contacts) over a period of two months.

### The Case of Stephen Wood

In many cases, a physican is the first professional to be consulted by parents, and the clinician is wise to enlist the support of local pediatricians in the early identification of children beginning to stutter. Stephen Wood, however, was referred to the clinic by his maternal uncle, who had received therapy for stuttering in a different community and knew of the senior author through his publications. Mr. Wood called us at home one weekend in midsummer and asked if we would see his son as soon as possible. He told us that Stephen had begun to stutter several months before—around the Christmas holiday, he thought. He added:

> At first he did it only occasionally. Even now it comes and goes in waves. Some days he will be talking along just fine and then, bang!—he stutters badly. We ignored it for a while, but when it persisted we told him to "take his time" and "think what he wanted to say." He doesn't like it when we give him advice; I noticed the other day he put his hand over his mouth and walked away when he got stuck. We are really worried that we may have waited too long.

We agree with Wyatt (1969) that the onset of stuttering is a crisis situation in which swift intervention is absolutely essential. It was arranged to see Stephen and his parents on Monday. We praised Mr. Wood for calling and suggested that Stephen did not need to know the real purpose of the visit to the speech clinic; we advised him simply to tell the child that his parents had to see some people at the university and he could come along and play a few of the interesting games they had for children.

In planning for the evaluation, we delineated several objectives that would guide our efforts:

1. Determine if the child is stuttering.
2. If he is, identify to what stage or level of development the disorder has progressed.
3. Obtain the parents' perception of the onset and current status of the problem.
4. Sample the child's general level of functioning in regard to auditory, motor, and language abilities.
5. Perhaps most important, commence the development of a counseling relationship with the parents.

We assigned an undergraduate student clinician to observe Stephen and his parents in the clinic waiting room. She was to watch unobtrusively the parent-child interaction and submit a descriptive report to us before we interviewed Mr. and Mrs. Wood. Here is what she wrote:

> The child is well dressed and well groomed. At first he sat on his father's lap, but when he saw the toy box he climbed down and played with the farm animals. He talked constantly, asking questions, commenting on what was taking place outside, and describing his animal parade. I heard some repetitions in

his speech, especially when he was trying to get his parents to attend to him. I noticed that Mrs. Wood always called him "Stephen," not "Steve" or "Stevie." Does that mean anything?

Before examining a child individually, we like to chat informally with both the youngster and the parents. We do this primarily to observe if the parents are reacting in an overt way to the child's speech. When the child is asked a question, do the parents attempt to answer for him? Do they point out instances of stuttering to the examiner? Do they signal their presence by nonverbal behavior—gestures, postures, and the like? How does the child respond to this?

We took the family on a brief tour of the speech clinic, ignoring Stephen and chatting with Mr. and Mrs. Wood. Ushering them into a playroom, we invited the child to sample the toys while we talked with his mother and father. Gradually, we edged closer to the boy and casually began to join his play, commenting on what his cars were doing, and asking him some questions. Soon he was chattering to the clinician. We noted several repetitions—all on small words, pronouns like "he," "I," "you"—but they were easy and rhythmical. When he attempted to utter the word "blue," however, he used the schwa vowel on the first two repetitions (bə-bə—blue-blue). Only one prolongation was heard, and occurred when he asked a question beginning with the word "how." Mrs. Wood tensed noticeably and looked at the examiner questioningly when Stephen repeated and hesitated. Once she finished a word for the child when he had repeated it five times. We could discern little overt reaction on the part of Mr. Wood, except he did slump in his chair and look out the window when his wife completed Stephen's utterance. We now needed a larger sample. Would his speech change if his parents left the room? How would be respond to stress?

On a prearranged signal, a graduate student came in and asked Mr. and Mrs. Wood if they would like to see the rest of the "school." Stephen glanced up briefly as his parents left, but continued playing and talking with the examiner. No increase in disfluency was noted.

Diagnosticians observe two clinical rules when examining young children thought to be starting to stutter: They use indirect means of obtaining a speech sample, and they never do anything that might bring the child's disfluency to his attention. Employing play as a vehicle, it was very easy to engage Stephen in conversation. With some more reluctant children we have used puppets, extended periods of self-talk, or projective drawings. But we also must have some idea of the impact of stress on the child's fluency. Slowly and subtly at first, we began to hurry the play and to interrupt Stephen in midsentence with our own message. We asked him a question, and before he could finish his answer, we asked another. Then when he tried to respond or direct the examiner's attention to some facet of our joint play, we looked away from him and purposely dropped toys on the floor and noisily scurried to pick them up. We gauged the communication stress carefully, watching for changes in the child's speech. Following this, we once again resumed an easy, relaxed style of interaction with the youngster. We abandoned the play for a moment, feasted on a salted peanut, and went to get a drink of water. Returning to the room with Stephen, the examiner pointed to a log building set and said, "We really should build a barn for the animals . . . but, golly, I have to do some school things first. Say, if you helped me, maybe we could get done faster, okay?" Stephen eagerly volunteered to "help" administer a hearing screening test, a measure of receptive vocabulary, and several tasks to assess motor skills. We thanked the child for coming in to see us, and started him on the barn-building project with a student clinician while we prepared for the interview with Mr. and Mrs. Wood. But first, while our impressions of Stephen were clear and fresh, we recorded these observations:

> The child is not a stutterer in the sense of a fully developed symptom pattern, but he did exhibit several forms of abnormal disfluency: multiple repetitions, an occasonal intrusive schwa vowel, and a few prolongations. The repetitions occurred most often on the initial word of an utterance. During a free-play situation, he repeated on approximately nine to eleven words per hundred; the number of repetitions per unit ranged from three to as many as nine. The repetitions were easy and rhythmical—in the same tempo and speed as the rest of his speech. The intrusive schwa vowel occurred when he repeated words beginning with blends—*bl*ue, *str*aw, and *tr*actor. Stephen prolonged only four times and always on vowels, always in the initial position. There is little tension, forcing, or gaps in his speech; nor is there obvious evidence of "awareness"—he speaks constantly with an excellent vocabulary and good grammar. When communication stress was introduced, the disfluency was exacerbated: The number of repetitions increased. My impression is that "listener loss" produced the most stress, then "interruption," "hurrying," and finally "questioning." Stephen's hearing is normal, and he scored in the ninety-ninth percentile on a measure of receptive vocabulary. Motor behavior seems adequate: gait, stance, throwing, block building, and skipping all appeared normal. At this point in time (note: *the diagnostician must be aware that at the onset of the disorder, stuttering is characteristically intermittent and he may see the child on a "good" day*), although Stephen shows several danger signs (see Figure 6.1) of developing stuttering, the problem can probably be dealt with by environmental intervention.

The clinician needs experience in distinguishing normal from abnormal disfluency in the speech of young children.[2] The clinician's task is twofold: to determine *how many* and *what kind* of speech interruptions the youngster exhibits. If he has more than fifty disfluencies in 1,000 words, there is cause for concern. However, we are more interested in the types of disfluency the child shows. Some diagnosticians employ the disfluency classification system devised by Johnson and his associates (Adams, 1982). There are seven forms of speech interruptions included in this scheme: part-word repetitions, whole-word repetitions, phrase repetitions, interjections, revisions, tense pauses, and disrhythmic phonations. We prefer to scrutinize the child's speech for certain signs of developing stuttering. An excel-

---

[2] It is not always possible to determine if a given speech disfluency is normal or abnormal (Bloodstein and Grossman, 1981).

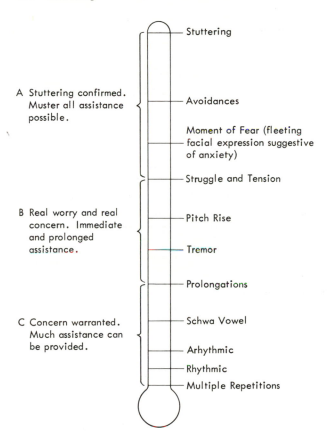

**FIGURE 6.1  The danger signs of developing stuttering.**

lent color film developed and narrated by Walle (1974) depicts each of eight danger signs of developing stuttering through the use of freeze-frames and slow-motion views; only children presenting actual fluency disorders were filmed. An unusually effective feature of the film is a gauge (see Figure 6.1) by which the diagnostician can judge the severity of the problem.

Before meeting with Mr. and Mrs. Wood, we checked our observations with those of a graduate student who had monitored the entire diagnostic session behind a one-way mirror. Her findings are summarized on a clinical worksheet (Figure 6.2) designed to facilitate identification of children beginning to stutter. (See Van Riper, 1982: 25, for a clinical schema to differentiate stuttering and normal disfluency; consult also the checklist devised by Cooper, 1973, and the work of Adams, 1977.)

*Initial interview with Mr. and Mrs. Wood.*  The initial interview with a parent of a child beginning to stutter is of critical importance. We must establish our professional competence, demonstrate our genuine interest, and convince the parents that we can be trusted. In short, our primary task in this initial contact is to build a

**FIGURE 6.2   Clinical worksheet: Onset of stuttering.**

Name:  Stephen Wood    Birthdate: 1/4/73   Date: 7/12/76   File: #76-271
Observer: M. Ruffatto    Situation:    "joint play"

1. Repetitions:   whole word  x   syllabic  x   phonemic

   a. Frequency of repetitions:    No. per word    3-10
                                   No. per hundred words    11
   b. Speed of repetitions:   same rate as fluent speech
   c. Tempo:  even, regular
   d. Co-articulation
        (is appropriate vowel used in repetition?):  schwa noted on
        blends--5 times
   e. Evidence of tension-struggle:     none
   f. How are the repetitions terminated:  no surge or stoppage

2. Prolongations:   syllabic  x   vocalic   x   consonant
                                 articulatory posture
   a. Frequency:    four
   b. Duration:  less than one second
   c. Change in pitch:   no
   d. Stoppage of air-flow/phonation:   no
   e. Repetitions end in prolongations or silent postures:   no
   f. Evidence of tension-struggle:   none
   g. Inappropriate articulatory postures:     no

3. Response to Communicative Stress:

   a. Type of stress:              b. Response:
      loss of listener                repetitions increased,
      hurrying him                    noted on pronouns
      interruptions
      overlapping questions

4. Awareness

   a. Eye contact:    seemed normal   b. Facial flushing no signs
   c. Eyeblink rate:      19                  26
                     (base rate)         (disfluency)
   d. Motor behavior:    no signs
   e. Verbalizes about speech problem:  not observed
   f. Behavior following disfluency:   continued talking and playing

5. Advanced features:

   a. Evidence of frustration:    none
   b. Evidence of avoidance:      none
   c. Breathing disturbance:      none
   d. Facial contortion, extraneous body movements:   none
   e. Tremor:   none

6. Other observations:  He appears somewhat small for his
   age but his movements are quick and well-coordinated.
   His articulation skills are excellent and he generates
   long, complex sentences.

relationship for subsequent counseling sessions. We also listen carefully to the parents' presenting story: How do they see the child and his problem? In their view, what might have caused it? What do they identify as their role in the onset of the child's stuttering? What expectations and apprehensions do they have regarding the nature and outcome of treatment?

Let us emphasize here that this is *their* story: Hear them out. This is not the proper time to take a lengthy case history; there will be plenty of time for a careful review of the background of the problem in subsequent interviews when the parents can then profit from an objective review of the situation. Guilt, which is almost always present in these sessions, must not be engendered by the interviewer's questions or commentary.

We prefer to record these initial interviews; this frees us from the onus of note taking, and we can devote our entire attention to the respondent. It also permits repeated review of the session. Here is a résumé of our initial interview with Mr. and Mrs. Wood:

At the outset of the interview, both parents pressed the examiner for his impressions of Stephen's speech problem. We told them that we were pleased with our findings and would explain in detail after we had a chance to hear from them. Mrs. Wood was the main informant; her husband corroborated dates and added minor details. Both parents appeared tense and uncertain— Mrs. Wood seemed especially anxious. Throughout the interview her vocal quality was querulous, and her eyes filled with tears several times as she related the onset of Stephen's speech problem.

The youngster began to stutter seven months ago, during the Christmas holidays. At this time both sets of grandparents were visiting and the home was filled with a great deal of excitement and confusion. Mrs. Wood even remembered the very first instance when she noted that Stephen was having trouble—when he attempted to name items in a picture dictionary book he had received as a gift. When we asked her to describe the child's speech at that time, she said he repeated letters—*k, m, n*. Mr. Wood added that Stephen also seemed to draw out some letters, but his wife insisted that this came later. After the holidays the problem seemed to go away, only to reappear a few weeks later; now, they agreed, there are fewer days when the child is free of speech interruptions. It was also during the holidays that Mrs. Wood discovered that she was pregnant with their second child (Philip, Jr., was born in early June 1976), and she wondered what impact this had on Stephen. She admitted that she has had very little time to spend with him since the baby was born.

The parents described Stephen as an active, inquisitive child. He began to talk early and enjoys describing events; he provides a running commentary when the family goes for a ride or on some other outing. Mr. Wood added that his son is very adult-oriented and, in fact, interacts with neighborhood children as if he were a parent instead of a playmate.

Mrs. Wood confided that she is very concerned about Stephen because her younger brother stuttered severely and she had observed how the disorder hampered his education and social life. She does not want the same thing to happen to Stephen. "Although I have tried to be permissive," she confessed, "I find myself adopting the same rigid perfectionism that characterized my own parents."

The parents have attempted to manage the fluency problem by asking

Stephen to "slow down," "take his time," and "think what he intends to say." They have also suggested that he whisper the word first before trying to say it out loud. These home remedies do not seem to help.

It is important that parents obtain some closure during these initial interviews, so we related our findings briefly:

> Stepnen does indeed have some breaks in his speech, more than normal for a child of his age. He is doing some stuttering but it is still the "good kind": He is not struggling or avoiding and, most important, he doesn't seem to be very aware that talking is tough (we drew a rough sketch of the stuttering gauge depicted in Figure 6.1 and showed them that Stephen exhibited only the three early danger signs of stuttering). We want to prevent the disorder from developing further and cannot do anything without your help. We need to find out why he is having speech breaks; we need to know when he does it, under what circumstances. In short, we have to start looking at behaviors, at what he *does,* not a condition he *has.* In many cases like this, if we identify and alter certain environmental situations, the child stops stuttering. Stephen's speech will likely get worse if we ask him to stop or change the way he is talking. Talking is automatic, and the more he tries to think and plan how he is speaking, the more tangled up he will get. You were very wise to bring him in now, before the fear and frustration had a chance to develop. Let's plan on meeting again tomorrow, and together we can begin to review Stephen's background and then decide how to gather information on what is happening now.

*Plan of treatment.*    The therapeutic management of children beginning to stutter is largely indirect: We work for changes in the environment through parental counseling and education.[3] In the case of Stephen Wood, our treatment plan included four basic goals:

1. To deal with parental emotions and resistance
2. To obtain a careful case history
3. To review the nature and onset of stuttering
4. To provide general and specific suggestions for altering the home situation and parent-child interaction

For purposes of discussion, we will consider each goal separately, although it is rarely possible to do this in clinical practice. Note the interplay of diagnosis and therapy as we review our activities relative to the four goals.

Handling Emotion and Resistance.    The first (and continual) task in a counseling relationship is to deal openly with the client's emotions. A person's feelings are primary. Consequently, at the outset of the second session with Mr. and

---

[3] Even if the evaluation shows that a child is normally disfluent, it is still important to initiate counseling. The clinician must help the parents look at the youngster's speech behavior as a temporary developmental phase.

Mrs. Wood we encouraged them to relate what impact our initial interview had had. Again, Mrs. Wood was the main respondent, and here, in part, is what she said:

> We were really dumbfounded—but relieved in a way too—when you said that Stephen does not need active therapy . . . but you would be seeing us today. Last night after the children were in bed, we sat down and reviewed what has happened the past seven months. There is a great deal of hurry and tension in our home, especially when we have to go somewhere; it seems like we are always trying to hasten Stephen along so we can make some deadline. We tend to talk too much, too swiftly, and in a complicated fashion to him— maybe we are expecting too much, too early because he is so bright and verbal. Anyway, we feel just sick that we may be responsible for his problem.

We let Mrs. Wood talk it out, nodding occasionally and expressing our interest and understanding. When she had finished, we searched for the right words:

> Most parents feel a bit guilty when their children begin to stutter. They sense that they may have caused the problem—a notion that unfortunately is reinforced by many laymen. Parents, especially the mother, are blamed for everything negative about their youngsters. And stuttering is such a highly visible problem; the neighbor kid might wet the bed every night, but no one else need know. No doubt you were a bit surprised when I indicated that I would be seeing you and not Stephen. I'm very glad that you told me how you feel and that you are open and honest, because it's difficult to deal objectively with a problem when feelings get in the way. An undercurrent of guilt or resentment makes the problem very difficult to clear up. As I pointed out yesterday, you were most wise to bring Stephen in now when we—you and I as a team—can sort out and eliminate those things that produce speech breaks. We can't change what happened, but that's not nearly so important as what's going on right now. We can alter the present. Here is the phone number of the Munsons; last year they were in the same situation you are, and they volunteered to talk with other parents. A problem shared is a problem lessened. Now, why don't we get started by reviewing all the aspects that we can think of?

The Case History.  We seek more than information when we compile a case history. A parent's careful review of the many factors involved in his child's problem tends to foster objectivity. It also shifts the focus away from a general impression of "trouble" to observation of specific behavior. Here are some questions we use as guides in assembling information from a parent:

—When did the child begin exhibiting disfluencies?
—What were the circumstances under which the disfluencies were noted?
—How long has the child been exhibiting the disfluencies?
—What changes have been noted in the frequency or form of the disfluencies?
—What factors seem to increase or decrease the child's disfluency?
—In what ways has the family tried to help the child?
—What is the child's reactions to the family's efforts to help him?

We include a portion of our case history of Stephen Wood:

*History of the speech problem.* Stephen began to "stutter" approximately seven months ago. Onset occurred, according to the parents, when he faltered at naming pictures in the presence of a group of relatives. No prior history of speech, language, or hearing difficulty. Both parents have offered various forms of advice with no lasting effect. Disfluency consists of syllabic repetitions and a few prolongations. No negative reactions from playmates or adult visitors. Disfluency has been cyclic but became more persistent in the last month.

*Developmental history.* Normal (first) pregnancy. No untoward conditions associated with delivery. Described as an "active" baby. Sat up at three months, walked at eleven months, and spoke first word at twelve months. Usual childhood colds and flu, but no high fevers. Father describes the child as "adult-oriented" and officious in his relationship with other youngsters.

*Family.* Glenda Wood, age twenty-eight. Married six years. Homemaker. Earned a two-year certificate in business management after completing high school and worked several years in a bank. Describes herself as perfectionistic and compulsive about order and cleanliness.

Philip Wood, age thirty-one. Federal health inspector. College degree, currently taking graduate work in health planning.

Additional items to assess in obtaining a case history include (1) a specific review of any familial incidence of stuttering; (2) the impact, if any, of relatives or babysitters upon the child; (3) a description of how the child spends a typical day; and (4) a description of any prior professional treatment.

**The Nature and Onset of Stuttering.**   The second interview with Mr. and Mrs. Wood was devoted mainly to obtaining a case history. By this time they were insistently curious: What is stuttering? What causes it? What did we mean when we said that Stephen still had the "good kind" of stuttering? We gave them a copy of a short pamphlet (Emerick, 1983) written for parents whose children are beginning to stutter and asked that they read it carefully and discuss its contents.[4] Perhaps, we warned, portions of the booklet might make them feel a bit guilty; we reminded the parents that our purpose was to convey information, not to point an accusing finger. Finally, we asked Mr. and Mrs. Wood to record their observations regarding Stephen's speech breaks.

It is often helpful if we put down on paper some of the things we see and hear about the way our child is talking. It will help obtain a clearer picture of the child's situation. Try to be as objective and honest as you can in making your observations. Use the chart (Figure 6.3) at the end of the pamphlet. In the first four squares you record what you observed (and the date) with respect to the questions listed along the border. For example: Mrs. Emery made an effort on January 19 to study Mary's nonfluency. She found that the child was mainly repeating first sounds of words (muh-muh-Mommy). Mrs. Emery put this information, with the date, in one of the four blocks

----

[4]Another reference that provides information for counseling parents of children who are beginning to stutter is Ainsworth and Fraser-Gruss (1977).

**FIGURE 6.3   Form for recording parental observations of speech interruptions.**

| SPEECH CHART | | |
|---|---|---|
| What type of speech inter-<br>ruptions did the child have<br>(repeating sounds or words;<br>hesitations, changing his<br>sentences)? | date:<br><br>..............<br><br>date: | date:<br><br>..............<br><br>date: |
| Did he appear to be tense<br>or struggle with the speech<br>interruptions? | date:<br><br>..............<br><br>date: | date:<br><br>..............<br><br>date: |
| Did he seem to be aware that<br>he was having the interrup-<br>tions; did he react to them?<br>If so, how did he react? | date:<br><br>..............<br><br>date: | date:<br><br>..............<br><br>date: |
| To whom was he talking when<br>the speech interruptions<br>were noted? | date:<br><br>..............<br><br>date: | date:<br><br>..............<br><br>date: |
| What was he talking about? | date:<br><br>..............<br><br>date: | date:<br><br>..............<br><br>date: |
| What had happened immediately<br>prior to his speaking (was he<br>interrupted, ignored, ex-<br>cited, frustrated, tired)? | date:<br><br>..............<br><br>date: | date:<br><br>..............<br><br>date: |
| What was happening--what was<br>the listener doing--when the<br>child was talking?  (Did<br>they offer advice, look<br>away, become tense, etc.?) | date:<br><br>..............<br><br>date: | date:<br><br>..............<br><br>date: |

| Record number of times: | | | | | | |
|---|---|---|---|---|---|---|
| 1. Demand for speech | | | | | | |
| 2. Child told "no" or "don't" | | | | | | |
| 3. Child was interrupted<br>while talking | | | | | | |
| 4. Parental conflict or<br>tension | | | | | | |
| 5. Gave child speech advice,<br>such as "stop and start<br>over," "take a deep<br>breath," "slow down." | | | | | | |

opposite the first question. She then followed down the page and put her other observations about Mary's reactions in the rest of the blocks opposite the questions.

It will be helpful to you to see under what circumstances the child is experiencing the most speech interruptions. To whom was he talking? What was he talking about? What happened immediately before he began to talk? What happened when he was trying to talk? If, for example, you note that the child's speech interruptions occur most frequently when he is competing with his brothers and sisters for speaking time, then you will readily see what needs to be corrected in order to help him. Using this chart, we will be able to find the reasons for an increase in the child's speech interruptions. Once we know *how* and *why* the child is hesitating, we are less apt to label his behavior as stuttering; we concentrate less on the speech and more on the circumstances. Also, we can then take steps to smooth out the circumstances that seem to increase the child's speech interruptions.

We find often that simply asking parents to monitor the antecedents and consequences of their child's speech disfluencies is sufficiently motivating to engender change. Environmental events that disrupt a child's flow of speech become obvious when parents begin to chart.

At the end of the second counseling session Mr. and Mrs. Wood were visibly relieved. Before they left, they asked what they could do to help besides observing. It is important that parents be provided with suggestions when they ask for them:

> Once we identify the factors associated with Stephen's fluency disruptions, we can act to eliminate or reduce them. In the meantime, however, there are several things you can do: (1) Be the best listener you can be—not all the time obviously, but arrange it so when you *can* listen to him, do it *totally*; (2) talk simply with him, using short sentences and a slow, relaxed tempo; throw in an easy repetition now and then—and if he asks about it, tell him even big people make mistakes when they talk; (3) arrange to have some quiet times alone with him where he has you one-on-one with no distractions; (4) try to relax the standards or expectations you have for his behavior, at least for now; he is still a small boy even though he seems so adultlike; and, finally (5) whenever he does have difficulty talking, make sure you complete the communication—let him know that the message, not the struggle, is paramount.

Altering Home and Parent-Child Interaction.     We held four additional counseling interviews with Mr. and Mrs. Wood during the remainder of the summer school session. These meetings were devoted to analyzing the parents' observations of Stephen's speech behavior; we also made a number of suggestions designed to reduce fluency disruptors. The best suggestions came from the parents themselves. The primary focus of this book does not permit a complete account of this phase of counseling with the family. We have included only fragments to illustrate the clinician's role in modifying the home and parent-child relationship:

> Mr. and Mrs. Wood held a conference each evening to review their observations of Stephen's speech disfluency. They slowed the pace of activity in the

home and reduced the demands upon the child. Mrs. Wood enrolled in a program of Parent Effectiveness Training offered through the local school system. They both agreed that the most effective modification they made was improving their listening habits; once the child realized that his parents were actively attending, his incessant chatter declined dramatically. Almost immediately the repetitions and prolongations disappeared.

It has been our experience that most parents are amenable to making changes that will benefit their child, if the rationale is explained to them and if it is obvious that the clinician is totally commited to the prevention of stuttering. In order to assist mothers and fathers in altering their interaction with youngsters beginning to stutter, we have offered a wide variety of suggestions. Here are just a few: Allow the child to express her fears and anger; count the number of times you say no each day and reduce these by half;[5] devise stable and consistent rules for behavior; and balance the ratio between demand and support so the balance shifts to the latter. We often made a home visit, not only to observe the child in a naturalistic setting, but also to demonstrate that our concern is far more than casual.

There are two additional tools that we have found helpful in parent counseling. Some parents are unaware of the impact of negative comments on their children, and we have had to show them how to analyze their verbal interaction. We lend them a portable tape recorder and ask them to collect samples of conversations with their child. Then, using the research of Egolf et al. (1972) and Kasprisin-Burrelli, Egolf, and Shames (1972), we show them how to categorize positive and negative statements. This graphic procedure helps them to become more creative, more supportive in their interaction with the child.

The other tool we use in helping parents are two excellent films: *Family Counseling* (Walle, 1975) and *Is It Me? Is It You?* (Walle, 1977). Both films are invaluable in helping parents understand how they can help children overcome the broken and hesitant speech they often display between two and six years of age.

### Outcome of Treatment

By the end of August, Stephen was exhibiting no signs of stuttering except occasionally when he was very excited. Once, when a large dog knocked him off his tricycle, he was disfluent for several hours; but Mrs. Wood managed the traumatic event in a calm, supportive manner. Mr. and Mrs. Wood met with the Munsons (parents who had undergone counseling when their child was beginning to stutter), and the women formed a close friendship. Now both mothers make presentations in our university classes. A frequent fringe benefit of counseling parents is the personal gains they derive; Mr. and Mrs. Wood report that they feel better, their home is more relaxed, and they enjoy their children much more.

---

[5] Savitsky and Hess (1975) found that an act of correction occurs between a mother and her two-year-old child on the average of every three minutes.

### Prognosis

We are very impressed with the efficacy of treatment for young children beginning to stutter. When the clinician can intervene before the child develops fear and avoidance reactions, and if the parents are amenable to counseling, the prognosis for recovery is excellent. Our own records on 209 cases, admittedly limited and incomplete, reveal an astounding success ratio of 86 percent. There are several factors that the clinician must consider when estimating a client's prospects for recovery:

1. How long has the child been stuttering? The older the child is and the longer his exposure to adverse environmental reactions, the poorer his prognosis.
2. What type and intensity of environmental reactions has the child been exposed to? Our cases who experienced slapping or other forms of physical abuse had the worst prognoses.
3. Is the child aware that she has difficulty speaking? (See Figure 6.2.) The more heedful the child is of her speech interruptions, the less positive the prognosis.
4. What type of speech disfluency characteristics are present? The more danger signs present (see Figure 6.1)—in particular, cessation of phonation, stoppage of airflow, moment of fear—the poorer the prognosis.
5. How amenable are the parents to counseling? The presence of parental psychopathology is an extremely poor sign for prognosis.
6. What is the child's level of intelligence? We have had more limited success with "slow" children.
7. Are there organic or neurotic factors that figure in the onset of stuttering? Chances for recovery are more limited if either is present.

Our clinical success or failure with children beginning to stutter is also related to the characteristic pattern of factors present at the onset of stuttering. Apparently, there are several ways of becoming a stutterer (Van Riper, 1982: 94; Yairi, 1983). We find the model developed by Myers and Wall (1982) useful for synthesizing diagnostic information and making a prognosis about a young disfluent child. The many variables that may be involved in the onset of stuttering are organized into three major categories: physiological, psycholinguistic, and psychosocial (Figure 6.4). Note how the three categories may overlap. For example, a child delayed in language development and deficient in motor skills could be particularly susceptible to high parental standards or communication competition with siblings.

We have often wondered how much we actually did for some of these cases. Would they have gotten better without our help, due simply to the passage of time and some internal recovery potential in the child? Did we do any good? In most instances, however, the recovery from stuttering occurred too swiftly after the initiation of therapeutic practices (two weeks to several months) to be attributed to spontaneous recovery (Wingate, 1964; Shearer and Williams, 1965; Sheehan and Martyn, 1970). Consult the work of Wyatt (1969: 310-312) for a list of variables contributing to and inhibiting progress.

PSYCHOLINGUISTIC FACTORS

Phonology
Prosody
Syntax
Semantics/Cognition
Propositionality of Utterance
Pragmatics

PSYCHOSOCIAL FACTORS

Parents
Other Significant Adults
Peers
Social "Load" of Discourse

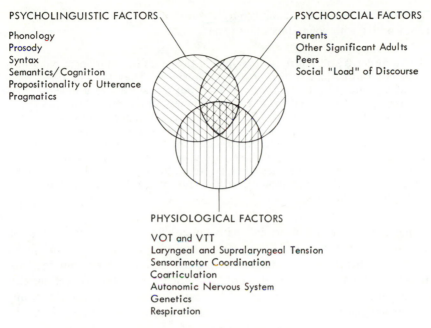

PHYSIOLOGICAL FACTORS

VOT and VTT
Laryngeal and Supralaryngeal Tension
Sensorimotor Coordination
Coarticulation
Autonomic Nervous System
Genetics
Respiration

FIGURE 6.4   Factors influencing early childhood stuttering.

## EVALUATION OF THE SCHOOL-AGED CHILD

Appraising and treating elementary school stutterers is particularly challenging. This group of children, approximately seven to twelve years old, is no longer beginning to stutter; they are not simply repeating and hesitating. They struggle noticeably when speaking and attempt to avoid or disguise their difficulty; they are frustrated and bewildered by their behavior. The self-perpetuating cycle has started and it is now necessary to deal directly with the stuttering.

The clinician is faced with several thorny problems when planning an examination of a young stutterer: (1) Young children frequently lack the insight and cooperation necessary to analyze their problem objectively and rationally. (2) Children are reluctant or unable to verbalize freely their internal feelings. (3) Children can face unpleasant and feared experiences only with great difficulty; they don't understand enduring temporary discomfort for a future payoff. (4) The speech clinician is associated in the child's mind with the teaching personnel, who may in some cases be penalizing or disturbing listeners. In addition, the clinician may find himself identified with authority figures; this tends to undermine a trusting relationship. (5) Last, and perhaps most significantly, the child usually has no choice about entering therapy; most likely she is brought for evaluation by her parents, referred by a teacher, or identified by a speech clinician.

As Van Riper (1973: 427) points out, however, there are several advantageous factors in working with youngsters who stutter:

> The disorder is still not fully developed in the child. Its component behaviors have not had as long a history of reinforcement. They are not fixed. The avoidance and struggle reactions are less complex. Morbidity is lower. Living primarily in the present, past trauma are less important in the design of therapy. The child stutterer forgets his unpleasant experiences more swiftly than the adult, who often nurtures them. The child's fears also seem more transitory and his malattitudes less severe. The clinician finds that the child's resistances are more open and direct; we do not find the ingenious sabotage which often characterizes the adult stutterer. And perhaps most important of all, the child has not interiorized the stuttering role to the degree manifested by the adult.

Some clinicians continue to deal with young stutterers as if their problem were incipient or onset in nature. They talk in hushed voices about rhythm problems and report that they are "watching" a child who stutters. Parents and teachers are advised to refrain from using the word "stuttering." Literature concerning the onset of stuttering is sent home, which, in the absence of counseling and follow-up, merely increases the parents' guilt. This leads to an elaborate conspiracy of silence that only makes matters worse:

> To pretend that there is no speech defect when it is obvious to the child and everyone else is folly, since this pretense will only make him feel he is doing something unclean, as well as unspeakable. (Van Riper, 1961: 114)

In their uncertainty lest they do something harmful and create "stuttering," such clinicians do nothing at all. The emperor has no stuttering problem. Perhaps this is one reason why the children, taking their cue from their elders, so frequently *act* as if they were not greatly concerned about their speech (Silverman, 1970).

The diagnostician will find that these youngsters respond to an honest, straightforward clinical approach. With preschoolers and early elementary school children, we use descriptive language—"tensing," "getting stuck"—to inquire about their speaking difficulty, not out of any fear of the word stuttering, but simply because the term either doesn't mean much to the child or, in some cases, is too negatively charged. It is better to refer to different ways of *talking* when assessing younger children (Williams, 1971). Here is a fragment taken from a recording of a recent diagnostic session with a seven-year-old child. The examiner is trying to elicit the little girl's own description of her fluency problem:

> These are your eyes. You use them for seeing. Do you have any trouble seeing? These are your ears. You use them for hearing. Do you have any trouble hearing? This is your mouth. You use it for talking. Do you ever have any trouble talking?

With older elementary school children, we use a frank, direct style. The clinician must establish trust and confidence by showing the client that she is competent, that she *knows* about the problem of stuttering. She does this by demonstrating that she understands what it feels like to stutter, by revealing a bit about herself, and by her willingness to touch stuttering without fear or distress. Notice how swiftly the clinician accomplishes those objectives in the following example:

> Hello, I suppose you're wondering what's going to happen today. You know that I am a speech-correction teacher and that my job is to help you get rid of your stuttering. But you don't know what kind of person I am except that I'm a stranger and you often have more trouble talking to a stranger. And you don't know how much I'll make you talk or how much stuttering you'll have. So you're probably a bit scared. You don't have to be, because today I'm going to do most of the talking.
>
> You noticed that I didn't ask your name. That's because I know that saying your name is often one of the hardest things there is to do. How did I know that? It's because I have worked with other kids who've stuttered—a lot of them. And it's because I had to do a lot of stuttering myself when I was learning to be a speech-correction teacher. I had to go into stores and stutter like this [Demonstrates] and like this . . . and like this . . . and many other ways, too. I had to know how it looked and how it felt. And at first, I was sure scared and embarrassed—especially when I had to do it on the phone or to one of my classmates. Once, it almost seemed to run away with me and I couldn't stop. So I think you'll find that I can understand how you feel when you stutter. I also learned how to help the stutterer and I want to help you. So let's get started.
>
> The first thing I've got to do is to know *how* you stutter. Let me give you some samples and ask you if you've ever had that kind of stuttering. How about this kind? [Therapist illustrates a very severe and unusual form of stuttering.] You don't have that kind? Good! One of the kids I worked with had that kind when we first started. How about this kind? . . . Or this? . . . [Therapist gradually shows models of decreasing abnormality and unfamiliarity.] But I bet you've often had some like this, haven't you? [Illustrates.] (Van Riper, 1964: 30–31)

### An Assessment Plan

The evaluation of a young stutterer does not differ greatly in substance from an assessment of an older individual (with children, environmental, parental, and school factors are more important); therefore, we will defer a detailed description of diagnostic procedures until a later section of this chapter.[6] In order to reveal the range of information generally sought, however, we have included an outlined assessment plan prepared by a diagnostic team composed of a faculty member and graduate students. The plan was compiled for the evaluation of a ten-year-old child referred to a university speech clinic by a public school clinician:

[6] For a complete evaluation kit, see Thompson (1982).

*Assessment Plan for Alan Schlicher*

I. *Identifying Information*

Obtain all the usual information regarding address, grade level, and so on. This can be obtained from Mrs. Hronkin, the referral source, or in the parent interview. Be sure to inquire about living arrangements: Ms. Hronkin mentioned that a parental grandfather may reside with the family and apparently he is a dominant force in the family (reportedly, he is against Alan receiving speech therapy and insists he overcame stuttering by eating mashed potatoes!).

II. *Description of Stuttering*

A. Global description: What are the salient descriptive features of Alan's stuttering behavior? Is it basically fixative or oscillative? Are there long silent periods of internal struggle, or does he exhibit a more overt pattern?

B. Core behaviors: Make an analysis of the repetitions and prolongations observed—the number of oscillations per unit, tempo, duration, and so forth.

C. Tension-struggle features: Using the items on the Summary Sheet (Figure 6.5), note the occurrence and location of any ancillary behaviors.

D. Freqency: This analysis will serve as our baseline for reevaluation of Alan, so we need to be especially precise. Collect data (count repetitions, prolongations, other salient features of his moments of stuttering) on at least three types of speech samples—reading, paraphrasing, and spontaneous speech. We can compute the relative frequency of stutterings per minute, or per total words uttered, by analyzing the videotape later. One word of caution: Stuttering is notoriously ephemeral and it is very difficult to obtain reliable baselines. Ryan (1969) recommends recording data in three different sessions in order to count reliably and define specific behaviors. (He also includes more speaking tasks—echoic, naming pictures, speaking with puppets, and so forth).

E. Severity: We will use the *Riley Stuttering Severity Instrument* (Riley, 1972); this instrument employs the three dimensions of frequency, duration, and physical concomitants and yields a score that can be converted to a percentile. A severity measure like this (particularly when it allows the examiner to score a client on a common scale of 0 to 100) is useful when communicating the results of the evaluation to the parents, teacher, even the child himself. The severity scales devised by Darley and Spriestersbach (1978: 313) and others (Andrews and Harris, 1964: 5; Wingate, 1976: 319) are also useful.

F. Variations in frequency/severity: Explore with the child and his parents whether his stuttering comes and goes in cycles, which situations or listeners provoke variations in his problem, and whether there are any words or sounds that are particularly difficult. Determine what impact delayed auditory feedback and masking noise have on his speech.

G. How does the child try to control his stuttering? What techniques has he devised for coping with speech interruptions? How effective are they? Additionally, we need to identify which speech-altering strategies—slowing, easy onset, and so forth—induce fluency. Use Cooper's (1982) *Disfluency Descriptor Digest* as a checklist to record observations.

H. Can the child predict when he is about to stutter? Ask him if he can; but also have him underline words he thinks he might stutter on as he

**FIGURE 6.5   Evaluation of young stutters: Summary sheet.**

1.   Identifying Information

   Name:_____ Birthdate:_____ Sex:_____ School:_____
   Address:_____ Teacher:_____ Grade:_____
   _____ Phone:_____ File Number:_____
   Family Structure:_____
   (Father)   (age) (education)        (occupation)

   _____
   (Mother)   (age) (education)        (occupation)

   _____
   (sibling)   (age) (sibling)            (age)
   Living arrangements:_____
   _____

II.   Description of stuttering
   A.   Global description:_____
   B.   Core behaviors:

   repetitions              prolongations        C.   Tension – Struggle
                                                               features:

   No./unit_____ duration_____ tremor_____
   Tempo_____ pitch change_____ avoidances_____
   Co-articulation_____ how terminate_____ retrials_____
   How terminate_____ _____ starters_____
   _____ _____ breathing_____
                                                        head_____
                                                        extremities_____

                                                        eyes_____

   D. Frequency:            E. Severity:
      reps.  prolong.  —  —  #words time  Riley scale_____
                                                other_____
   read
   para-
   phrase
   sponta-
   neous

   _____
   _____

   F. Variations in frequency/severity:   G.   How does client contorl?_____

   cycles_____   _____
   situations/listens                       H.   Can client predict?_____
      when worst_____
      when best_____           _____
      ever absent_____           I.   Post-stuttering behavior:___
      (e.g. alone,_____
      singing,_____           _____
      with pets)_____

   words/sounds_____
   DAF/masking_____

**FIGURE 6.5  (cont.)**

III.  Attitude dimension

    A.  Client's attitude  
        To stuttering:_____  
        _____  
        To treatment:_____  
        _____

    B.  Parental attitude:_____

    C.  Others:

        Siblings:_____  
        _____  
        Other children:_____  
        _____  
        Other adults:_____

IV.  Case History

    A.  General development (motor, language, social):  
    B.  Onset and development of stuttering:  
        Parental explanation_____client's_____  
        How has it changed?_____  
        Treatment_____

    C.  Medical History  
    D.  Family History

                    Paternal                Maternal

      stuttering    _____   _____  
      speech defects_____   _____  
      twinning     _____   _____  
      diabetes     _____   _____  
      others       _____   _____

V.  Present functioning

    A.  Personality:

        description_____  
        special features:  
          sensitive_____  
          tics_____  
          fears_____  
          others_____  
          _____  
        interests/hobbies:_____  
        _____

    B. School:

        academic_____  
        social_____  
        _____

    C.  Related testing:

        psychological referral_____  
        _____  
        medical referral_____  
        _____  
        motor_____  
        hearing_____  
        language_____  
        other_____

    D.  Diagnostic session:

        response to examiner_____  
        estimate of motivation_____  
        response to stress_____  
        trial therapy_____  
        _____

      E.  Prognosis and recommendations:_____  
         _____  
         _____  
         _____

reads silently a simple passage. Have him read it aloud and determine the degree to which he can accurately predict his stuttering.
  I.  What is the client's poststuttering behavior? Does he continue talking, give up, become angry, or cry? Does he appear indifferent?
III.  *Attitude Dimension*
This is the most difficult and least reliable aspect of the evaluation. Some information can be obtained through observation of Alan and his parents and by what they say about the problem. We can also administer several self-inventory scales (see particularly Chapman, 1959, or the more recent A-19 Scale developed by Guitar[7]) or have him do some projective drawings (Bar, 1973). What is the child's attitude toward treatment? How much does he know about stuttering? Has he been teased at school or home because of his problem?
IV.  *Case History*
We will want to obtain background information with respect to four basic areas: history of general development (motor, language, social), onset and development of stuttering, medical history, and family history. These areas can be explored in the parent interview.
 V.  *Present Functioning*
  A.  Personality: Describe the child's personality in general terms (shy, aggressive, and so on) and identify any special features (fears, tics, nail biting, and the like) that may apply to him. Ascertain his special interests or hobbies.
  B.  School: Obtain information relevant to his academic and social adjustment in school.
  C.  Related testing: Is a psychological or medical referral indicated? Perform screening evaluations on the child's motor behavior, hearing, and language ability. The latter is particularly important, as there is some evidence that children who stutter may have a language disability (Wyatt, 1969; Andrews and Harris, 1964), although the research is equivocal (Perozzi and Kunze, 1969; Perozzi, 1970; Williams and Marks, 1972; Manning and Riensche, 1976). Plan to use the testing format suggested by Riley and Riley (1982). They advocate evaluating the following skills:
   1.  *Attending behavior.* Is the child distractible? Does he perseverate?
   2.  *Auditory processing.* Does he delay in responding to tasks? Does he request repetitions of instructions?
   3.  *Sentence formulation.* Is there any evidence of a breakdown in word order?
   4.  *Oral motor.* What is the child's diadochokinetic rates for $/p/$, $/k/$, and $/t/$? Is there any evidence of articulatory imprecision?
  D.  Diagnostic session: How did the child behave during the diagnostic session? What could be discerned about his level of motivation? How did he respond when put under communicative stress? How did he respond to trial therapy?

### Prognosis

Since 1962 when we set out to devise a therapy program for young stutterers (Emerick, 1970), we have seen a total of 155 children and have consulted with public school clinicians about many others. According to our records, and they are

[7]Copies of the experimental version of this scale are available from B. Guitar, Department of Communication Science and Disorders, University of Vermont, Burlington, Vt. 05405.

frankly incomplete in follow-up, 113 children made a total recovery and are no longer considered stutterers by parents, peers, or teachers; an additional 24 children made considerable improvement or are still undergoing treatment; the 18 remaining youngsters made little or no improvement. What factors are crucial for improvement? What variables should the diagnostician consider when making a prognosis?

According to our records, the most significant improvement in therapy was noted in those cases where the following factors obtained:

1. No prior record of unsuccessful treatment (children identified and treated unsuccessfully as "primary" stutterers did poorly in our program; an absence of treatment seems more conducive to success than a history of therapeutic failure)
2. *Cooperative parents, willing to participate meaningfully in a program of counseling*
3. More severe stuttering pattern; mild stutterers showed little improvement
4. *A predominantly clonic stuttering pattern featuring struggle and escape* (children who had become adept at avoidance generally had more difficulty)
5. Cooperative teachers and other school personnel
6. *No other significant problems* (reading difficulty, a scholastic problem independent of stuttering, and so on)
7. When *the child has other resources* (expertise in scouting, athletics, music)
8. When group therapy can be utilized
9. *When it is possible to schedule intensive therapy* (at least three, preferably four, contacts a week)
10. When the child can tolerate imitating various stuttering patterns (not necessarily his own) demonstrated by the examiner

All of the factors listed are significant prognostically; however, items 2, 4, 6, 7, and 9 loom as the most critical to recovery. According to research already cited, a large number of individuals apparently outgrow stuttering between its onset and young adulthood. Certain variables, severity and family history among others, are related to spontaneous recovery, and we suggest that the reader review these investigations carefully (see Emerick and Hamre, 1972). For a convenient checklist of variables that are related to prediction of chronic stuttering, see the work of Cooper (1973) and others (Fowlie and Cooper, 1978; Riley, 1981).

For an account of therapy for young stutterers, including case studies of clinical successes and failures, see Emerick (1970). You will find much that is helpful in the contributions of Chapman (1959) and others (Willis, 1965; Van Riper, 1964; Goven and Vette, 1966; Simpson, 1966; Stennett, 1967; Anderson, 1970; Fox and Connelly, 1970; Savage, 1970; Williams, 1971; Violon, 1973; Silverman, 1974; Polow, 1975; Heistad, 1977; Dell, 1979; Emerick, 1981; Thompson, 1982).

## ASSESSMENT OF THE ADULT STUTTERER

The disorder is fully developed in the adult (adolescent and older) client: Speech interruptions are more complex and characteristically compulsive; fears and apprehensions become chronic; avoidance, disguise, and negative attitudes hamper and distort the individual's relationships with others. At this stage a speech breakdown is not simply a response, it is also a stimulus—the problem has become cyclic and self-reinforcing. Clinicians agree that the treatment of stuttering at this advanced stage is complicated and exceedingly difficult.

There is a bewildering array of treatment approaches, each with a diagnostic strategy for the problem of stuttering.[8] It is our position that no legitimate form of therapy should be denigrated, because all types of remediation have been effective with certain clients. On the other hand, no form of therapy is successful with *all* clients. On balance, then, it is reasonable to conclude that a multidimensional approach, a form of assessment and treatment that includes as many features of the disorder as possible, will yield the most lasting results.

In fact, there is overwhelming advocacy in the literature for a broad-based program of treatment for persons who stutter; clinician-investigators from all theoretical persuasions support a form of therapy that attends to the needs of the total person (Prins, 1970; Cooper, 1971; Egolf, Shames, and Blind, 1971; Perkins, 1973; Perkins et al., 1974; Andrews and Cutler, 1974; Ingham, Martin, and Kuhl, 1974; Ingham, 1975; Guitar, 1976; Klevans and Lynch, 1977; Miller, 1982). Typically, the authors cited concluded that no single conceptual framework can cope adequately with all aspects of a stutterer's problem. Miller's comments are representative:

> The establishment of fluency is only a part of the larger treatment program involving desensitization, attitudinal changes, and coping strategies. (1982: 198)

Williams's conclusions are more specific:

> Keep in mind that all a clinician can do is to help a stutterer learn to change his way of *speaking,* to change his *emotional reactions* toward himself and his listeners, and, most important, to *adjust* to those changes. (1974: 9) (Italics ours)

There appears to be a great deal of agreement, then, that the best, the most successful treatment for stuttering includes activities that help the individual alter his habitual ways of *behaving, feeling,* and *thinking*—as those three elements relate to communication in general and fluency breakdown in particular.

We believe that the same triad—speech disfluencies, emotional reactions, and mental constructs—also offers the best focus for assessment of the adult stutterer (Figure 6.6). Quite obviously, our classification is arbitrary, and there is considerable overlapping among the three dimensions. For example, a tremor can be *described* as an aspect of speech disfluency; the number of times it occurs can be counted; the anatomical locus, its duration, and release characteristics can be documented. A tremor "happens" to a person, and we also need to obtain a subjective report of what she *experiences* (panic, frustration, anger) before, during, and after its occurrence. Finally, it is important to ascertain what meaning the struggle

---

[8] Apparently, even being on a waiting list for treatment tends to reduce stuttering. See Andrews and Harvey (1981).

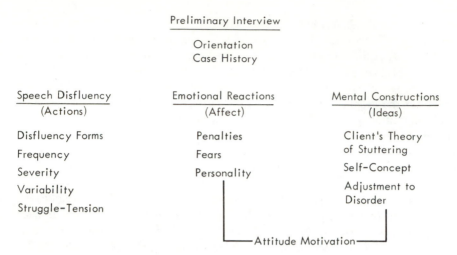

**FIGURE 6.6   Overview of assessment of adult stutters.**

pattern has for her—What is her *intent* or purpose in attempting to speak the way she did? Does she believe that talking requires a ritualistic pattern of tensing and forcing?

The evaluation process described below may seem unnescesarily lengthy and complicated.[9] We believe that the more information we have about a client, the more complete our picture of how he acts, feels, and believes, the better will be our prospects for therapeutic success. Remember, too, that we are presenting an ideal, comprehensive assessment procedure, and the clinician may, in many situations, adumbrate the outline to fit the needs of a particular individual. By all means, the evaluation delineated here can, and no doubt should, be conducted over several clinical sessions.

### Preliminary Interview

Prior to undertaking formal observation and testing, we like to perform an intake interview. This preliminary clinical session is designed to accomplish five objectives: (1) to inform the client what to expect in the diagnostic session; (2) to obtain routine information; (3) to determine why he is coming to treatment at this particular time; (4) to assemble historical information; and (5) to establish a working relationship.

Because we want the client to be a partner in the exploration of his problem, we feel it is important for him to know *what* we intend to do and *why* we propose to do it. By structuring the clinical transaction so the stutterer knows what role he is to play in his own recovery, we are establishing a therapeutic contract. Eliminating the mystery also reduces anxiety. The clinician will find it helpful to ver-

---

[9]Some clinicians, particularly those advocating a behavioral orientation, limit assessment to description and quantification of stuttering under several different speaking situations.

balize the apprehensions, embarrassment, and reservations that clients often bring to a diagnostic session.

Routine information includes the client's name, address, phone number—all the relevant identifying information (see Figure 6.5). Although generally we obtain this information by direct inquiry, in some instances when interviewing very severe stutterers, we have them fill out a standard questionnaire form. There will be sufficient opportunity later, when the client feels more comfortable with the examiner, to elicit speech samples.

The third objective of the intake interview is to determine why the client is coming (or being sent) to a speech clinician at this particular point in time. Has the individual undergone a "bottoming-out" experience, a severe crisis in her social, occupational, or educational life? What does she expect from treatment? What do others expect of her? Answers to these questions are useful in determining the client's motivation and in making a prognosis.

We feel that it is important to assemble historical information in the following areas: onset and development of stuttering; type and success of previous therapy; education; social adjustment; vocation; and avocation. In order to implement changes in a client, we need to know as much as possible about who he is and how he came to be the person he is now. If we ignore the salient features of the client's case history, we are likely to repeat old mistakes without knowing it.

Finally, the initial contact with a client is of inestimable importance in establishing a working relationship. We tried to discern the critical factors involved in an unusually swift rapport established with a client we worked with in a treatment demonstration project (Starkweather, 1972). The preliminary interview had been held in the stutterer's hometown:

> (1) The clinician demonstrated his interest by coming to the stutterer's home base. (2) The clinician is also a stutterer—we did mention this source of identification but we did not dwell on it. (3) We talked straight and tough to Joe, told him exactly what the institute entailed. Some clinicians think that a velvet-glove, Pollyanna approach is effective, but stutterers suspect this tactic, for they know deep inside that solving their problem will not be easy. (4) We invited him to take a chance, we extended a challenge which implied faith in his capabilities; everyone needs an open horizon to aim for in life's journey, and maybe we simply showed Joe the beckoning mirages ahead. Other features could be listed—we somehow revealed our competence even in that brief exchange, we showed him that we could be trusted, and we verbalized for him the lack of hope we saw in his sad features.

### Analysis of Disfluency

The clinician's primary mission in evaluation of a stutterer is to perform a careful analysis of the individual's speech disfluency behavior. An analysis should include a thorough description of the stuttering pattern (topography) and measures of the relative frequency with which various features of the pattern occur. The disfluency assessment accomplishes two basic purposes: It delineates the behaviors to be altered and it provides a base measure to which the worker can refer when monitoring the impact of treatment.

The first step in the disfluency analysis is to obtain a representative sample of the client's speech. The operative word here is *representative*; stuttering is an intermittent disorder, and the amount of difficulty an individual has is contingent on the speaking task. the situation, and other variables. If it is possible, there are obvious advantages to collecting samples of the client's "real" communication in naturalistic settings—the playground, informal group situations, the family dinner table. Generally, however, clinicians rely on data obtained from three speaking tasks: oral reading, paraphrasing, and conversation. A standard passage can be used for the reading and paraphrasing tasks. Be sure to tape-record, or better videotape, the session and note the time elapsed for each segment of the total sample; it will then be easier to specify rather precise frequency and severity values. We always ask the stutterer to discuss both neutral topics (hobbies, sports, vacations) and threatening topics (family, school, dating) to ensure that we obtain a range of speaking difficulty. It is important also to know what produces stress and how the individual responds to it; we experiment in the session with things like hurrying the client, feigning listener loss, and asking him to repeat.

*An overall description.* We commence the analysis with a global description of the individual's speech behavior. What is his normal speech like in terms of rate, rhythm, degree of tension, articulation, and voice? What are the salient features of his stuttering pattern? Here is how we described one client's disfluency:

> Predominantly fixative blocks, almost on every word (except a few stereotyped social ritual expressions or trite asides, which are generally uttered fluently) with little variation in frequency or severity in three types of talking—reading aloud, paraphrasing, and spontaneous conversation. Overall impression is of extreme tension as he moves slowly and deliberately from word to word.

*Core behaviors.* The lowest common denominators of the problem of stuttering are repetitions (oscillative phenomena) and prolongations (fixative phenomena). Although most individuals have either predominantly clonic or predominantly tonic disfluency patterns, all stutterers exhibit both forms of speech interruption. A key feature of the disfluency analysis, therefore, is a precise description of these core behaviors.

With respect to *repetitions,* we want to identify the size of the unit (phrase, whole word, syllable), the number of oscillations per unit, their tempo and degree of tension involved, and how they are terminated. Are there silent oscillations of articulatory postures? Does the client perform an articulatory posture—does he assume, for example, a bilabial valving posture prior to emission of air and sound when attempting to utter the word "bat"? Does he have difficulty finding the proper vowel during the course of the repetitions? Here is a checklist we use for observing repetitions:

*Size of unit* (record examples)
1. Phrase _____
2. Whole word _____
3. Syllable _____
4. Articulatory posture (silent oscillation)
    a. pre-forming _____
    b. incorrect posture
Coarticulation _____
Tempo _____
Tension _____
How terminated _____

In terms of *prolongations,* we are interested in the anatomical site of the fixations, whether they are silent or audible, how long they last, degree of tension involved and how they are terminated. Here is a description of the fixations of a client with very severe stuttering; note the delineation of a sequence of behaviors:

> *Fixations* of articulatory postures: silent plosives and affricatives, or audible prolongation on semivowels and fricatives; fixations may last as long as thirty seconds and be as brief as three seconds with an average duration of eight seconds; airflow shut off initially at lip or tongue-tip and gum-ridge valves, and as tension increases the locus of fixation shifts to the larynx; a fixation may be released with a surge of tension or with a deep breath and a retrial. If neither works and the tension increases, a tremor is noted.

*Struggle-tension features.*  Very rarely does a client exhibit *only* repetitions and prolongations. Anyone who has observed stutterers know that they appear tense and often make irrelevant sounds and movements while attempting to speak. Stutterers display a wide variety of these mannerisms, and they may vary in frequency of occurrence and degree of involvement in particular clients; some individuals manifest an astounding array of eye blinking, head jerking, postponement rituals, and other behaviors, whereas others appear relatively quiescent, at least overtly. Most, if not all, of these mannerisms seem to be artifacts of the individual's efforts to speak smoothly, to disguise or eliminate fluency breakdowns. Some of the behaviors no doubt arise from following bad advice (long delays may follow from continual admonitions to "think what you are going to say and then say it"); others seem to stem from automatic arousal overflow, from efforts at self-help, or from superstitious conditioning. Regardless of their origin, all the "accessory features" appear to be a variety of coping behavior that is designed either to avoid or escape from the core forms of speech interruption. It is ironic that they make the individual's problem all the more obvious.

Clinical assessment of a client's struggle-tension features has two facets: a catalog of specific mannerisms and a description of the behaviors in a time sequence. The first task is basically taxonomic—identification of the specific mannerisms displayed by the individual. The diagnostician can either devise her own checklist (see Figure 6.5 for a beginning) or choose from several published inventories. Borrowing from the "physical concomitants" portion of the *Riley Severity Instrument,* a clinician could create a simple form for recording observations of a client's pattern:

*Extraneous sounds*
  Speech related _____

  _____

  Not related _____

  _____

*Facial expressions*
  Jaw jerking _____
  Tongue protrusion _____

  _____

*Head movements*

  _____

  _____

*Extremities movement*
  Arms and hands _____

  _____

The Iowa form (Darley and Spriestersbach, 1978: 307–308) is a good choice, but we prefer the *Southern Illinois Behavior Checklist* (Brutten and Shoemaker, 1974) because it is very comprehensive (it lists ninety-seven different behaviors) and is designed so that both the client and the clinician can record the presence of various mannerisms. The Behavior Checklist is one part of a comprehensive diagnostic procedure, the *Behavior Assessment Battery,* prepared by Brutten and his associates.

Regardless of the particular format employed, it is obvious that the diagnostician will not be able to identify all of the stutterer's struggle-tension characteristics in a single session. We recommend that the worker pay particular attention to four common forms of escape behavior, and document as many of the client's avoidance techniques as possible.

The following four tension-struggle features are especially noxious to both the stutterer and his listeners:

Tension.  Identify the *site* of excess tension, its *extent* (devise a simple rating scale), and *impact* (distracting, impeding) on the act of speaking. Does the stutterer have any voluntary control over the tension? Some forms of excess muscular activity will be obvious to the examiner; in some instances, however, the clinician will have to rely on the client's report.

Tremor.  A stuttering tremor—rapid vibratory activity of various muscle groups that often follows a surge of energy to a fixated articulatory posture—is a devastating experience for the stutterer. Real panic is precipitated by a sudden loss of self-control. We must specify the anatomical *site* (the trigger points), measure the *duration,* and specify how the tremors are *released.* We include the following description of one client's tremor (again note the specification of a behavioral time sequence):

> The tremor starts at the right corner of his mouth, spreads rapidly down the right side of his face and neck; if the fixation is long (over five seconds), the tremor may extend into Joe's right arm to his index finger, which is extended in a gesture that seems to say, "just a minute."

**Release Behaviors.**  What are the stutterer's strategies for terminating strings of repetitions and escaping fixative blocks? Does she time the utterance with a movement of her head, hands, or feet? Does she redouble her efforts and blurt out the word in a sudden surge of energy? Or does she wait interminably for the "right" moment to proceed? Here is a description of releasing behaviors observed in a severe stutterer:

> *Release behaviors* included in order of frequency of use: sudden surge of tension, often accompanied by postural shift; a tongue-sucking sound ("tsk"); sucking and lip-licking movements; a spitting motion that may or may not be accompanied by saliva. The latter three release devices are infrequently used to initiate a speech attempt or as transitions between fixations seemingly to keep his oral mechanism moving.

**Stoppages of Airflow and Phonation.**  Inspect the client's speech performance for evidence of momentary occlusions of the airway. Where do these take place—the lips, velum, larynx? Are there indications of abnormal breathing—rapid, shallow respirations, flaring of the nostrils, attempts to speak on the last bit of exhaled air?

Some research (Webster and Furst, 1975; Schwartz, 1976; Hillman and Gilbert, 1977; Freeman, 1979; Zimmerman, 1980) suggests that persons who stutter may have basic physiological difficulties in the coordination of respiration, phonation, and articulation. Hutchinson (1975) found several distinct and unusual aerodynamic patterns associated with stuttered speech; the implication is that stuttering may be an anomaly in the initiation, timing, and maintenance of airflow and phonation. Schwartz (1976) describes the respiratory abnormality observed in stutterers as the primitive airway dilation reflex; a laryngospasm with complete abduction of the vocal folds is triggered by "kinks" or stoppages of the airway by the core repetitions and prolongations. Further research is needed to clarify the possible role of "glottal spasms" and aerodynamic anomalies in the onset and perpetuation of stuttering. At present the instrumentation employed by investigators in this area is impractical for diagnostic purposes; however, biofeedback (EMG) techniques may be one method of detecting the location of airflow and phonation stoppages.

We are also interested in *how much* and *what types* of avoidance behavior the client exhibits. Clinically, avoidance behavior is an important feature to deal with because it tends to reinforce and compound the stutterer's difficulty. Rather than diminishing, fears tend to incubate and grow when a person recoils from them; avoidances keep the apprehension high and the problem expanding.

Avoidance behavior may take several forms. It is useful, we feel, to identify two broad categories which we have termed *primary* and *secondary*. Primary avoidance is characterized by the speaker's attempts to alter the act of speaking per se: Although evading, the individual is still utilizing oral communication as his battleground. Several types of primary avoidance may be identified:

Starters.   Starters are words, sounds, gestures, or rituals that stutterers use to get the flow of speech initiated. Often a series of starters may become chained together in an elaborate delaying tactic.

Postponement.   Some stutterers attempt to delay the act of speaking or of uttering a specific word by utilizing periods of silence (pretending to think what they intend to say), by ritualistic devices (licking of lips, stereotyped body movements), or with verbal stalling or filibustering.

Retrials.   A retrial is another form of postponement whereby the stutterer lets the needle stick on the part of the sentence that he has uttered fluently. Some stutterers back up and repeat a sentence or phrase over and over again in a vain attempt to hurdle the barrier of a feared word.

Circumlocutions.   Some stutterers become very adept at selecting words on which they feel they will not stutter, at rearranging sentences to evade encounter with their anticipation of impending difficulty. Often this makes the individual sound stupid and silly.

Antiexpectancy.   In this type of avoidance, the stutterer attempts to alter the communication context to reduce or eliminate his anticipation of difficulty. He may do this by talking in an accent, speaking in a rhythmic manner, or with overprecise articulation; he may do it by making a joke of everything, or even by singing. One stutterer told us that he usually pulled into a gas station, rolled down the window, and sang brightly, "Fill 'er up to the brim." Antiexpectancy is the most malignant type of primary avoidance because it (1) produces more fluency than the other types, thus increasing the dread of stuttering, (2) lets the stutterer masquerade as a fluent speaker, and (3) tends to distort the individual's self-concept.

Secondary avoidance is characterized by reduction in or cessation of communication: the stutterer retreats from the act of talking. Although many clients manifest both primary and secondary avoidance behavior, some individuals in the more advanced stages of the disorder employ the latter almost exclusively. There are two basic types of secondary avoidance:

1.  *Reducing verbal output or not talking at all*—Silence is viewed as protective, and some stutterers would rather sit silently and be thought a fool than to open their mouth and betray their disorder.

2. *Depending on others for communication*—Many stutterers have had, at one time or another, a relative or friend who talked for them and protected them from verbal demands. We have even seen a few stutterers who were almost totally dependent on another person for communication with the outside world.

*Frequency of disfluency.* How often does the client stutter? After making an inventory of the specific behaviors that comprise a client's pattern of stuttering, the diagnostician will want to determine the frequency with which moments of stuttering (a global measure) and components of the block (a molecular analysis) are emitted. More specifically, the clinician seeks answers to the following four questions:

1. We like to obtain a global measure first: *On how many words did the client stutter relative to the total number of words uttered?* This procedure yields a ratio (or percentage) of stuttered words to the total number of possible words. Some workers use the syllable as the unit of measure and record the number of stuttered syllables relative to the total number of syllables uttered. Another way to obtain a frequency measure is to compute the number of moments of stuttering for a given time segment; the worker divides the number of stuttered words by the time spent talking and obtains a simple ratio of stutterings per minute.

Some stutterers talk very slowly; a range of 130 to 250 words per minute is considered normal; Wingate (1976) suggests that 200 syllables per minute be used as a normative frame of reference if the diagnostician prefers to use syllables as the unit of measure. Although they emit very few moments of stuttering, their speech patterns are clearly abnormal. It is helpful to record the rate of each client's speech, as one index of recovery from stuttering is an increase in the number of words uttered for a given time segment.

Beginning diagnosticians may find it difficult to count reliably moments of stuttering, and we suggest they make several assessments of the same speech sample; it is also helpful to compare results with those of other clinicians.

2. *What is the relative rate of emission of the various components of the moment of stuttering?* A simple frequency count of moments of stuttering masks differences in the extent to which the elements of a block vary (Brutten, 1975). A moment of stuttering is, after all, a process, not a static entity, and its components—core behaviors and coping mannerisms—are probably different kinds of events. Here is a portion of a molecular analysis:

**Tasks**

| COMPONENTS | READING | CONVERSATION | TOTAL |
|---|---|---|---|
| Part-word reps | /// | ⊥HT /// | 11 |
| Fixations | | /// | 3 |
| Retrials | | /// | 3 |
| Lip smacking | // | ⊥HT //// | 11 |
| Head movement | | / | 1 |
| Eyes closed | / | //// | 5 |

3. *Do the various components that comprise the moments of stuttering vary together in any regular manner?* Do the subelements increase or decrease simultaneously? As one component increases, do others decrease in rate of occurrence? Does there seem to be a sequential pattern of behaviors—first an eye blink, then a head movement, and so on.

4. *Does the frequency of moments of stuttering—or its components—vary by time segments?* Does it vary by type of speaking task—reading, paraphrasing, conversation? Is there evidence of adaptation or consistency in successive reduplications of the same material?

It is important to remember that we are counting instances of behavior for specific purposes—as one measure of severity and, more important, to establish a base rate for monitoring the impact of treatment. Some workers we know carry the counting aspect to an absurd level and tend to obscure the client with all their charts.

*Severity.*   There are several extant measures of stuttering severity (already cited), but none has achieved a high degree of precision. Clinically, in our work with adult stutterers, we prefer to use the Van Riper Severity Equation (1982: 200–203) because it includes so many of the pertinent variables:

$$S = aF + bD_1 + cD_2 + dT_1 + eT_2 + fA + gE$$

where

$F$ = frequency of stuttered words as a percentage of spoken words
$D_1$ = average duration of a stuttering moment
$D_2$ = duration of the longest stuttering moment
$T_1$ = average tension of a stuttering moment
$T_2$ = amount of tension in the stuttering moment of greatest tension
$A$ = amount of avoidance
$E$ = amount of emotional involvement

Van Riper includes a profile of stuttering severity that we find useful in assessment of an adult client:

| SCALE | FREQUENCY | TENSION-STRUGGLE | DURATION | POSTPONEMENT-AVOIDANCE |
|---|---|---|---|---|
| 1 | Under 1% | None | Under ½ sec. | None |
| 2 | 1– 2% | Rare but present | Average ½ sec. | Less than 5% |
| 3 | 3– 5% | Usual but mild | Average 1 sec. | 5–10% |
| 4 | 6– 8% | Severe | Average 2 sec. | 11–12% |
| 5 | 9–12% | Very severe | Average 3 sec. | 21–31% |
| 6 | 13–25% | Overflow to eyes and limbs | Average 4 sec. | 31–70% |
| 7 | More than 25% | Overflow to trunk | Average longer than 5 sec. | More than 70% |

Any estimate of severity should also include the client's own perceptions of the magnitude of her problem. The clinician can obtain the stutterer's self-rating of severity in the interview or by administering the *Perceptions of Stuttering Inventory* (Woolf, 1967). The *PSI* is an instrument devised to assess three dimensions of stuttering behavior—struggle, avoidance, and expectation—as perceived by the stutterer; it yields a profile that the examiner can then compare to scores obtained by a reference group of stutterers.

*Variation in frequency and severity.*  We have alluded several times to the fact that stuttering is an intermittent disorder. Variations in the frequency and severity of stuttering are of interest to the diagnostician for several reasons. There may be specific cues (sounds, words, speaking situations) associated with exacerbation or remission of stuttering, and the identification of these variables may be useful for treatment. It may be possible to commence arraying the various cues in a hierarchy desensitization; it demonstrates to the client that his disorder is subject to variation and that change is possible. Finally, by knowing what factors reduce stuttering, the clinician will be able to distinguish between temporary fluency and genuine remedial gains.

When evaluating an adult who stutters we search for evidence of several types of variability:

Cycles of Stuttering.  Does the individual report daily, weekly, or monthly variations in the frequency and severity of his stuttering? If so, do these swings seem to be related to personal or environmental variables? We asked five stutterers to keep careful records of the frequency and severity of their stuttering for several months and compared the results to computerized charts of their intellectual, emotional, and physical biorhythms. Although the correlations were low, we did observe a negative relationship between frequency of stuttering and the emotional dimensions for four of the clients. See the work of Quarrington (1956) and Sheehan (1969) for information on cyclic variations in stuttering.

Situation-Listener Variables.  The diagnostician should review the types of speaking situations and listeners that increase or decrease the client's stuttering. This can be accomplished by interviewing the person or by having her fill out a checklist. The clinician can devise a form for recording data (simply list different speaking situations, topics of conversation) or use a published inventory (Darley and Spriestersbach, 1978: 317-319). The *Speech Situation Checklist* prepared by Brutten and Shoemaker (1974) is particularly useful; the client is asked to rate herself on the degree of emotional response and severity of speech disruption in fifty-one life situations; Shames and Egolf (1976: 40-41) list various circumstances (audience size, specific people, different talking situations) and suggest tactics for sampling actual speech behavior under those conditions.

In addition to listing the conditions under which stuttering is increased or reduced, the diagnostician should ask the client to rank-order the items in terms of speech difficulty and emotional impact.

**Word and Sound Fears.** Many stutterers report that they have particular difficulty with certain words and speech sounds. We make a list of these items and then determine later, by examining the speech sample, if he does in fact stutter more on some sounds or words. During trial therapy we like to show the client how he can ameliorate his stuttering by picking his most feared word or sound; it can be a very vivid demonstration of the efficacy of treatment.

**Response to Altering Listening-Speaking Set.** The final aspect of an assessment of variability involves a determination of the impact of altering the client's listening-speaking set. There are several ways to do this: delayed auditory feedback, masking noise, biofeedback, choral reading. We even have the client try to suppress voluntarily either moments of stuttering or particular subelements (avoidances, grimaces, or other mannerisms). The ease with which a client's pattern of disfluency is altered is related to prognosis: The more resistant the stuttering is to change, the less favorable the predicted outcome of treatment. Some clients are startled, and heartened, to learn that their stuttering pattern is not immutable, that they can change the way they talk.

*Expectancy.* Most stutterers can tell—on some level of awareness—when they are going to stutter; some can predict quite accurately when they will have difficulty, as this illustration shows:

> Joe read a passage silently, marking words on which he thought he would stutter if he read the same passage aloud; when he did read it aloud, his prediction was 93 percent accurate. He described his anticipation of stuttering in this manner: "I know I am going to have trouble getting the word out, and I feel inside like someone is going to jump on me." His posture is consonant with his report—his shoulders bend forward and sag down in a cowed, shrinking manner.

Anticipation of stuttering is unpleasant, to put it mildly, and acts as a trigger to release a chain of coping behaviors—tension, avoidance, struggle. Thus, it is important to discern a client's level of expectancy.

*Efforts at self-therapy.* Sometimes it is difficult, if not impossible, to distinguish between the stuttering behavior and the things the person does to help himself talk without stuttering. We have already described how the clinician makes an inventory of the core behaviors and the struggle-tension features. In this section we are concerned with the most salient methods the client employs to "help himself talk without stuttering." Do they really help, or do they impede the flow of speech? How committed is he to these techniques as a "solution" to his difficulty? Keep in mind that all these behaviors, which we classify as self-defeating, represent his best efforts at solving the dilemma of his disfluency. They have been successful on occasion and he will resist their removal in treatment.

*Poststuttering behavior.*   How does the client behave after he has stuttered? Does he report feelings of guilt, hostility, embarrassment, or shame? Does he withdraw? Does he experience relief? Here is how a clinician described the poststuttering behavior manifested by one stutterer:

> He lowers his eyelids, feigns a relaxed or indifferent posture, and may spit silently several times (as if saying, "I just stuttered, but so what, I am still cool and it does not bother me."). Covertly, however, the client reports feeling "stupid" and "inferior" after stuttering.

The facets of a complete disfluency analysis are summarized in Figure 6.7.

### Evaluation of Emotional Reactions

According to several authoritative reviews of available research (Sheehan, 1970; Bloodstein, 1981; Wingate, 1976), as well as extensive clinical evidence, stutterers are not psychologically different from nonstutterers; the fluency breakdown is not symptomatic of neurosis or psychosis. Nor do stutterers as a group exhibit a "typical" personality.

We are not insinuating, however, that persons who stutter are undisturbed or emotionally quiescent about their speech problem. In fact, because oral communication is such a significant human attribute, an impairment of speech, particularly one that has no obvious overt basis and is intermittent in nature, affects a person in a very human sort of way. It is a common clinical observation that stuttering does contaminate, to varying degrees, how clients *feel* about themselves and about persons with whom they interact. Would it not be rather unusual for the individual to have no or very little emotional reaction to a disorder that disrupts his personal, occupational, educational, and social functioning? Experienced clinicians report that stutterers exhibit the same range of emotions seen in persons afflicted with other disorders that disrupt significant aspects of human functioning.

**FIGURE 6.7   Summary of disfluency analysis.**

| | |
|---|---|
| 1. *Global Description* | 5. *Severity* |
| 2. *Core Behaviors*<br>—Repetitions<br>—Prolongations | 6. *Variability*<br>—Cycles<br>—Situation-listeners<br>—Word-sound fears<br>—Trial therapy |
| 3. *Struggle-Tension Features*<br>—Tension<br>—Tremor<br>—Release<br>—Airflow-phonation<br>—Avoidances | 7. *Expectancy* |
| | 8. *Efforts at Self-Therapy* |
| | 9. *Poststuttering Behavior* |
| 4. *Frequency*<br>—Molar<br>—Molecular | |

Although there is no "typical stuttering personality," a number of emotional reactions are commonly observed during diagnosis and treatment. Stutterers, on the average, are not as well adjusted as nonstutterers; they have lower levels of aspiration and lower self-esteem; they tend to exhibit patterns of social withdrawal, sometimes associated with feelings of anger, resentment, shame, and fearfulness. Feelings of frustration, embarrassment, and hostility are also common. We are not impugning that stuttering is *caused* by emotional factors—except in the sense that they compound the individual's problem—but rather that they are a *consequence* of stuttering. Our position is that the clinician must recognize the importance of the negative feelings associated with stuttering and deal with them openly in diagnosis and treatment.

It is generally wise for the diagnostician to regard her observations and test scores as tentative, working assumptions. This guideline is particularly relevant when evaluating a client's emotional reactions to stuttering. Because of the sensitive and personal nature of the clinical tasks, the examiner should be aware that assembling data with respect to feelings may extend well beyond the boundaries of one or two sessions. A complete evaluation in this area includes information from five sources: the client's report; informal tests and observations; formal tests; physiological measures; and referral for psychological appraisal.

*The client's report.* The easiest and most direct way to determine how a person feels about something is to ask him. We find that we got better responses from clients who stutter by *leading into* questions about feelings. Instead of asking directly about how he feels—a generic question he may find difficult to answer—we commence with queries like these: What is he aware of in the process of stuttering—before, during and right after it occurs? Is he more aware of the reactions of his listeners or his own internal state? What bothers him the most about stuttering? The least? What are his major satisfactions, hopes, deprivations?

It may be easier for the client to write her responses. In this case, the diagnostician can use an inventory, such as the *Fear Survey Schedule* devised by Brutten and Shoemaker (1974); this device contains fifty-one items to which the stutterer can respond employing a five-step rating scale. Some clinicians prefer to have the stutterer prepare an autobiography or prepare a vignette in which she describes herself as if she were a character in a play. Whatever method is used, the diagnostician attempts to delineate the range of emotions, arrange them into thematic content categories, and begin the process of establishing rankings or hierarchies.

Like normal speakers, persons who stutter vary in their ability to *express* their feelings verbally. The key word is *express,* as many stutterers learn to hide their disorder, to pretend that it doesn't bother them, to wear a mask of indifference. Genuine expression of feelings is discouraged for cover-up, image making, or retreating behind a facade. Perhaps we are too harsh, but it is hard to ignore the extreme popularity of encounter groups, pop psychology fads, and telephone-listening services. It seems apparent that something is lacking in our day-to-day relationships.

The point we are making is this: Strong forces augur against a person talking openly about his hopes and fears, and we may have to help the client learn to accept and express his feelings in relation to his problem of stuttering. There are several techniques for assisting the person to get in touch with himself. First, the clinician should consult the large body of information about enhancing self-awareness (Stevens, 1971). The adjustment inventories and self-inspection checklists published by Fox and Connelly (1970) and Chapman (1959) are also useful, especially when the results are analyzed in a group setting. Finally, we often ask our clients to keep daily logs of their moods in relation to their stuttering and listener reactions. This provides a body of information that is useful for counseling.

*Informal tests and observation.*  A significant amount of information about the client's personality and emotional adjustment can be obtained by direct observation, interviews with her relatives, scrutiny of documents in her school file, and the administration of various indirect and nonstandardized testing procedures. From these data, the diagnostician tries to assemble answers to the following questions:

1. What are the salient features of the client's personality? Is he basically shy, aggressive, anxious, guilty, or do other adjectives apply? How does he confront problems? Are there special features of his personality—phobias, obsessive-compulsive behavior, nervous tics, enuresis—that may confound treatment? What are the client's major assets and liabilities?

2. How does the client perceive himself relative to his stuttering problem? That is, how salient is his problem in regard to his self-image and day-to-day functioning? We have seen some clients whose stuttering problem completely dominates their life; it dictates their occupation, their friends, even their choice of a marriage partner. There are several ways, all very limited in their scientific rigor, to gain some insight into a client's self-view: the use of free drawing (Bar and Jakab, 1969), open-ended sentences (Griffith, 1969) and queries such as "What would you do differently if you woke up in the morning and no longer stuttered? How might the diagnostician use word association tasks or the W-A-Y (Who are you?) technique (Zelen, Sheehan, and Bugental, 1954) to gain additional information?

3. How does the client handle the moment of stuttering? Although there are no significant personality differences between stutterers and the rest of the population, when the stutterer is struggling in a block he feels very different from everyone else:

What is it like to stutter? Think of yourself on a highway. It's dark. You're in a hurry. No traffic. You squeeze on the gas. Suddenly, out of nowhere, directly in front of you, looms the terrifying back of a huge truck. Horror! Slam on the brakes, spin the wheel, swerve, pray. Anything to keep from colliding. The truck is the word that looms ahead of a stutterer. You can't always tell what word it will be. But suddenly you see one that could spell trouble.

Each moment of stuttering is a miniature crisis (Goraj, 1974). Fear and panic flood the person's consciousness; the autonomic nervous system is triggered into action, increasing pulse rate and blood pressure; the individual feels trapped, helpless, and disoriented. Some stutterers actually "tune out" from their surroundings temporarily.

Is there any meaning in the way a client goes about his stuttering? Is the act of stuttering revealing of self? Some stutterers feign bewilderment; others an uneasy amusement; some appear to whimper and moan; a few stutter in an aggressive, hostile manner, and others remain inert, frozen until the panic passes. At present, all our attempts to read the meaning of how a person "chooses" to stutter are highly speculative.

*Formal tests.*    There are several personality inventories that purport to assess some facets of an individual's psychological adjustment. We believe that, for the most part, these inventories are of limited value in the evaluation of an adult stutterer. The *Minnesota Multiphasic Personality Inventory, Bell Adjustment Inventory* and *Eysenck Personality Inventory* are probably the most useful for clinical purposes (Ellis, 1946; Wiener, 1947; Eysenck and Eysenck, 1963).

*Physiological measures.*    Another method of identifying emotional reactions to stuttering is to measure indices of autonomic arousal. The palmar sweat index, galvanic skin response, blood pressure and pulse rate changes, and variations in respiration are all useful if the clinician has access to the appropriate equipment. These measures assist in planning a regimen of desensitization.

*Referral for psychological appraisal.*    Although few stutterers require psychological appraisal, from time to time such a referral is indicated. (See Chapter 3 for general guidelines.) Be sure to inform the client *at the outset* of a diagnostic session that it may be necessary to look at his problem from many perspectives, including the psychological. A consultation of our clinical files revealed a number of reasons for referral of individual stutterers: conflicting information (the client says that stuttering doesn't bother him and yet restricts his life severely because of the disorder); presence of other problems (marital, academic, familial); repeated failures in professional treatment programs; and a significant amount of secondary gain (pity, excuse for failure, attention) derived from the disorder.

### Appraisal of Mental Constructs

In this final section we are concerned with how the client *thinks* about her stuttering problem: What type of mental images does she have about oral communication in general and disfluent speech in particular?

To a great extent, humans process the universe and direct their behavior by reference to mental constructs or analogs of reality. Through the use of language symbols, we can create cognitive models that filter or mediate between the environment and ourselves. The meaning of an experience for a person, and the intent and nature of his responses, can be understood more clearly by examining his mental images (Werner, 1982).

A person's images can be altered significantly by an anomaly. Criminals, alcoholics, and obese individuals not only *act* and *feel* different; they also come to *think* in different ways. In order to help them change their behavior, it is also necessary to modify their mental constructs. The same situation prevails in dealing with the stutterer (though we are *not* saying that stuttering is the same type of problem as obesity or alcoholism); repeated failures in oral communication create a host of negative images that hamper his ongoing performance. He comes to believe that there are certain things he must do in order to speak, and his intentions become new obstacles. Gradually, the stutterer's self-image as a talker becomes almost totally infiltrated with these abnormal mental schema. At this point, stuttering is perpetuated because he becomes highly skilled at it:

> No wonder the stutterer keeps on exercising this skill of his. He knows how to relate to people when he stutters but they are a mystery to him when he does not. (Fransella, 1972: 70)

We maintain that a form of treatment that identifies and alters cognitive components of stuttering—as well as overt speech behavior and emotional reactions—is far more effective than those that focus on only one aspect. We could cite many others, but a single example will illustrate: Desensitization, a popular form of therapy for negative emotion, is far more potent when rational elements are included (Kazdin and Wilcoxon, 1976; Moleski and Tosi, 1976).

HIGHLIGHT   *Cognitive Therapy*

It is rather easy to get an adult stutterer to speak fluently in certain situations—almost anyone can do it. With appropriate therapy, in many cases, the client even reduces his panic and anxiety about talking. But it is difficult to maintain these gains; relapse is a common problem in the treatment of persons who stutter. Why is the problem so persistent? Although many variables are involved in therapeutic relapse, the most common culprit, in our clinical experience, is the client's mental attitude.

Long after the speech and affect dimensions of a client's problem have improved, she may still have deeply imbedded, negative, self-defeating mental images. Sometimes, particularly when she encounters a difficult speaking situation, the stutterer unwittingly sets herself up for failure with old, irrational automatic thoughts. In short, although her speech may be relatively fluent, she still *thinks* like a stutterer. We include here a portion of a weekly report prepared by a client that illustrates the importance of positive mental imagery:

> I was really bummed out for a while last night. We, my fiancée and me, went to a movie with another couple. I had never met either the

guy or the girl. But things were going pretty well. I was talking O.K., until we decided to stop for chow at a fast-food place. When I went with the other guy to the counter to order, I got hung up on the *h* in hamburger. No sound, not a squeak. The counterperson filled in for me, of course. I acted like a real nerd the rest of the evening—quiet, withdrawn, a bit sullen. Later, when I thought about the situation the way you suggested, I think I figured out what happened. It wasn't the stuttering that caused me to be anxious and angry, it was the internal imagery, how I *interpreted* the event that bugged me. It surprised me, in retrospect, how fast I started playing my old "tragedy tapes." "Damn," I thought automatically, "I'm having a relapse." There I was in the middle of Burger King acting like Chicken Little: One out-of-control block and I make a catastrophe out of it. The stuttering sky is falling! A single slip and I no longer see myself as capable. You know, I'm going to listen carefully for more of those old thoughts and devise some better self-messages.

## Three Steps of Therapy

In cognitive therapy, we attempt to deal directly with the stutterer's incorrect premises and distorted mental imagery. Three steps are utilized: identifying the faulty thought patterns, subjecting them to reality testing, and then formulating more positive substitutes.

*Identification.*    First, the stutterer must make an inventory of his negative images, thoughts, and expectations. Here are instructions we gave to one adult client to study his mental imagery:

We all have certain ideas that may or may not be helpful—these are the automatic thoughts that intervene between an event (A) and how we feel about it (C). We will call these mental constructs (B).

Some mental constructs are *general* and may or may not relate to stuttering. Here are some examples:

—Making mistakes is terrible.
—My emotions cannot be controlled.
—Everyone must like me or I will be miserable.

But some, and these are of more interest to us right now in therapy, are *specific* to stuttering. Again, here are some examples:

—If I stutter, people will think I'm dumb.
—I must talk in a hurry because the listener's time is very important.
—I must play the quiet role in a group.

Now, during the next week, try to keep track of those little automatic thoughts. Use this simple format to record your observations:

*Event* (A)        *Thoughts* (B)        *Emotional Response* (C)

*Reality testing.*    After the client has assembled her repertoire of mental constructs, we help her assess each of them on a logical basis. We teach her to evaluate and challenge the automatic thoughts rather than blindly accept them. Here are only three of the questions that can guide the reality testing:

— Do they (the mental constructs) help accomplish the therapy goals?
— Do they make me feel better?
— Do they help me get along better with other people?

*Formulating substitutes.* The third and final step in cognitive therapy is the development of new, positive mental imagery. The stutterer is taught to tell himself "stop!" when he uses a self-defeating thought and then consciously shift to some alternative, more therapeutically helpful statements.

This brief description does not do justice to the wide range of methodology employed by cognitive therapists, but it does illustrate the basic strategies. For more information on the cognitive approach, consult the work of Beck (1976) and others (Goldfried and Merbaum, 1973; Mahoney, 1974; Emery, Hollon, and Bedrosian, 1981; McMullin and Giles, 1981; Maxwell, 1982; Werner, 1982; Turk, Meichenbaum, and Genest, 1983).

Diagnostically, we explore four dimensions of a client's mental constructs regarding stuttering: his theory about his stuttering, his attitude, his motivation, and the type of adjustments he has made to the disorder. To illustrate the scope of activity in assessment of these four dimensions, we include a memorandum prepared by a diagnostic team:

There is, of course, a great deal of overlapping in the four areas we will explore with the client. In addition, you should have some good clinical hunches regarding the answers to the questions posed in each area on the basis of other contacts with the client. Here are some guidelines for the assessment.

*The client's theory.* We are interested in his theory about the onset and nature of his stuttering because it influences his personal and social adjustment, propels him to undertake certain forms of self-therapy, and may interfere with the treatment program we devise. How does he talk about his stuttering? Does the way in which he talks reflect personal responsibility for his behavior, or does he infer that stuttering is somewhere inside him, that words won't come out (Williams, 1957)? Does he confuse the consequences of stuttering—nervousness, excitement—for what causes it? Do his assumptions about his problem compound it; for example, does he worry that he is psychologically disturbed? What can be discerned about his *intent* or purpose when he uses various mannerisms during speech attempts? Does he believe he can improve? Does he exhibit a form of helplessness, an attitude that his life and actions are simply beyond his control (Adams, 1983)? What does he think he needs to do in order to improve?[10]

[10]Silverman (1980) has prepared the *Stuttering Problem Profile* to assist both client and clinician in identifying the goals of therapy. This instrument features eighty-six statements ("I am usually willing to stutter openly"; "I am usually willing to use the telephone") that the stutterer would like to be able to make at the end of treatment.

*Attitude.* The client's attitude toward her disorder—a composite of both emotional and cognitive elements—is pivotal to her recovery (Quesal and Shank, 1978; Guitar and Bass, 1978). To a significant extent, a stutterer's attitude about her problem may reflect attitudes of the nonstuttering population toward the disorder. A strong, unfavorable stereotype does exist and apparently it is unaffected by exposure to stuttering (Woods and Williams, 1976); there is even evidence that speech clinicians share this negative image of stutterers (Tracy and Hood, 1976).

There are two popular inventories of a stutterer's attitude. The *Iowa Attitude Scale Toward Stuttering* (Johnson and Ammons, 1944) samples a client's reaction to questions like "A husband who stutters should try to have his wife answer the doorbell or telephone." The respondent indicates his degree of agreement or disagreement by circling one of five scale values. If the *Iowa Scale* is used, look for the following things: the intensity of the client's reactions, the relationship between scale scores and his observed behavior, evidence of projection or paranoid responses, and whether his responses are equivocal.

The instrument devised by Erickson (1969) is a more objective measure of attitude. The final form of his thirty-nine-item *S-Scale* evaluates the extent to which a stutterer's communication attitude deviates from those of nonstutterers. Andrews and Cutler (1974) analyzed the relationship between speech-fluency changes and attitude using a short version of the Erickson scale. They found that the subjects' attitudes did not change after they achieved fluency and conclude that "it may be important that successful treatment requires not only that stutterers speak normally but also that they believe themselves to be as effective as normal speakers in their interaction with others" (Andrews and Cutler, 1974: 317).

*Motivation.* How much does the stutterer want to get better—what is she willing to sacrifice in terms of time, expense, energy, and temporary discomfort? Is she being pushed into treatment by others (fiancé, parent, employer)? Can various forms of resistance (denial, intellectualization, and so forth) be seen during the diagnostic session (Starkweather, 1974)?

To broaden the concept of motivation, use the following paradigm. Prepare a chart with three categories, *motivation, opportunity,* and *capacity,* and then list as many factors as possible under each category. Try to assign a weight or priority ranking to the factors. See if you can extend on this heuristic model:

| MOTIVATION | OPPORTUNITY | CAPACITY |
|---|---|---|
| Utility of the speech change | Family cooperation | Personal adjustment |
| Cost to the client | Frequency of therapy | Social adjustment |
| Self-estimate regarding probability of success | Distance to be traveled for therapy | Severity of problem |
| History of achievement | | |
| Current level of aspiration | Others | Attitude |
| Secondary gains derived from defective speech | | General health and vitality |
| Others | | Others |

*Adjustments to the disorder.* We need to determine the degree to which the client has adjusted to the problem of stuttering. For a number of adults, stuttering becomes a way of life, a familiar means of structuring responses to his social environment. When he is uncertain or anxious about a particular situation, he can gain a measure of self-control—in the sense that the results are predictable—by returning to old habits of disfluency (Fransella, 1972). But habits are like fences: they provide a modicum of protection but limit an individual's range of freedom. We have seen stutterers who had considerable difficulty adjusting to fluency; speech without stuttering was not a facet of their personal system of mental imagery. Almost without exception, the stutterers who achieved lasting improvement in their speech also underwent significant changes in their lifestyle.

Now, more specifically, seek answers to the following questions in the diagnostic-therapeutic sessions:

1. What does she do because she stutters? In what respects does she narrow or limit her life, her choice of roles? One client reported that he waited outside a coffee shop every morning until a particular waitress to whom he could speak freely came on duty. Another said he always ordered fish in fast-food restaurants because that is what he could say fluently.
2. How realistic is the client's view of his potential as a person if he acquires fluent speech? Many stutterers harbor a Demosthenes fantasy: If only they were fluent speakers, they could do mighty deeds. A few even seem to look at life as if it were a dress rehearsal and believe that someday they will have a chance to play it over again. It is sometimes difficult to relinquish a dream for the demanding labor that speech therapy requires.
3. What advantages accrue to the client because he stutters? Does he use his speech problem as a ready excuse for failure? Does he use it as an excuse to get out of responsibility? To what extent is stuttering an attention-attracting device for the client? Does he use his problem as a badge or an ornament?

A more formal testing technique for assessment of the cognitive dimensions of stuttering is the *Role Construct Repertory Test* (Fransella, 1972). This instrument evaluates the nature of an individual's adjustments to a disorder by tapping his responses to queries regarding social interaction, forcefulness, self-sufficiency, and other aspects. The client is asked to rate himself "when he is stuttering," "when he is fluent," and "as others see me."

One final admonition: Remember that most everyone's adjustment is relatively fragile; do not attempt to break through a client's protective shell too soon or too forcefully.

### Prognosis

Making a prognosis of success and failure in stuttering therapy is a little like predicting next season's fashions—even though the territory to be covered has finite limits, the possible variations make precise forecasting impossible. In the past eighteen years, we have seen more than 300 adult stutterers, and for each client we made a private prognosis about the outcome of treatment. Our accuracy is only slightly better than 50 percent, which, interestingly enough, corresponds almost exactly with our ratio of therapeutic success. Some of the most disabled clients have made startling recoveries, often despite an awesome array of negative environmental factors. On the other hand, stutterers with an impressive number of personal advantages have failed to make a significant shift in their behavior. Even more confusing, many clinicians have been startled, as we have been, when a stutterer with whom we had only minimal success later returns and, talking easily, offers his thanks for our help. (For a fascinating account of success and failure in stuttering therapy, see the Speech Foundation booklet edited by Luper, 1968.) But perhaps we have overstated the dangers of prophecy in clinical work with stutterers; there are, in fact, a number of considerations that therapists find useful in predicting a client's potential for treatment.

The following is an incomplete and heuristic list of factors that help in making prognoses. (See the articles by Boberg, Howie, and Woods, 1979; and Perkins, 1983.) The items are presented in random order, for at present we have no data that would allow us to assign weight to them.

*Severity.*   Paradoxically, the more severe stutterers, other factors being equal (which they seldom are), seem to make better progress than do milder stutterers. Perhaps the reason is that contemporary therapy is especially designed for the more involved cases. The only way they have to go is up; they have nothing to lose but their blocks. The mild stutterers, on the other hand, do get by, and it is difficult for them to relinquish their symptoms for the dubious sanctuary of "fluent stuttering."

*Motivation.*   You can lead a client to the therapy room, but you can't make him follow the plan of treatment. Motivation is, of course, a most significant variable in all types of therapy.

*Timing.*   A client's motivation for treatment is often related to crucial life experiences; stutterers who have reached a critical stage and feel blocked by their disordered speech, barred from job advancement, education, or marriage, and voluntarily seek therapy have a more favorable prognosis.

*Age.*   Adolescents, particularly between the ages of thirteen and sixteen, are especially resistant to therapy. Similarly, clients over forty tend to do poorly in treatment, probably because older individuals are more rigid, and somehow, they have made an accommodation with stuttering.

*Sex.*   Women seem to be more difficult to treat in stuttering therapy than men. Our own records show not a single therapeutic success with adolescent girls.

*Nonstuttered speech.*   The more well integrated the client's nonstuttered speech (in terms of prosody), the better the prognosis.

*Type of stuttering.*   Predominantly repetitive stutterers make more rapid progress than do predominantly fixative stutterers; clients who feature escape reactions are easier to work with than chronic avoiders. Interiorized stutterers—especially those manifesting laryngeal blocking—are very resistant to therapy.

*Attitude.*   The better the client's pretreatment attitude, the more successful will be the outcome of treatment (Guitar, 1976).

*Organic or neurotic concomitants.*   Clients presenting organic complications (sensory impairment, motor slowness) or neurotic symptoms (compulsions and conversion symptoms) require more prolonged treatment and do less well than stutterers who do not have those characteristics.

*Identification.*   The interpersonal relationship is crucial in stuttering therapy; the stutterer and clinician must come to share a common set of values, at least regarding the solution of the fluency problem. Clients who exhibit unusual lifestyles (social withdrawal, compulsivity, overcompensation, and so on) tend to see participation in therapy as an act of submission.

*Prior therapy.*   It is far worse to have tried and failed than never to have tried at all. Clients with a history of therapeutic failure have a poor prognosis.

*False fluency.*   Sudden, dramatic fluency early in treatment—we have even seen the phenomenon in trial therapy—is a poor prognostic sign. It rarely lasts and the client is often devastated upon the return of his symptoms. A rapid "flight to health" is generally attributed to suggestion.

*The stutterer's environment.*   The prospects for successful treatment are enhanced by a supportive environment (Tharp and Wetzel, 1969). However, be wary of relatives or friends who say, when change is discussed, "But we love him just the way he is now. We don't notice the stuttering." Secondary gains—benefits from being a stutterer—are tough therapeutic competitors. In some instances, clients with good social adjustments find it more difficult to change than persons who are socially maladjusted (Prins and Miller, 1973).

*Inconsistency.*   Variability in the client's stuttering pattern and fluctuation in her self-concept are good prognostic signs. Clients who exhibit cycles in the frequency and severity of their stuttering seem to make better progress than those who do not. Perhaps they can see the possibility for change.

*Assets and liabilities.*   Except in cases of overcompensation, clients who have acknowledged expertise or talent in some area make better progress than individuals with an excess of liabilities.

*Intensive therapy.*   Token treatment is worse than no treatment at all. When intensive therapy (minimal daily contact of at least one hour) is available and the client can participate in a comprehensive program, the prospects for recovery are significantly more favorable.

## BIBLIOGRAPHY

ADAMS, M. (1977). "A Clinicial Strategy for Differentiating the Normally Nonfluent Child and the Incipient Stutterer." *Journal of Fluency Disorders,* 2: 141-148.
—— (1982). "Fluency, Nonfluency, and Stuttering in Children." *Journal of Fluency Disorders,* 7: 171-185.
—— (1983). "Learning from Negative Outcomes in Stuttering Therapy. I. Getting Off on the Wrong Foot." *Journal of Fluency Disorders,* 8: 147-153.
AINSWORTH, S., and J. FRASER-GRUSS, eds. (1977). *If Your Child Stutters: A Guide for Parents.* Memphis, Tenn.: Speech Foundation of America.
ANDERSON, E. (1970). *Therapy for Young Stutterers.* Detroit: Wayne State University Press.
ANDREWS, G., and J. CUTLER (1974). "Stuttering Therapy: The Relationship Between Changes in Symptom Level and Attitude." *Journal of Speech and Hearing Disorders,* 39: 312-319.
ANDREWS, G., and M. HARRIS (1964). *The Syndrome of Stuttering.* Clinics in Developmental Medicine No. 17. London: William Heinemann.
ANDREWS G., and R. HARVEY (1981). "Regression to the Mean in Pretreatment Measures of Stuttering." *Journal of Speech and Hearing Disorders,* 46: 204-207.
ANDREWS, G., et al. (1983). "Stuttering: A Review of Research Findings and Theories circa 1982." *Journal of Speech and Hearing Disorders,* 48: 226-246.
BAR, A. (1973). "Increasing Fluency in Young Stutterers versus Decreasing Stuttering: A Clinical Approach." *Journal of Communication Disorders,* 6: 247-258.
BAR, A., and I. JAKAB (1969). "Graphic Identification of Stuttering Episodes as Experienced by Stutterers," in *Art Interpretation and Art Therapy,* ed. I. Jakab. New York: S. Karger.
BECK, A. (1976). *Cognitive Therapy and the Emotional Disorders.* New York: International Universities Press.
BLOODSTEIN, O. (1981). *A Handbook on Stuttering.* Chicago: National Easter Seal Society for Crippled Children and Adults.
BLOODSTEIN, O., and M. GROSSMAN (1981). "Early Stutterings: Some Aspects of Their Form and Distribution." *Journal of Speech and Hearing Research,* 24: 298-302.
BOBERG, E., P. HOWIE, and L. WOODS (1979). "Maintenance of Fluency: A Review." *Journal of Fluency Disorders,* 4: 93-116.
BONFANTI, B., and R. CULATTA (1977). "An Analysis of the Fluency Patterns of Institutionalized Retarded Adults." *Journal of Fluency Disorders,* 2: 117-128.
BROWN, C., and W. CULLINAN (1981). "Word-Retrieval Difficulty and Disfluent Speech in Adult Anomic Speakers." *Journal of Speech and Hearing Research,* 24: 358-365.
BRUTTEN, E. (1975). "Stuttering: Topography, Assessment and Behavior Change Strategies," in *Stuttering: A Second Symposium,* ed. J. Eisenson. New York: Harper & Row.
BRUTTEN, E., and D. SHOEMAKER (1974). *The Southern Illinois Behavior Check List.* Carbondale: Southern Illinois University.
CHAPMAN, M. (1959). *Self-Inventory.* Minneapolis: Burgess.
COOPER, E. (1971). "Reflections on Conceptualizing the Stuttering Therapy Process from a Single Theoretical Framework." *Journal of Speech and Hearing Disorders,* 36: 471-475.
—— (1973). "The Development of a Stuttering Chronicity Prediction Checklist: A Preliminary Report." *Journal of Speech and Hearing Disorders,* 38: 215-223.
—— (1982). "A Disfluency Descriptor for Clinical Use." *Journal of Fluency Disorders,* 7: 355-358.
DARLEY, F., and D. SPRIESTERSBACH (1978). *Diagnostic Methods in Speech Pathology.* 2nd ed. New York: Harper & Row.
DEAL, J. (1982). "Sudden Onset of Stuttering: A Case Report." *Journal of Speech and Hearing Disorders,* 47: 301-304.
DeFUSCO, E., and M. MENKEN (1979). "Symptomatic Cluttering in Adults." *Brain and Language,* 8: 25-33.
DELL, C. (1979). *Treating the School Age Stutterer.* Memphis, Tenn.: Speech Foundation of America.

DONNAN, G. A. (1979). "Stuttering as a Manifestation of Stroke." *Medical Journal of Australia*, 1: 44–45.

DOUGLASS, E., and B. QUARRINGTON (1952). "The Differentiation of Interiorized and Exteriorized Secondary Stuttering." *Journal of Speech and Hearing Disorders*, 17: 377–385.

EGOLF, D., G. SHAMES, and J. BLIND (1971). "The Combined Use of Operant Procedures and Theoretical Concepts." *Journal of Speech and Hearing Disorders*, 36: 414–421.

——, et al. (1972). "The Use of Parent-Child Interaction Patterns in Therapy for Young Stutterers." *Journal of Speech and Hearing Disorders*, 37: 222–232.

ELLIS, A. (1946). "The Validity of Personality Questionnaires." *Psychology Bulletin*, 43: 385–440.

EMERICK, L. (1970). *Therapy for Young Stutterers*. Danville, Ill.: Interstate Printers and Publishers.

—— (1981). *A Casebook of Diagnosis and Evaluation in Speech Pathology and Audiology*. Englewood Cliffs, N.J.: Prentice-Hall, Inc.

—— (1983). *With Slow and Halting Tongue*. Danville, Ill.: Interstate Printers and Publishers.

EMERICK, L., and C. HAMRE (1972). *An Analysis of Stuttering*. Danville, Ill.: Interstate Printers and Publishers.

EMERY, G., S. HOLLON, and R. BEDROSIAN (1981). *New Directions in Cognitive Therapy*. New York: Guilford Press.

ERICKSON, R. (1969). "Assessing Communication Attitudes Among Stutterers." *Journal of Speech and Hearing Research*, 12: 711–724.

EYSENCK, H., and S. EYSENCK (1963). *The Eysenck Personality Inventory*. London: University of London Press.

FARMER, A., and E. BRAYTON (1979). "Speech Characteristics of Fluent and Dysfluent Down's Syndrome Adults." *Folia Phoniatrica*, 31: 284–290.

FIEDLER, P., and R. STANDOP (1983). *Stuttering: Integrating Theory and Practice*. Rockville, Md.: Aspen Systems Corp.

FOWLIE, G., and E. COOPER (1978). "Traits Attributed to Stuttering and Nonstuttering Children by Their Mothers." *Journal of Fluency Disorders*, 3: 233–246.

FOX, D., and E. CONNELLY (1970). *Exiting the Circle*. Houston, Tex.: University of Houston.

FRANSELLA, F. (1972). *Personal Change and Reconstruction*. London: Academic Press.

FREEMAN, F. (1979). "Phonation in Stuttering: A Review of Current Research." *Journal of Fluency Disorders*, 4: 79–89.

GAVIS, L. (1946). "Bombing Mission No. 15." *Journal of Abnormal and Social Psychology*, 41: 189–198.

GOLDFRIED, M., and M. MERBAUM, eds. (1973). *Behavior Change Through Self-Control*. New York: Holt, Rinehart & Winston.

GORAJ, J. (1974). "Stuttering Therapy as Crisis Intervention." *British Journal of Communication Disorders*, 9: 57.

GOVEN, P., and VETTE, G. (1966). *A Manual for Stuttering Therapy*. Pittsburgh: Stanwix House.

GRIFFITH, F. (1969). "Use of the Sheehan Sentence Completion Test in Speech Therapy for Stuttering." *Journal of Speech and Hearing Disorders*, 34: 342–349.

GRINKER, R., and J. SPIEGAL (1945). *War Neuroses*. Philadelphia: Blakiston.

GUITAR, B. (1976). "Pretreatment Factors Associated with the Outcome of Stuttering Therapy." *Journal of Speech and Hearing Research*, 19: 590–600.

GUITAR, B., and C. BASS (1978). "Stuttering Therapy: The Relation Between Attitude Change and Long Term Outcome." *Journal of Speech and Hearing Disorders*, 43: 392–400.

HEISTAD, M. (1977). *Stuttering and Respiration*. Brandon, Vt.: Brandon Gap Publishing Co.

HILLMAN, R., and H. GILBERT (1977). "Voice Onset Time for Voiceless Stop Consonants in the Fluent Reading of Stutterers and Nonstutterers." *Journal of Acoustical Society of America*, 61: 610–611.

INGHAM, R. (1975). "A Comparison of Covert and Overt Assessment Procedures in Stuttering Therapy: Outcome and Evaluation." *Journal of Speech and Hearing Research*, 18: 346–354.

INGHAM, R., R. MARTIN, and P. KUHL (1974). "Modification and Control of Rate of Speaking by Stutterers." *Journal of Speech and Hearing Research,* 17: 489–496.

IRVINE, T., and R. REIS (1980). "Cluttering as a Complex of Learning Disabilities." *Language, Speech and Hearing Services in Schools,* 11: 3–14.

JOHNSON, W., and R. AMMONS (1944). "Studies in the Psychology of Stuttering. XVIII. The Construction and Application of a Test of Attitude Toward Stuttering." *Journal of Speech Disorders,* 9: 39–49.

KASPRISIN-BURRELLI, A., D. EGOLF, and G. SHAMES (1972). "A Comparison of Parental Verbal Behavior with Stuttering and Non-Stuttering Children." *Journal of Communication Disorders,* 5: 335–346.

KAZDIN, A., and L. WILCOXON (1976). "Systematic Desensitization and Nonspecific Treatment Effects: A Methodological Evaluation." *Psychology Bulletin,* 83: 729–758.

KENT, R., and L. LaPOINTE (1982). "Acoustic Properties of Pathological Reiterative Utterances: A Case Study of Palilalia." *Journal of Speech and Hearing Research,* 25: 95–99.

KLEVANS, D., and G. LYNCH (1977). "Group Training in Communication Skills for Adults Who Stutter: A Suggested Program." *Journal of Fluency Disorders,* 2: 11–20.

KOLLER, W. (1983). "Disfluency (Stuttering) in Extrapyramidal Disease." *Archives of Neurology,* 40: 175–177.

LaPOINTE, L., and J. HORNER (1981). "Palilalia: A Descriptive Study of Pathological Reiterative Utterances." *Journal of Speech and Hearing Disorders,* 46: 34–38.

LeBRUN, Y., J. RETIF, and G. KAISER (1983). "Acquired Stuttering as a Forerunner of Motor Neuron Disease." *Journal of Fluency Disorders,* 8: 161–167.

LEITH, W., and H. MIMS (1975). "Cultural Influences in the Development and Treatment of Stuttering: A Preliminary Report." *Journal of Speech and Hearing Disorders,* 40: 459–466.

LUPER, H., ed. (1968). *Stuttering: Successes and Failures in Therapy.* Memphis, Tenn.: Speech Foundation of America.

McMULLIN, R., and T. GILES (1981). *Cognitive Behavior Therapy.* New York: Grune & Stratton.

MADISON, D., et al. (1977). "Communicative and Cognitive Deterioration in Dialysis Dementia: Two Case Studies." *Journal of Speech and Hearing Disorders,* 42: 238–243.

MAHONEY, M. (1974). *Cognition and Behavior Modification.* New York: Ballinger.

MANNING, W., and L. RIENSCHE (1976). "Auditory Assembly Ability of Stuttering and Non-Stuttering Children." *Journal of Speech and Hearing Research,* 19: 777–783.

MARTYN, M., J. SHEEHAN, and K. SLUTZ (1969). "Incidence of Stuttering and Other Speech Disorders Among the Retarded." *American Journal of Mental Deficiency,* 74: 206–211.

MAXWELL, D. (1982). "Cognitive and Behavioral Self-Control Strategies: Applications for the Clinical Management of Adult Stutterers." *Journal of Fluency Disorders,* 7: 403–432.

MILLER, S. (1982). "Airflow Therapy Programs: Facts and/or Fancy." *Journal of Fluency Disorders,* 7: 187–202.

MOLESKI, R., and D. TOSI (1976). "Comparative Psychotherapy: Rational and Emotive Therapy versus Systematic Desensitization in the Treatment of Stuttering." *Journal of Consulting Psychology,* 44:309–311.

MYERS, F., and M. WALL (1982). "Toward an Integrated Approach to Early Childhood Stuttering." *Journal of Fluency Disorders,* 7: 47–54.

PERKINS, W. (1973). "Replacement of Stuttering with Normal Speech. I. Rationale." *Journal of Speech and Hearing Disorders,* 38: 283–294.

—— (1983). "Learning from Negative Outcomes in Stuttering Therapy. II. An Epiphany of Failures." *Journal of Fluency Disorders,* 8: 155–160.

PERKINS, W., et al. (1974). "Replacement of Stuttering with Normal Speech. III. Clinical Effectiveness." *Journal of Speech and Hearing Disorders,* 39: 416–428.

PEROZZI, J. (1970). "Phonetic Skill (Sound-Mindedness) of Stuttering Children." *Journal of Communication Disorders,* 3: 207–210.

PEROZZI, J., and L. KUNZE (1969). "Language Abilities of Stuttering Children." *Folia Phoniatrica,* 21: 386–392.

POLOW, N. (1975). *A Stuttering Manual for the Speech Therapist.* Springfield, Ill.: Chas. C Thomas.

PRINS, D. (1970). "Improvement and Regression in Stutterers Following Short-Term Intensive Therapy." *Journal of Speech and Hearing Disorders,* 35: 123–135.

PRINS, D., and M. MILLER (1973). "Personality Improvement and Regression in Stutterin; Therapy." *Journal of Speech and Hearing Research,* 16: 685–690.

QUARRINGTON, B. (1956). "Cyclical Variations in Stuttering Frequency and Severity and Some Related Forms of Variation." *Journal of Psychology,* 10: 179–183.

QUESAL, R., and K. SHANK (1978). "Stuttering and Others: A Comparison of Communication Attitudes." *Journal of Fluency Disorders,* 3: 247–252.

RAGSDALE, J., and J. ASHBY (1982). "Speech-Language Pathologists' Connotation of Stuttering." *Journal of Speech and Hearing Research,* 25: 78–80.

RILEY, G. (1972). "A Stuttering Severity Instrument for Children and Adults." *Journal of Speech and Hearing Disorders,* 37: 314–322.

—— (1981). *Stuttering Prediction Instrument for Children and Adults.* Tigard, Oreg.: C. C. Publications.

RILEY, G., and J. RILEY (1982). "Evaluating Stuttering Problems in Children." *Journal of Childhood Communication Disorders,* 6: 15–25.

ROSENBEK, J., et al. (1978). "Stuttering Following Brain Damage." *Brain and Language,* 6: 82–96.

RYAN, B. (1969). *Behavior Modification Techniques with School Age Children Who Stutter.* Tulare County, Calif.: Scicon School.

ST. LOUIS, K., and N. LASS (1981). "A Survey of Communication Disorder Students' Attitudes Toward Stuttering." *Journal of Fluency Disorders,* 6: 49–79.

SAVAGE, A. (1970). *Straight Talk: A Manual for Use by Therapists in Working with Elementary School Age Stutterers.* Pittsburgh: Stanwix House.

SAVITSKY, J., and T. HESS (1975). "A Child's Emotions and Adult Authoritarianism as Determinants of Punishment." *Journal of Genetic Psychology,* 126: 249–256.

SCHWARTZ, M. (1976). *Stuttering Solved.* Philadelphia: Lippincott.

SHAMES, G., and D. EGOLF (1976). *Operant Conditioning and the Management of Stuttering.* Englewood Cliffs, N.J.: Prentice-Hall, Inc.

SHEARER, W., and J. WILLIAMS (1965). "Self-Recovery from Stuttering." *Journal of Speech and Hearing Disorders,* 30: 288–290.

SHEEHAN, J. (1969). "Cyclic Variation in Stuttering." *Journal of Abnormal Psychology,* 74: 452–453.

—— (1970). *Stuttering: Research and Therapy.* New York: Harper & Row.

SHEEHAN, J., and M. MARTYN (1970). "Stuttering and Its Disappearance." *Journal of Speech and Hearing Research,* 13: 279–289.

SHEEHAN, J., and K. KILBURN (1968). "Speech Disorders in Retardation." *American Journal of Mental Deficiency,* 73: 251–256.

SILVERMAN, F. (1970). "Concern of Elementary-School Stutterers About Their Stuttering." *Journal of Speech and Hearing Disorders,* 35: 361–363.

—— (1974). *Bibliography of Literature Pertaining to Stuttering in Elementary School Children: Tentative Edition.* Milwaukee: Marquette University.

—— (1980). "Stuttering Problem Profile: A Task that Assists Both Client and Clinician in Defining Therapy Goals." *Journal of Speech and Hearing Disorders,* 45: 119–123.

SILVERMAN, F., and D. WILLIAMS (1972). "Prediction of Stuttering by School Age Stutterers." *Journal of Speech and Hearing Research,* 15: 189–193.

SIMPSON, B. (1966). *Stuttering Therapy: A Guide for the Speech Clinician.* Danville, Ill.: Interstate Printers and Publishers.

STARKWEATHER, W. (1972). *Stuttering: An Account of Intensive Demonstrative Therapy.* Memphis, Tenn.: Speech Foundation of America.

—— (1974). *Therapy for Stutterers.* Memphis, Tenn.: Speech Foundation of America.

STENNETT, N. (1967). *A Workbook for Stuttering.* Chicago: King.

STEVENS, J. (1971). *Awareness: Exploring, Experiencing, Experimenting.* Moab, Utah: Real People Press.

THARP, R., and R. WETZEL (1969). *Behavior Modification in the Natural Environment.* New York: Academic Press.

THOMPSON, J. (1982). *Assessment of Fluency in School-Age Children.* Danville, Ill.: Interstate Printers and Publishers.

TRACY, K., and S. HOOD (1976). "An Investigation of Responses from Speech Clinicians and Lay Public to the Concept 'Typical Adult Stutterer.'" *Ohio Journal of Speech and Hearing,* 12: 58-68.

TURK, D., D. MEICHENBAUM, and M. GENEST (1983). *Pain and Behavioral Medicine: A Cognitive-Behavioral Perspective.* New York: Guilford Press.

TURNBAUGH, K., B. GUITAR, and P. HOFFMAN (1979). "Speech Clinicians' Attribution of Personality Traits as a Function of Stuttering Severity." *Journal of Speech and Hearing Research,* 22: 37-45.

―― (1981). "The Attribution of Personality Traits: The Stutterer and the Nonstutterer." *Journal of Speech and Hearing Research,* 24: 288-291.

VAN RIPER, C. (1961). *Your Child's Speech Problems.* New York: Harper & Row.

―― (1963). *Speech Correction: Principles and Methods.* Englewood Cliffs, N.J.: Prentice-Hall, Inc.

――, ed. (1964). *Treatment of the Young Stutterer in the School.* Memphis, Tenn.: Speech Foundation of America.

―― (1973). *The Treatment of Stuttering.* Englewood Cliffs, N.J.: Prentice-Hall, Inc.

―― (1982). *The Nature of Stuttering.* 2nd ed. Englewood Cliffs, N.J.: Prentice-Hall, Inc.

VIOLON, A. (1973). "In Regard to a Case of Stuttering in the Child: Methodologic and Therapeutic Aspects," in *Neurolinguistic Approaches to Stuttering,* ed. Y. Lebrun and R. Hopps. The Hague: Mouton.

WALLE, E. (1974). *The Prevention of Stuttering. I. Identifying the Danger Signs* (a film). Memphis, Tenn.: Speech Foundation of America.

―― (1975). *The Prevention of Stuttering. II. Parent Counseling and Elimination of the Problem* (a film). Memphis, Tenn.: Speech Foundation of America.

―― (1977). *The Prevention of Stuttering. III. SSStuttering and Your Child. Is It Me? Is It You?* (a film). Memphis, Tenn.: Speech Foundation of America.

WEBSTER, L., and L. FURST (1975). *Vocal Tract Dynamics and Dysfluency.* New York: Speech and Hearing Institute.

WEINER, A. (1981). "A Case of Adult Onset of Stuttering." *Journal of Fluency Disorders,* 6: 181-186.

WERNER, H. (1982). *Cognitive Therapy: A Humanistic Approach.* New York: Free Press.

WIENER, D. (1957) "Individual and Group Forms of the Minnesota Multiphasic Personality Inventory." *Journal of Consulting Psychology,* 11: 104-106.

WILLIAMS, A., and C. MARKS (1972). "A Comparative Analysis of the ITPA and PPVT Performance of Young Stutterers." *Journal of Speech and Hearing Research,* 15: 323-329.

WILLIAMS, D. (1957). "A Point of View About Stuttering." *Journal of Speech and Hearing Disorders,* 22: 390-397.

―― (1971). "Stuttering Therapy for Children," in *Handbook of Speech Pathology,* ed. L. Travis. New York: Appleton-Century-Crofts.

―― (1974). "Evaluation," in *Therapy for Stutterers,* ed. C. Starkweather. Memphis, Tenn.: Speech Foundation of America.

WILLIS, B., ed. (1965). *A Speech Therapy Workbook for the Child Who Stutters.* Chicago: Board of Education.

WINGATE, M. (1964). "Recovery from Stuttering." *Journal of Speech and Hearing Disorders,* 29: 312-321.

―― (1976). *Stuttering: Theory and Development.* New York: Irvington.

WOODS, C., and D. WILLIAMS (1976). "Traits Attributed to Stuttering and Normally Fluent Males." *Journal of Speech and Hearing Research,* 19: 267-279.

WOOLF, G. (1967). "The Assessment of Stuttering as Struggle, Avoidance, and Expectancy." *British Journal of Disorders of Communication,* 2: 158-171.

WYATT, E. (1969). *Language Learning and Communication Disorders in Children.* New York: Free Press.

YAIRI, E. (1983). "The Onset of Stuttering in Two- and Three-Year-Old Children: A Preliminary Report." *Journal of Speech and Hearing Disorders,* 48: 171-177.

ZELEN, S., J. SHEEHAN, and J. BUGENTAL (1954). "Self-Perception in Stuttering." *Journal of Clinical Psychology,* 10: 70-72.

ZIMMERMAN, G. (1980). "Articulatory Behaviors Associated with Stuttering: A Cinefluorographic Analysis." *Journal of Speech and Hearing Research,* 22:108-121.

# CHAPTER SEVEN
# THE ASSESSMENT
# OF APHASIA IN ADULTS

When an adult suddenly loses the easy use of words, it must be a devastating experience. Indeed, perhaps only the person abruptly deprived of language—and thus his communicative bond to others—really understands aphasia. A former client described his difficulty understanding speech in this way: "It's a little like trying to read by the flickering light of a single firefly."

Aphasia is the most common disorder of communication resulting from brain injury. The adult client with aphasia does not have a *speech* problem, but rather a more basic interference with her comprehension and use of *language*. The linguistic code, the substance of messages shared interpersonally, is deficient. Aphasia, then, is a disturbance in the very attribute that is so uniquely human, a person's ability to symbolize. More specifically, aphasia is a syndrome of language impairment resulting from destruction of cortical tissue, and is characterized by one or more of the following symptoms:

1. Disturbance in receiving and decoding symbolic materials via auditory, visual, or tactile channels. Although the individual can still hear and see, he has difficulty deciphering the learned associations of messages.
2. Disturbance in central processes of meaning, word selection, and message formulation.
3. Disturbance in expressing symbolic materials by means of speech, writing, or gesture.

Rarely is a client totally impaired in the use of language, and hence the term *dysphasia* may be more appropriate. Indeed, there is a rather wide range of disturbance extending from the mild impairment suffered by former President Eisenhower (1965) to the almost total loss of language described by McBride (1969). In keeping with traditional writing, however, we shall use the term *aphasia* to refer to this total range of impairment.

It is important to remember that the improverishment of language observed in aphasia is not due to loss of mental capacity, impairment of sensory organs, or paralysis of the speech apparatus.[1] Aphasia is not, however, simply a loss of words. It can generally be shown clinically—by the use of open-end sentences, oral opposites, or other forms of cueing—that even severe aphasics are capable of uttering words. The problem seems to be in *retrieving* words—that is, translating internal idiosyncratic symbols into convenient language forms. The more common a word, the more probable that it will be retained. For example, an aphasic may understand or use the words "kiss" or "rain" but not "osculation" or "precipitation," even though all four might have been in his premorbid vocabulary.

Although there is still some controversy as to whether the language disturbance in aphasia is uni- or multidimensional, careful clinical assessment of patients fails to reveal subtypes with isolated linguistic deficits (Smith, 1971; Brookshire, 1983); in fact, aphasics typically show some degree of disturbance in all areas of language usage. Aphasia is a multimodality language impairment (Darley, 1982):

> Early students of aphasia concerned themselves with an elaborate taxonomy based upon symptomatology. There was a compulsion to name and classify every possible phenomenon, even to the last anosmia. At the present time, many workers recognize two primary patterns of aphasia: (1) *Broca's,* or "motor" (nonfluent) aphasia, is due to damage to the anterior portion of the brain. Patients have halting, groping speech. (2) *Wernicke's,* or "sensory" (fluent), aphasia is due to a lesion in the posterior part of the brain. This patient has difficulty understanding speech. (See Figure 7.1.)

**FIGURE 7.1    Left cerebral hemisphere showing sites of two major types of aphasia.**

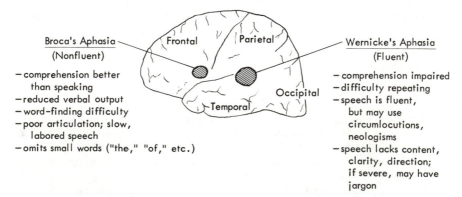

Broca's Aphasia
(Nonfluent)

— comprehension better
   than speaking
— reduced verbal output
— word-finding difficulty
— poor articulation; slow,
   labored speech
— omits small words ("the," "of," etc.)

Wernicke's Aphasia
(Fluent)

— comprehension impaired
— difficulty repeating
— speech is fluent,
   but may use
   circumlocutions,
   neologisms
— speech lacks content,
   clarity, direction;
   if severe, may have
   jargon

[1]An overview of motor speech disorders is presented in the Highlight for this chapter.

Most neurologists agree, however, that there is a great deal of inconsistency of brain organization from person to person. Because the site of lesion usually can be determined by brain scan and computed tomography, we prefer to focus our attention on the client's communication abilities. When evaluating aphasic clients, we try to describe carefully what the individual can and cannot do with respect to language. Instead of using esoteric labels, the clinician can delineate the client's ability to talk, listen, read, and write.

In our zeal to identify the psycholinguistic dimensions of aphasia, it is possible to forget that brain injury is a grave health problem. The individual has suffered a major life crisis that has profound medical, psychological, and social consequences. In addition to the language impairment, the client may present paralysis or paresis of the extremities (generally the right side, sometimes including the face), sensory abnormalities, and behavioral disturbances. There seems to be little, if any, relationship between these difficulties and the extent of the language impairment. Above all, the diagnostician must remember that asphasia is both a personal catastrophe and a family crisis, as Buck (1968) so eloquently points out.

## DIFFERENTIAL DIAGNOSIS

The clinician is called upon occasionally to distinguish between aphasia and a number of other conditions involving abnormality in language. We include below a brief discussion of three disorders that might be confused with aphasia. However, keep in mind that impairment of symbolic functioning can coexist with any of these anomalies.

### Psychosis

Although it is rather easy for the professional to distinguish aphasia from psychosis, it is understandable why laypersons are often confused. The aphasic may say yes when he means no, use obscenities and other antisocial language or gestures freely, laugh or cry often, lapse into euphoria, deny his symptoms, or withdraw into severe depression and despair. The distinguishing features of psychosis are, however, rather obvious: severe personality decomposition—not just frustration or emotional overflow when trying to comprehend or speak—and distortion of, or loss of contact with, reality. The vast majority of aphasic patients do not show evidence of mental deterioration or gross disturbances in processing reality. Additionally, the aphasic generally will try hard to communicate with others, whereas for the psychotic interpersonal contact is irrelevant.

Considering all the frustrations aphasics encounter, we have often wondered why they do not behave in a more abnormal manner than they do. Indeed, their demeanor and social interaction, aside from the language impairment, are remarkably normal. Nevertheless, some individuals with aphasia do experience psychotic episodes, particularly periods of severe depression (see Hodgins, 1964, for a personal account of an involutional depression following aphasia).

### Language Confusion

Persons suffering from diffuse brain damage manifest a number of cognitive disfunctions that, on cursory appraisal, might be mistaken for aphasia. Because the injury to the brain is widespread (and often due to trauma), many higher intellectual capabilities are d:-*··rbed, as the following case example illustrates:

> Tom Snively, a twenty-year-old college junior, suffered a closed head injury in a skiing accident. He was in a coma for two weeks. Now, two months post onset, he is an inpatient in the Marquette Rehabilitation Center. When evaluated with a standard test of aphasia, Tom showed no disturbance of vocabulary or syntax; he did have some limited word-finding difficulty. The examiner noted, however, that the young man had trouble attending and staying in touch with the test situation. The patient tended to give responses that, although syntactically correct, often were irrelevant. Additionally, Tom was disoriented and, particularly, in response to open-ended questions, gave rambling, fabricated answers. Here is a portion of an interview conducted by a medical social worker that reveals the patient's disorientation and tendency to confabulate:

> WORKER:  Where are you?
> TOM:  Ah, in training camp. Colorado Springs. And tomorrow we do time trials for the giant slalom.
> WORKER:  But, what is this place?
> TOM:  A training center. I had a hamstring pull and need whirlpool treatments.

As the label suggests, patients with language confusion do not think clearly, have memory loss, and tend to be disoriented. In many cases, they show changes in personality as well. The confusion may range from mild and temporary, such as in concussion or hypothermia, to profound, as in head injury or drug overdose.

### Dementia

Dementia refers to a group of disorders all of which feature generalized intellectual decline. The deterioration of emotional control, cognitive skills, and language use is caused by diffuse, bilateral subcortical and cortical brain injury or atrophy. Dementia is caused by, among other factors, infectious diseases, tumor, multiple strokes, and Parkinson's and Alzheimer's diseases. Unlike language confusion, dementia often has a gradual, insidious onset.

Before a clinical diagnosis of dementia can be confirmed, several key features must be present (Berg et al., 1982):

1. A sustained deterioration of *memory,* plus a disturbance in at least three of the following areas: (a) orientation in time and place; (b) judgment and problem solving (dealing with everyday situations); (c) community affairs (shopping, handling finances); (d) home and avocations; and (e) personal care.

2.  A gradual onset and progression.
3.  A duration of at least six months or longer.[2]

In order to illustrate the salient behavioral and communicative symptoms observed in dementia, we include a portion of a diagnostic report on a patient in the second phase of Alzheimer's disease (Powell and Courtice, 1983):

> This 64-year-old patient manifested the following behaviors: lowered drive and energy level; memory loss; slow reaction time; and difficulty making decisions. Her personality has changed in the past year so that now she typically is dull, bland, and unresponsive socially.
>
> Mrs. Davis' language abilities are only mildly impaired at this time. She can match objects, point to and name pictures, and repeat words, phrases, and short sentences. Phonologically and syntactically her speech is within normal limits. She does have limited output, however, and restricted usage. The patient's speech performance is slow and often, after trying to respond to a task, she will say, "I don't know."
>
> The patient's language disturbance was more evident on tasks requiring greater intellectual effort and abstraction. For example, Mrs. Davis was unable to find and correct semantic errors in sentences ("My sister is an only child") or discern the ambiguity in sentences ("Visiting relatives can be a nuisance"). (Bayles and Boone, 1982)

Additional material on aphasia and the differential diagnosis of language disorders may be found in the work of Wertz (1978) and others (Jenkins et al., 1975; Kertesz, 1979; Benson, 1979; Albert et al., 1981; Sarno, 1981; Darley, 1982; Davis, 1983; Eisenson, 1984).

## INCIDENCE AND ETIOLOGY

Aphasia is always caused by damage to the brain. Brain damage, however, will not *always* result in aphasia. Automobile accidents in which head injury is incurred, infectious diseases (such as meningitis), tumors, or certain degenerative diseases are all possible sources of cortical damage and aphasia. The most frequent cause of aphasia, however, is a disturbance of the blood supply to the brain, commonly called a stroke. The cerebral vascular accident (CVA) is a relatively common illness that affects approximately a million persons each year. In the United States, stroke now stands in third place as a cause of death, outdistanced only by heart disease and cancer. No one knows precisely how many surviving stroke victims are left with language impairment; estimates suggest at least a quarter of a million or more individuals present some degree of aphasia that warrants treatment.

---

[2]The professional must be very careful not to assume that when an older person shows signs of confusion, he is "senile," while a person in his thirties or forties with the same difficulties is considered to have a specific cause for his confusion. Dehydration, medication, and depression can cause temporary or pseudodementia in the elderly.

Information regarding the etiology of aphasia may be found in the following sources: Buchanan (1957), Netter (1958), Page et al. (1961), Grinker and Sahs (1966), Chusid and McDonald (1967), Vick (1976), and Adams and Victor (1977).

## CASE EXAMPLE

In order to portray the nature and scope of the clinician's involvement in the evaluation of adults with language impairment, we now present an extensive case example. The account is chronological and delineates our role from the moment we were first alerted by the physician until a treatment plan was devised. We are aware that this illustration is but a single case and that there is a great deal of variability from individual to individual. Yet we are also aware that speech and language clinicians see their clients in this manner—one at a time. My purpose in focusing on an individual client is to remind the reader of the saliency of the human variables in assessment. We work with *persons* who have aphasia, not aphasia.

A comprehensive evaluation of an adult aphasic includes several clinical tasks: (1) a review of pertinent medical information and the sequence of events leading up to the referral; (2) a preliminary interview with the client's spouse or other close relative; (3) a case history, including information about the impact of brain injury on the client and how much natural or spontaneous recovery has taken place; (4) an inventory of the client's language performance; (5) observation and related testing—oral peripheral examination, hearing test, a vocabulary measure, and, if indicated, a specific assessment of speech fluency and auditory abilities; and (6) a determination about the type and form of treatment to employ and a judgment about the individual's prospects for recovery.

### Prologue

A series of events transpired prior to our entry into the case, and the following account was pieced together—from limited fragments Mr. Tenhave could tell us, descriptions offered by his wife, and hospital records—only after we began to work with the client. Compare the following account with those by Hodgins (1964), Whitehouse (1968), Moss (1972), and Wulf (1973).

> Roy Tenhave arose abruptly at 11:30 P.M. soon after retiring, muttering something about an idea he must write down or he would surely forget it. His wife, familiar with her husband's late flashes of insight, turned over and dozed. Padding through the darkened house and into his study, Mr. Tenhave noticed that his right leg was somewhat stiff and felt a tingling and creeping numbness as if his limb were going to sleep. Turning on his desk lamp, he found his notebook and selected a pencil. Mr. Tenhave had been working on a manuscript dealing with bird migration in Upper Michigan, and just as he was drifting off to sleep, he had suddenly divined a novel way to illustrate flight routes. (Later, Mr. Tenhave could not recall the idea; that page of his notebook contained only an illegible scrawl.) As he bent over his desk and started to write, he felt dizzy and watched in curious fascination as the pencil slid

slowly out of his hand. Then the room became a fuzzy blur, and he felt himself cascade over the swivel chair and crash to the floor in a grotesque heap. "This is silly," he thought; as he was struggling to arise, he discovered that his right arm and leg stubbornly refused to function. After several unsuccessful attempts to get up, he called for his wife—at least, he meant to call—but all he heard was a strange vowel sound, almost like an animal bleating. In that instant, Mr. Tenhave knew what was happening to him: he was having a stroke. Mrs. Tenhave immediately summoned the city ambulance and alerted her husband's physician, Dr. Roger Wilson, a specialist in internal medicine. In the emergency room, the resident physician worked swiftly to insure the patient could breathe easily, carefully measured his blood pressure, and administered antibiotics.

### Early Intervention

We entered the case five days later, when Dr. Wilson's nurse called and requested consultation. A note from Dr. Wilson followed:

> Roy Tenhave, fifty-two-year-old high school biology teacher, suffered a moderately severe CVA on January 19. Left cerebral hemisphere, clinically diagnosed as thrombotic. Right hemiplegia: The leg is responding to physical therapy but, though it is early yet, the arm is doubtful. He may also have a visual field cut on the right—his responses are inconsistent. A neurological workup is being done, and the results will be in his record when you get to the hospital. He is having a great deal of difficulty communicating. I talked briefly with his wife, but she needs more information about aphasia.

We cannot overemphasize the critical importance of early intervention in the clinical management of aphasic clients; this position becomes obvious when we consider the broader definition of aphasia as a personal and family catastrophe (Buck, 1968). A little bit of early support and counseling is much more effective than a great deal of help later. By prompt involvement, we do not necessarily mean initiating language therapy, although if accomplished indirectly in the form of general stimulation, it is certainly a wise recommendation. Rather, we refer to the following: (1) Nurses and others who work with the patient should receive in-service training. Hospitals in small, isolated communities are not generally equipped or staffed to deal adequately with aphasic patients during the primary stage of recovery (Twamley and Emerick, 1970). (2) There should be information-sharing and planning conferences with professional team members—the physician, physical therapist, occupational therapist, social worker, and others concerned with the rehabilitation of the patient. Consult the work of Leutenegger (1975) and Haynes and Greenberg (1976) for useful material for in-service training. (3) Supportive monologue interviews with the aphasic patient should be conducted to provide release of feelings and to reassure him that a professional worker is concerned and attempting to do something about his language problem. (4) Finally, family counseling is most important. The maintenance of a supportive, nonthreatening environment for the brain-injured patient is crucial to his recovery (Evans and Northwood, 1983).

### Interview with Mrs. Tenhave

In order to adequately understand the aphasic patient, it is necessary to understand something about the people close to him, their prior relationships with him, their present fears and reactions, and their hopes for the future. Families are confronted with a crisis when an adult member is suddenly afflicted with a deadly, often mysterious illness that results in such profound physical and psychological alterations. A serious illness disrupts communication patterns, dissolves or shifts roles, and forces family members to assume unfamiliar responsibilities. The resolution of the crisis situation, the manner in which members reorganize the family structure, will have profound implications for the patient and the prospects for rehabilitation (Kinsella and Duffy, 1978).

As we planned our initial counseling session with Mrs. Tenhave, we reviewed the many difficulties with which the family of an aphasic must cope—often, unfortunately, without professional guidance (Derman and Manaster, 1967; Porter and Dabul, 1977):

> In terms of life cycle, at what stage is the family? Are there young or adolescent children? Is it a middle-aged couple, now alone and with leisure and peak earning power? What premorbid marital problems existed? Will they be exacerbated or will the family unit draw more closely together to meet the threat? Does the spouse have health problems? How does the family handle the fear of recurring strokes? Are there financial difficulties? Is there any guilt? How are they coping with the communication impairment? What are their impressions of the physical changes?[3]

We arranged to meet Mrs. Tenhave in the speech clinic, assuming that she had become satiated with the aseptic atmosphere of the hospital during her prolonged vigil. She arrived early for the interview, a petite, attractive women in her late forties. She was well dressed and groomed but looked haggard and worn. Despite her subdued manner, however, we sensed almost immediately her basic strength of character.

We directed Mrs. Tenhave to a comfortable chair and offered her a cup of coffee. Recalling Derman and Manaster's (1967) advice that relatives of aphasics need information, reassurance, and an outlet for frustration, we invited her to tell us about her husband's illness. We began by acknowledging quietly that the past few days must have been very difficult for her. She seemed to welcome the opportunity to pour out some of her pent-up thoughts and fears:

> Yes, it certainly was a shock. Roy was perfectly well and then, suddenly, he was struck down like this. At first I was terrified he was going to die; then, when I saw he was paralyzed and couldn't talk, I found myself praying that he would. That made me feel so terribly guilty—but an active life means so much to him. What will he be able to do now? If only I would have insisted

---

[3]For a review of how families cope with stress, see the work of Rollin (1984) and Sheehy (1976).

that he see Dr. Wilson earlier when he had the dizzy spells and the tingling in his arm and leg; I just attributed it to arthritis and the fact that he had been working so hard on his bird migration manuscript. I feel so . . . so alone. No . . . (she raised her hand to politely reject our murmur of reassurance), I don't mean to play the little housewife in a quandary. I have taught elementary children for almost twenty years. I mean, Roy and I did so much together— hikes, I edited all his writing, went on field trips with his students, I even went hunting with him. Now I don't know what will happen. The doctor talks about brain damage . . . but will he be normal? What can I expect? What will he be able to do? Here I am feeling sorry for myself when I should be thinking about him. He must be so upset.

At this point Mrs. Tenhave began to weep softly. We gently suggested that it was good to let the tension and uncertainty come out, that we understood how she felt, and that it was certainly normal to have the feelings she reported. When she recovered her composure, Mrs. Tenhave was full of questions:

Dr. Wilson said that Roy is aphasic. I looked that up in the dictionary and found it meant loss of power to use and understand speech. But how much can he understand? Can he write? I gave him a pencil the other day when he was trying to tell me something, and he just pointed to his right arm and shook his head. What can I do to help him? A colleague of mine at school gave me a child's first alphabet book and suggested I start teaching Roy with it. She said that it had helped her father when he had a stroke. When I tried with Roy, he threw the book and knocked over a vase of flowers. He never was a violent man. He swears so much now and cries so easily. He was always such a reserved and quiet person and now he seems so exposed. Perhaps that's why he doesn't want to see any of his colleagues or students. They come to the hospital, but I can tell Roy is terribly embarrassed. How can I make his friends understand when I don't myself?

Mrs. Tenhave had much more to say during this initial interview; we have included only a portion to show some of the concerns she reported. In many respects, she was an unusually easy respondent. Often we have had to be much more directive and reassuring with less educated and perceptive spouses. By the end of the hour, she was eager to receive the information we provided:

Aphasia is more than a disturbance in speech. It is an impairment of language that is coded and stored in the brain. When a person has a stroke, a portion of the brain dies. Initially, because of the swelling that occurs around the specific area of injury, the patient shows more disturbance in language and other respects than he will later. No one really knows how much recovery will take place spontaneously, or how long it will continue. Usually, however, spontaneous improvement occurs within the first three months after the stroke. The pamphlet I will give you at the end of our chat will explain this more fully.

I want to mention a bit more about language. As you know from teaching elementary children to read, language is an elaborate system of symbols. The word "cow," for example, stands for, or is used as, a shorthand way of identifying a Holstein or Hereford. It would be impossible to run out in the pasture and lead in a furry, lactating quadruped every time we wanted to use the word "cow." We use symbols, as you know, in four basic ways—talking, listening, reading, and writing. Usually an aphasic patient has difficulty in all four areas, although he generally seems to have more trouble generating language—that is, speaking and writing. So Mr. Tenhave's reluctance to write may not just be due to his paralyzed arm. Often people think that the aphasic person seems to understand everything spoken to him. But it usually can be shown that the patient indeed cannot understand everything but rather detects certain nonverbal cues or makes some socially approved gestures that give the impression of accurate listening. As Mr. Tenhave seems to, many aphasics have some oral expression that we can call automatic speech. They may be able to count, recite letters of the alphabet (and other items occurring in a series), swear, and repeat memorized prayers and poems. It is important to remember that this language is mostly involuntary, it does not involve the conscious search for and use of words. Some patients can even imitate words uttered by others. This, too, is not true language. Most aphasics have a low threshold of frustration—and a horde of frustrations! Small wonder that they cry so frequently. What should you do when this happens? The best response is to acknowledge his feelings, let him know you understand, and then divert his attention to something else.

We advised Mrs. Tenhave to avoid the role of teacher with her husband; he needed her support and affection, not tutoring. We explained that children's books are insulting to aphasics, who, even though severely retarded in language usage, retain an adult outlook. It is essential, we added, that people continue to deal with the aphasic on an adult level; it is infantilizing enough to be physically helpless, to have lost the power of speech, and to be utterly dependent on others for satisfaction of all one's needs. Finally, we stressed the importance of maintaining lines of communication with her husband. Human contact and stimulation appear to be vital deterrents to withdrawal and depression (Buck, 1968; Farrell, 1969; Knox, 1971). We concluded:

> Keep talking to him, even if the responses are negligible. In some cases, because the patient is more or less silent, the persons surrounding him cease to talk. They assume that because he does not verbalize, he does not want to hear conversation. It is obvious, of course, that no one should talk *about* Mr. Tenhave in his presence. Don't bombard him with questions that demand a response, for this will only serve to point up his lack of verbal ability and further frustrate him. Experiment with different ways to communicate with him—gestures, printed cards, anything. I plan to give your husband a brief screening test soon, and then we can get together again to discuss the best ways of communicating with him.

In order to further her understanding of Mr. Tenhave's problem, we lent Mrs. Tenhave a copy of a well-known pamphlet on aphasia (Taylor, 1958) and promised we would meet at a later date to discuss its contents. There are several other excellent publications written for relatives of adult patients with aphasia (Horowitz, 1962; American Heart Association, 1965; Longerich, 1955; Boone, 1961; Peterson and Olsen, 1964). The book by Griffith (1970) describes a rather complete home treatment plan; Broida (1979) offers suggestions for coping with strokes.

Thinking she might need additional support, as well as an emotional outlet, we gave Mrs. Tenhave the phone number of the wife of a former patient who had recently started a discussion group for relatives of adult aphasics. The clinician can also refer relatives to a local or regional stroke club (McCormick and Williams, 1976) for information and guidance on how to deal with persons who have suffered brain injury.

### The Screening Test

We went to St. Luke's Hospital to make a preliminary appraisal of Mr. Tenhave's language problem. Although he had been in the hospital only eight days, his physical recovery, according to Dr. Wilson, had been remarkable. Mr. Tenhave now sat up in a chair twice daily for almost an hour, had regained bowel and bladder control, and seemed alert and responsive to his environment. We questioned the nurses on the floor, and they revealed that although he was still swearing and labile when he tried to communicate, he appeared to understand short, simple sentences, responded with a reliable yes or no, and was using more words spontaneously. He also manifested considerable "reactive language"—words and short phrases that seemed to be prompted by the situation or a verbal stimulus but that he could not repeat voluntarily.

Checking Mr. Tenhave's medical file, we noted the neurologist's report:

> This alert, oriented adult male suffered a CVA on 1/19/70. Expressive-receptive aphasia. Right hemiplegia. Babinski sign on the right. Gross motor functioning of involved leg is returning; arm and hand are doubtful. Electroencephalography revealed a focal lesion in the left parietal-temporal region. Site of lesion confirmed by brain scan and angiography. Right side astereognosis. Right hemonymous hemianopsia.

This report told us several important things about the patient: The brain damage was apparently localized and was not widespread; the aphasia was probably not transitory, as lesions in the region cited generally result in more persistent language impairment; he could not identify objects by touch when they were placed in his right hand; and he could not see in the right field of vision. This last anomaly would require that we present testing materials from the patient's left side. Information assembled by the neurologist is, of course, very useful to the clinician. In addition to the size and locale of the lesion, the nature of the injury may be pertinent diagnostically. Patients incurring traumatic brain injury often experience a different course of recovery than persons suffering vascular episodes. The clinician should be familiar with the terms and tests employed in a neurological examination—EEG, brain scan, angiography, computed tomography, and others.

*Administering the screening test.* An adult aphasic, especially during the primary stages of recovery, has little or no means of communication. He is, in a very real sense, isolated. Investigations in sensory deprivation have shown what a frightening and devastating experience isolation can be; in aphasia it can lead to

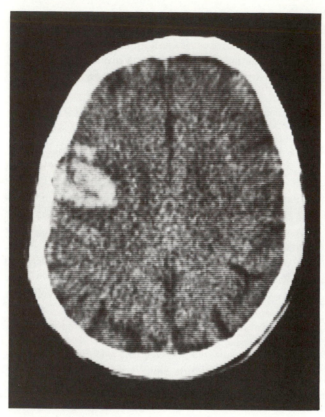

FIGURE 7.2 Computed tomographic (CT) scan (x-ray pictures taken from many angles and computerized) showing a lesion in the left hemisphere. The patient had a Broca's aphasia. (Photograph courtesy of D. Shah, M.D., Hines V.A. Hospital)

profound depression and withdrawal as well as nonverbal habits that make subsequent therapy difficult. Therefore, by early testing, we must discover ways to establish bonds of communication with the client. In order to assess rapidly a client's language capacity, a short screening test was devised (Emerick and Coyne, 1972).[4]

This instrument is designed to evaluate swiftly a patient's language abilities before the administration of a more lengthy inventory. It assesses a patient's communication abilities in two broad areas: *input,* or the evaluation of stimuli from an external source, and *output,* the generation of verbal responses. Although patients change rapidly during the first month following brain injury, it is important that the workers in the helping professions have some preliminary notion of the individual's communication abilities so they can (1) advise relatives about the best means of communicating with the patient; (2) assist other professional workers in the management of the patient; and (3) chart the patient's progress or lack of prog-

---

[4]Shortened versions of published language inventories may be used for early screening (Eisenson, 1954; Sklar, 1966; Wepman and Jones, 1961; Porch, 1967). See also the work of Orgass and Poeck (1969), Spellacy and Spreen (1969), Powell, Bailey, and Clark (1980), and Whurr (1983).

ress during the early stages of recovery (prognostically, of course, early improvement is a good sign).

It is not *necessary* to use a "test" at all; some clinicians prefer to rely on observation of the client in his natural environment. The *Functional Communication Profile* (Taylor, 1963) and the informal assessment tasks prepared by Ultaowska et al. (1976) are useful in providing a structure for observing the client's communication abilities in real situations.

When I entered his room, Mr. Tenhave was sitting up in bed, looking idly out the window; his right arm lay useless in his lap. Approaching from his left side, I extended my hand and introduced myself as a speech clinician. He pointed to his paralyzed arm and shook his head in a gesture of futility. I sat down next to his bed, opened the kit of testing materials, and immediately came to the point.

I would like to find out in what ways you are having difficulty talking and understanding. I will ask you some questions and have you look at some pictures. Some of the tasks will be simple; others will be more difficult. Just answer the best you can. Okay?

I talked slowly and distinctly, pausing often and watching carefully for any signs of confusion. Mr. Tenhave looked curiously at the testing kit, pointed to his mouth, and made a motion that seemed to say, "Let's get on with it." Testing need not be traumatic if the patient is approached in a friendly, humane, and adult manner. In fact, as Schuell, Jenkins, and Jimenez-Pabon (1964) point out, most aphasics expect that the clinician will want to determine what they can and cannot do with regard to language. We prefer not to refer to the tasks as "tests," but rather encourage the patient to explore his problem with us so we can determine where to begin helping him.

Rather than beginning directly with the items on the screening test, we decided to check Mr. Tenhave's auditory comprehension by using several verbal disparities. This procedure would allow him time to "tune up" his input circuits and also permit us to check the reliability of his yes and no responses. Keeping in mind Buck's (1968) advice that it is important to provide links with a client's former life, and remembering that Mr. Tenhave was an accomplished ornithologist, we named several real birds and some imaginary ones, and asked him to indicate which were real by nodding or answering.

We then turned to the screening kit and, starting with the input tasks (why do we begin with the input portion?), moved through the various items. The completed test protocol form is included (Figure 7.3) in order to show the types of tasks employed and the patient's responses to them. The total test took less than ten minutes to administer, but even that brief period of concentration left Mr. Tenhave somewhat fatigued.

As I thanked him and collected my things to leave, Mr. Tenhave seemed to be upset. He pointed to the testing kit and then his mouth; his eyes glistened with

**FIGURE 7.3  Screening test protocol: Mr. Tenhave.**

SCREENING TEST OF APHASIA

Test Protocol

by

Lon Emerick, Ph.D.
J. Michael Coyne, M.D.


Roy O. Tenhave          January 4, 1918
    patient              date of birth


I. INPUT

   A. Auditory (to be answered "yes" or "no" or in some
      manner of signaling affirmative and negative)

      1. Disparities:

         a. Is your name Mr. (use incorrect name)          "yes"
         b. Are you in the hospital? "yes"--disgusted look
         c. Are you 20 years old? shook head "no," smiled
         d. Is this the year 19 "yes" "yes"
         e. Do you take a bath in a teacup? "no," emphati-
            cally, waved as if wishing to move to more
            difficult tasks.

      2. Commands (the patient is instructed to point to
         appropriate objects and pictures after hearing a
         verbal cue):  Card I

| a. match | + | f. bed | + | |
|----------|---|--------|---|---|
| b. coin | + | g. pencil | + | |
| c. key | + | h. knife | + | swift, certain |
| d. pen | + | i. chair | + | responses |
| e. books | + | j. hammer | + | |

      3. Understanding multiple commands (avoid gestures
         that reveal the appropriate response):

         a. Put the key on the bed picked up the key--asked
            for repetition
         b. Put the pen on the table              +
         c. Put the coin in my hand put the coin on the table
         d. Put the match on the table            +

**FIGURE 7.3 (cont.)**

B. Visual (matching tasks):

1. Matching identical objects (The objects--pens, keys, coins, and matches--are arrayed in random fashion on the table before the patient, and he is instructed to place like objects together.)  The examiner can demonstrate if necessary.

        +                      +
_____  _____
all correct--swift
certain responses
        +                      +
_____  _____

2. Matching pictures and written words (the patient is instructed to place the word cards on the corresponding picture):  Card I, Card Series Ia

   a. books   +     d. car   +
   b. pencil   +    e. bed   +     All correct
   c. knife   +     f. hammer   +

II. OUTPUT

A. Automatic speech (have the patient perform the following tasks):

1. Count from 1 to 10 _____ + _____
2. Say the letters of the alphabet stopped at "m," refused to continue
3. Repeat the days of the week when cued
4. Does the patient exhibit other forms of automatic language, for example, swearing? _yes_
5. Does the patient use gestures? points; expressive gestures (wave of dismissal; shoulder shrug); no complex pantomime

B. Simple repetition (have the patient repeat after the examiner):

1. Say "methodist episcopal"    "methdist piscopal"
2. Say "ah"   +
3. Say "puh"   +       no abnormality noted
4. Say "tuh"   +
5. Say "luh"   +
6. Say "puh-tuh-kuh" several times _____ refused

**FIGURE 7.3 (cont.)**

C. Repetition of words (have the patient repeat after
   the examiner):

   1. car     "drive"      4. paper   "write"
   2. snow    "snow"       5. rake    "rake"
   3. clock   "time"       6. leaves  "rake"

   7. Winter is cold "it's winter" (looked out window)
   8. In fall the leaves turn many colors "leaves
            turn . . ."
   9. She had a face that launched a thousand ships
            "Troy!"

D. Open-end sentences (have the patient complete the
   sentences):

   1. You pound nails with a "wood, no, no, pound . . ."
   2. You chop wood with a "ah, ah, oh, shit, no, wood--
         chop--axe!"
   3. You read a "book"
   4. When you want to stop a car you step on the
            "pedal"
   5. Don't change horses in the middle of the "...shit"
   6. Don't put all your eggs in one (no response)

E. Spontaneous speech (the patient is asked to name
   objects that the examiner points to about the room):

   1. bed      "sleep"        4. light  "lamp"
   2. table    (no response)  5. door   (no response)
   3. window   "window"       6. chair  "sit"

F. Self-formulated responses: (not tested)

   1. Is it good to get an education?  Why or why not?
   2. What is democracy?
   3. What does it mean to say "one swallow doesn't make
         a summer?"

Comments: visual field cut; lots of struggle behavior; self-
          correction attempts noted.  See attached report.

tears and his chin quivered slightly. Sitting down again beside his bed, I realized my error: Aphasic patients need closure like any other client. Remembering that monologue interviews are often helpful in providing an outlet for language-impaired adults, I began to verbalize his feelings, speaking slowly and carefully:

> This is tough for you. You have words inside and you can't seem to get them out. Some people talk down or too loudly; some talk too fast and don't give you a chance to understand. It's booming and buzzing; your own language is like a foreign one. You get mad and want to fight, but your arm and your leg are holding you back. You swear and sometimes can't stop crying. But it is going to get better. I am encouraged by how you did today. Oh, sure, the tasks were simple ones, but the point is, you could do them. You recognized false bird names; you matched pictures and words; you were even able to repeat some words when I provided the model. These are all good signs, especially so soon after the stroke. I also like the way you were able to tell when you do make a mistake. I am going to talk to Dr. Wilson and arrange to come back again.

During this brief monologue, Mr. Tenhave sighed, nodded, and appeared to relax considerably.

Before leaving the hospital, we wrote this short note to Dr. Wilson:

> The results of the screening test are encouraging. Mr. Tenhave has good auditory recognition (pointing to objects and pictures when named) and his comprehension for auditory materials is good within his limited auditory memory span. His listening is accurate for simple, short messages. He seems to understand more than he really does because he is alert, well oriented, and he picks out a crucial word in a sentence. He has a good supply of automatic (counting, emotional language) and reactive speech. He frequently gives associations when asked to name objects or pictures; for example, he said "pedal" for "brake." His gestures are not more complex than his verbal output. We did not ask him to write at this time, but it is my impression that his language deficit cuts across all modalities. No dysarthria was observed, although he did "simplify" complex words such as "Methodist." He is making a great many attempts at self-correction. On balance, then, I would say that he has a good prognosis.

### The Case History

Language therapy for an adult aphasic has to be very personalized. Therefore, we need to know as much as possible about the individual when planning a program of treatment. What sort of person was she before the stroke? How did she meet her problems? What educational level did she achieve? What was her occupation? Her avocations? What changes in her behavior, if any, have occurred following the brain injury? The style, pace, and content of therapy will be based on the answers to these and many other questions.

Unfortunately, the aphasic patient himself is in no position to provide the kind of detailed information we seek. In some instances, official records (educational tests, military records) and personal documents (diaries, letters) are helpful. Usually, however, we must rely on the accuracy and veracity of informants who presumably are familiar with the patient. The most common method of assembling information about the language-impaired individual is a case history form that is filled out by a spouse or other close relative. Ideally, the clinician also interviews the respondent to clarify any ambiguities in the written information and to permit additional questioning. Keep in mind, however, that a long-term marriage partner typically sees the client as less impaired than objective language testing may show (Helmick, Watamori, and Palmer, 1976); Holland (1977) points out, however, that acontextual tests of language do not measure communication and the client may, in fact, perform better in a "real" setting.

In addition to the case history, the diagnostician may wish to prepare an index that reflects the severity of the client's total disability. The clinician can choose from several published scales, among them the *Maryland Disability Index, Communication Status Chart* (Wisconsin Division of Health, 1966), the *Pulses Profile and Barthel Index* (Granger and Albrecht, 1979), the *Functional Performance Assessment* (Harvey and Jellinek, 1983), and the *Functional Life Scale* (Sarno and Sarno, 1973). We prefer the latter device because it provides a quantitative measure of the individual's ability to participate in all phases of daily activity—in the home, outside the home, and in social interaction.

On the basis of our initial contact with Mrs. Tenhave, we decided that she would be a detailed and objective reporter. We therefore gave her an aphasia case history form and simply requested that she answer the various queries to the best of her ability. The entire form follows (see Figure 7.4).

We then had a rather detailed description of the salient aspects of Mr. Tenhave's premorbid personality, health history, and social orientation. We knew a lot about the man he had been, but what impact had this sudden illness wrought? How much change could we expect, and in what areas? Would his responses to the language impairment and physical disabilities merely be an exaggeration of earlier behavior patterns?

There are only limited answers to these questions. We suspect, however, that the nature of the illness, the treatment the patient receives, and his interpretation of both these aspects (as well as premorbid factors) are all crucial in determining the impact of the problem upon the individual. Understandably, the literature is limited in this area.[5] Some workers refer to the aphasic's altered behavior patterns with handy labels, for example, "egocentricity," "catastrophic response," "concretism." It is often inferred that these nonlanguage "deviations" are a direct product of the brain damage. The designation of "organicity" then excuses the clinician from identifying any further the dynamics behind the labels.

We do not deny that many aphasics become obsessed with themselves and their situation, that they often respond emotionally to seemingly minor barriers, that they have difficulty dealing with abstractions, or that they often become depressed (Robinson and Benson, 1981). However, it is our position that *an*

---

[5] Despite the tremendous frustration and alteration in self-concept that aphasia produces, most of our clients did not exhibit much change in their basic personality traits. For ways to assess the psychosocial impact of adult language impairment, see the work of Evans and Northwood (1983) and Müller, Code, and Mugford (1983).

**FIGURE 7.4  Aphasia case history: Mr. Tenhave.**

```
General Information

Name  Roy O. Tenhave     Birthdate  Jan. 4, 1918     Sex  M

Address  211 Radisson                    Phone  226-3801

Person filling out this form  Mary Tenhave (wife)
                              (name and relationship to client)

Address      -----          Phone  -----  Date  Feb. 3, 1970

Person(s) or agency who referred you to the Clinic
             Dr. Roger Wilson

Personal and Family History

Marital status:   single __  married X  separated __
                  divorced __  widowed __  remarried __ .

Spouse's address                                  Phone

Children:    Names:           Addresses:              Ages:
          Raymond        APO San Francisco             28
                         (in Viet Nam)

          _____     _____           ____

          _____     _____           ____

Grandchildren:  Number  ------           Ages  _____

Father's Name:  Ogden Tenhave    Living  ____  Deceased  x

If deceased, give cause of death   heart disease

Mother's name:  Bertha Trezona Tenhave  Living ___  Deceased  x

If deceased, give cause of death   cancer

Medical Information

Date of injury (accident, illness, stroke)   January 19, 1970

What caused the injury?   C.V.A.

Was the client unconscious?  Yes   If yes, for how long?
      less than two hours

Was the client paralyzed?  yes   Describe  right arm and leg

Did the client have convulsions?  no  Have they been
      controlled?  ____

Does the client complain of dizziness, fainting spells,
headaches?  did have several dizzy spells prior to the stroke
```

**FIGURE 7.4 (cont.)**

Does the client have any visual or hearing problems?
_Myopia, corrected_

Has the client been treated for other illnesses? _____
heart condition ___ stroke ___ others _Skin disorder_
_(herpes zoster), kidney stones, arthritis_

Name and address of physician _Dr. Roger Wilson, Ishpeming,_
_Michigan_

Has the patient been seen for any of the following services:

|                               | DATE      | PERSON/AGENCY        | ADDRESS   |
|-------------------------------|-----------|----------------------|-----------|
| Speech Therapy                |           |                      |           |
| Psychological counseling or testing |     |                      |           |
| Vocational counseling         |           |                      |           |
| Physical Therapy              | Presently | St. Luke's Hospital  | Marquette |
| Occupational Therapy          |           |                      |           |

Speech and Language Information

Describe what the client's speech was like at the onset of
the problem _couldn't say anything but "ah"_

How has it changed? _says some words_

Check the appropriate column as it applies to the patient
now.  Add comments on the right if needed to qualify the
answers.

CAN  CANNOT

| CAN | CANNOT | | |
|-----|--------|---|---|
| x | ___ | Indicate meaning by gesture | some |
| ___ | x | Repeat words spoken by others | |
| x | ___ | Use one or a few words over and over | swearing |
| x | ___ | Use emotional speech (swear words); (count or use other words that occur in a series, days of week, prayers) | |
| x | ___ | Use some words spontaneously | bird names |
| ___ | x | Say short phrases | |
| ___ | x | Say short sentences | |
| x | ___ | Follow requests and understand directions | |

**FIGURE 7.4 (cont.)**

| | | |
|---|---|---|
| ___ | ? | Follow radio and television speech |
| ? | ___ | Read signs with understanding |
| ? | ___ | Read numbers with understanding |
| x | ___ | Read single words |
| ___ | x | Read newspapers, magazines |
| ? | ___ | Tell time |
| ___ | x | Copy numbers, letters |
| ___ | x | Write name without assistance |
| ___ | x | Write single words |
| ___ | x | Write sentences, letters |
| ___ | x | Do simple arithmetic |
| ___ | x | Personal care (dressing, shaving, etc.) |
| ___ | x | Handle money |

How did the client react when he discovered that speech was difficult? very frustrated

What was your reaction? thought it was temporary, then concerned

What do you do when the client cannot answer or when he tries to talk? try to give him a "yes - no"

How does the client react when he cannot say what he wants to? swears; tries to use signs or gestures; scribbles with left hand

How does the client respond to personal contacts other than family members (friends, associates)? he does not seem to want to see them--or have them see him like he is.

Personal and Social Information

A.  Before the injury:

Where did the client spend his childhood? Upper Peninsula, White Pine, L'Anse

Where did he go to school? L'Anse, Michigan

How far did he go in school? M.A. degree, plus extra course work

What is his occupation? biology teacher
Did he like his work? yes, very much

**FIGURE 7.4 (cont.)**

How long has he worked at this job? <u>24 years</u>
What other work has he done?
 <u>naturalist in summers at state parks (11 summers)</u>
    (give dates and length of time)

What is the client's native language? <u>English</u>
Does he speak any other? <u>some Finn</u>

What hobbies or special interests does he have? <u>bird</u>
 <u>study; photography; hiking and canoeing; hunting and</u>
 <u>fishing</u>

What did he like to read? <u>all types--ecology, philosophy,</u>
 <u>biographies</u>

Which television programs did he enjoy? <u>movies; news</u>
 <u>programs</u>

Did he do much writing (if so, what **kind**)? <u>yes; pamphlets,</u>
 <u>a science unit</u>

Which hand did he prefer? <u>right</u>

Describe the client's personality A. <u>Before the injury</u>:

Nervousness <u>not especially</u>

Shyness <u>basically a private person although he liked</u>
 <u>small groups</u>

Moods <u>no</u> Getting along with others <u>good</u>

Meeting problems: gave up easily <u>  </u> kept on trying <u>x</u>
other <u>he always tried to approach things rationally</u>

B. <u>After the injury</u>:

How has the client reacted to the injury? <u>very frustrated.</u>
 <u>I think he feels that his body is letting him down.</u>

What seems to bother him the most? <u>can't make himself</u>
 <u>understood</u>

What personality changes have you noted? <u>he is so</u>
 <u>emotional now</u>

What is his attitude toward speech therapy? <u>I don't know</u>

Has the physician talked to you about the client's
speech difficulty? <u>briefly</u>

Any further information which may aid in the examination?
 <u>Roy always prided himself in his ability to think and</u>
 <u>reason. He is a skilled naturalist, especially in the</u>
 <u>area of ornithology. He is an expert in bird calls,</u>
 <u>and he has written a widely used pamphlet on attracting</u>
 <u>birds. He was an excellent teacher, and his students</u>
 <u>seem to have great respect for his quiet strength and</u>
 <u>wry humor.</u>

*aphasic's behavior is largely a product of his drastically altered life experience, not merely a result of damaged brain cells.* Further, we contend that if the experience of being aphasic is carefully examined, the basis for many of the so-called non-language deviations becomes evident. Let us consider briefly two important inter-related factors: *isolation* and *infantilization.*

The parallels between the experience of sensory (and perceptual) deprivation and asphasia are startling. It is surprising, then, that to the best of our knowledge, the results of research dealing with subjects' responses to isolation have not been applied to the situation of the adult aphasic. Consider this sampling of findings from sensory deprivation studies (Solomon et al., 1961; Zubek, 1969):

1. Subjects show regression in perception and cognition to more primitive modes.
2. Subjects manifest a marked reduction in motivation.
3. Subjects tend to create internal images, experience hallucinations.
4. Subjects, after adjusting to a severely restricted environment, may exhibit severe emotional reactions to increments in sensation.

Now, consider again the aphasic patients: There is an abrupt reduction in sensory stimulation; the sensory input they do receive may be severely distorted or lack variety; their physical activity is restricted; there are prolonged periods of enforced rest in quiet, darkened rooms. Several publications that describe the recovery of adults with aphasia stress the importance of continued stimulation, especially during the primary stage of recovery (McBride, 1969; Hodgins, 1964; Farrell, 1969; Luria, 1972; Moss, 1972).

The bland, dependent existence of the aphasic tends to be *infantilizing.* At least four overlapping factors are responsible:

*The nature of the disorder.* Aphasia generally has a very sudden onset; the individual has no chance to prepare herself for the experience. The illness destroys or alters drastically those attributes most critical to human functioning—communication, control of body functions, and physical ability. Abruptly, the person is stripped of her identity, and without identity an individual is without humanity.

Holmes and his associates (Holmes and Rahe, 1967) have prepared a scale that assigns an "impact value" to the relative amount of adjustment required to cope with life events. For example, loss of a work role is rated at 47 points; personal injury or illness, 53 points; change in eating habits, 15 points. The more life-change units a person experiences in a given period of time, the greater the impact in terms of his biological, psychological, and social functioning. Behavior patterns break down as the individual attempts to cope with the changes. According to Holmes, change—either good or bad—causes stress to a person and leaves him more susceptible to disease. Stress reactions also elevate blood cholesterol, and this may exacerbate the vascular disease that caused the stroke. (For an illuminating discussion of hospital-induced stress, see Cousins, 1983.)

*The sick role.* Minor illness is a socially acceptable excuse for the temporary abandonment of normal adult decorum and responsibilities. The gravely ill person, such as the aphasic adult, is exempted from all former role requirements and demands—work, family responsibilities, and social obligations. Because he is not responsible for his condition (although one middle-aged aphasic patient who suffered a stroke while shoveling snow, an activity forbidden by his physician, was severely and continually blamed for his condition by his family), he cannot be held accountable for anything except being a "good patient." A good patient submits without question to the hospital routine and treatment program; he forfeits reliance upon his family and follows orders given by strangers; his existence is passive, and he is always in a horizontal posture; he must not complain about his lost roles or the rules of the institution. In short, many hospitalized persons manifest EPB—environment pleasing behavior.

*The hospital routine.*   Another closely related source of regression is the hospital experience. Note the possibilities for infantilization in this vivid description of the hospital experience by Duff and Hollingshead (1968: 269):

> Between admission to and discharge from the hospital, the patients were subjected to orders of the staff. They were separated from their families. Their street clothes were shed. They were assigned beds, given numbers, and dressed in bedroom apparel. They had to permit strangers access to the most intimate parts of their bodies. Their diet was controlled, as were the hours of their days and nights, the people they saw, and the times they saw them. They were bathed, fed, and questioned: they were ordered or forbidden to do specific things. *As long as they were in the hospital they were not considered self-sufficient adults.* (Italics ours.)

In some hospitals, nurses and aides are instructed to call patients by their first names, apparently to simulate personal involvement. It is ludicrous and an insult to his dignity when a fifty-two-year-old biology teacher is referred to as "Roy" by a twenty-year-old student nurse. Consider, finally, the impact on a seriously ill and profoundly frustrated patient of the determined cheerfulness and casual bonhomie that often seem to be the main features of nurses' professional character armor. One of our colleagues who suffered a moderately severe cerebral vascular episode and has experienced a good recovery made this comment:

> Whenever I tried to find out something about myself, the nurses just smiled benignly and, using the title without an article, suggested that DOCTOR will let *us* know how everything is going. That's the worst cut of all, that dreadful hospital "we." "How are *we* today?" "How is *our* patient?" "Time for *our* bath." My wife told one nurse's aide that only the Pope and people with tapeworms should use the pronoun "we." She just smiled and said that *we* were following doctors' orders.

*The style of interaction.*   But perhaps the most devastating and pervasive source of infantilization the aphasic experiences comes with the altered style of interaction—verbal and nonverbal—used with impaired individuals. Persons do not (indeed, often cannot) talk to the patient the same way they did before the language disturbance:

1. They talk more loudly, more precisely.
2. They ask simple, obvious questions.
3. They frequently answer their own queries.
4. They talk around the person to others.
5. They may talk about the person in his presence.
6. They may overrespond to his infrequent verbalizations or minor communication successes.

Note that each instance is a typical (but even so, unfortunate) mode of communicating with a child.

Physically, the aphasic patient is often dependent on others. His wife, or someone else close to him, must help him bathe, dress, and perhaps even eat. It is easy to slip back into childhood when one is hovered over, insulated, and guarded.

> And I had seen so many begin to pack their lives in cotton wool, smother their impulses, hood their passions, and gradually retire from their manhood into a kind of spiritual and physical semi-invalidism. In this they are encouraged by wives and relatives, and it's such a sweet trap. Who doesn't like to be a center for concern? A kind of second childhood falls on so many men. They trade their violence for the promise of a small increase in life span. In effect, the head of the household *becomes the youngest child.* (Steinbeck, 1961: 19) (Italics ours.)[6]

But is all of this discussion relevant to the assessment of an adult aphasic patient? We think it is. Any information about the individual is important because it might bear upon the responses to the examiner and to the tests employed. What does it mean if a client fails to respond to a test item? A simple minus designation? A scoring category value of one? Rejection of the task? Fear of failure, anxiousness? Severe depression? Hostility? Auditory comprehension difficulty? Reduced auditory memory span? Perhaps a combination of any or all of these?

The point is that we must attempt to understand the person and what has happened to him as completely as possible; the more time spent in this regard, the better a diagnostician we become. Otherwise, it is dreadfully easy to be seduced by a particular diagnostic tool to the point that we come to see aphasia and the aphasic solely through a test. Indeed, if it is worth forty hours of study to acquire proficiency in scoring a patient's language responses according to the multidimensional scale, then certainly it is worth at least as much time trying to appreciate the impact of aphasia on an individual's humanity. A patient is more than a neat array of carefully charted profiles, as significant and desirable as those measurements may be. We must not mistake *measurement* for understanding.

---

[6]For a comprehensive review of family therapy in aphasia, see the chapter by Rollin (1984).

### The Language Inventory

Mr. Tenhave was discharged from the hospital on February 16. He wore a brace on his lower right leg and walked with the aid of a tripod cane; his right arm was held up in a sling. Each day he returned to the hospital as an outpatient for physical and occupational therapy. Although he was using some voluntary speech, including a few short phrases, his attempts to communicate were still extremely frustrating.

In order to devise a plan of treatment for Mr. Tenhave, as well as to predict the probable course and outcome of treatment, we would need a comprehensive appraisal of his present language abilities. Where is he having difficulty? Which modalities are working best? How does he make his errors? Are there discernible patterns to his errors? To answer these and other questions, we had to administer a language inventory.

The clinician has several published tests of aphasia from which to choose. (See Figure 7.5.) These instruments have been reviewed by Leutenegger (1975) and others (Buros, 1978; Darley, 1979; Davis, 1983; Tikofsky, 1984) and there is no need to duplicate their efforts here.

Beginning clinicians often ask which aphasia inventory they should select for examining clients. We prefer not to advocate any particular instrument but instead ask the clinician to specify her purposes in testing. What does she want the test to show? If she wants to be able to predict the course of the client's recovery, the *PICA* (Porch, 1967) is the instrument of choice; if she is more interested in the site of lesion, the *Boston Examination* (Goodglass and Kaplan, 1983) or the *Western Aphasia Battery* (Kertesz, 1980) are indicated; if she wishes to identify how the client performs on basic language functions, then the *Minnesota Test* (Schuell, 1965) is the best choice. In the hands of a skilled and perceptive clinician who is thoroughly familiar with the materials, any of the tests cited above will provide a detailed description of an aphasic's language disturbance.

Most diagnosticians prefer to administer a battery of tests rather than limit themselves to one particular instrument. Each sample of a client's performance permits another glimpse of her underlying language competence. Several workers (Wepman, 1972; Bliss, Guilford, and Tikofsky, 1976; Ultaowska et al., 1976) advocate a method of assessment that samples a client's communication ability in her natural environment. Only two of the extant tests—the checklist devised by Taylor (1963) and the instrument prepared by Holland (1980—elicit genuine communication:

> The PICA, or any other aphasia test, to the best of my knowledge makes no claim for measuring how a person communicates; it claims rather to address his or her ability to perform on a set of fairly stereotyped tasks which have only a tangential relationship to give and take of everyday communicative interaction. (Holland, 1977: 307)

As we pointed out in Chapter 3, a test is only a tool, a way to help the examiner make relatively precise observations of a particular client. None of the published aphasia inventories is pure, none is sacrosanct, not even the three most popular tests, the *Boston,* the *Minnesota,* and the *PICA.*

The PICA is perhaps the most popular tool at present for evaluating adult aphasics. It is a good test, very well constructed, and features a thorough scoring system employing a sixteen-step scale. The instrument allows the examiner to make precise observations and accurate predictions. It is not, however, the Holy Grail of aphasiology that some overly zealous diagnosticians impugn it to be. For example, we dislike the rigidity with which the test is used; we feel that the so-called standard procedure breaks down the client-clinician relationship, inhibits the client, and creates "noise" in his system. We agree with Keenan and Brassell (1975: 36) that "a badly presented item is a minor error, far less important than an impersonal or mechanical response to the patient." Additionally, we find that starting the examination with the

**FIGURE 7.5   Most commonly used language inventories.**

| | |
|---|---|
| *Minnesota Test for Differential Diagnosis of Aphasia* (1965; 2nd ed., 1973) | H. Schuell<br>University of Minnesota Press,<br>   Minneapolis, Minn. 55455 |
| *Sklar Aphasia Scale* (1966) | M. Sklar<br>Western Psychological Services,<br>   12031 Wilshire Blvd., Los Angeles, Calif.<br>   90025 |
| *Porch Index of Communicative Ability* (1967) | B. Porch<br>Consulting Psychologists Press,<br>   577 College Ave., Palo Alto, Calif. 94306 |
| *Functional Communication Profile\** (1969) | M. T. Sarno<br>Institute of Rehabilitation Medicine,<br>   New York University Medical Center,<br>   400 E. 34 St., New York, N.Y. 10016 |
| *Boston Diagnostic Aphasia Examination* (1983) | H. Goodglass and E. Kaplan<br>Lea and Febiger, 600 Washington Sq.,<br>   Philadelphia, Pa. 19106 |
| *Aphasia Language Performance Scales* (1975) | J. Keenan and E. Brassell<br>Pinnacle Press, P.O. Box 1122,<br>   Murfreesboro, Tenn. 37130 |
| *Neurosensory Center Comprehensive Examination for Aphasia* (1977) | O. Spreen and A. Benton<br>Neurosensory Laboratory,<br>   University of Victoria, Victoria, B.C., Canada |
| *Western Aphasia Battery* (1980) | A. Kertesz<br>Department of Clinical Neurological Sciences,<br>   University of Western Ontario,<br>   London, Ont., Canada |
| *Communicative Abilities in Daily Living* (1980) | A. Holland<br>University Park Press, 233 E. Redwood St.,<br>   Baltimore, Md. 21202 |

\*The FCP is not a test but rather a checklist that describes and quantifies a client's language performance in an informal setting.

most difficult task often overwhelms the aphasic and disturbs his subsequent performance. Although we have often used the instrument, and find it extremely valuable, the PICA offers only limited information about a client's verbal ability: only four of the eighteen subtests elicit verbal behavior; only one of the four, "describing how objects are used," affords any insight into how the client talks. Finally, we don't feel that a diagnostician should abrogate her personal clinical responsibility for judgment by deferring to a test or the numerical scores it generates. Perhaps this reveals our disenchantment with the accountability fad—which has often been used as an accusation (Siegel, 1975)—but we believe it is a poor trade to lose the richness in descriptive detail for the convenience that comes from manipulation of numerical data.

Nation and Aram (1977: 258) state the issue succinctly: "A good diagnostician relies on the feelings that have resulted as much as on the tools that were administered."

To evaluate Mr. Tenhave, we selected an instrument of our own construction (Emerick, 1971). The *Appraisal of Language Disturbance (ALD)* was developed as a product of the senior author's clinical experience with aphasic patients in Veterans Administration hospitals, private medical settings, and an active outpatient speech-and-hearing center.

> The *ALD* is a clinical tool designed to permit the clinician to make a systematic inventory of a patient's communicative abilities both in the modalities of input and output and the central integration processes. It enables the worker to make a careful appraisal of all possible linguistic tranmission factors—gesture to oral, aural to gesture—delineated in the research of Wepman and his associates. In this manner, the clinician receives a precise description of the patient's capacity with respect to the various pathways for stimulation and response. In addition, tasks are arranged in an ascending order of linguistic complexity within each subtest assessing input and output factors; this permits the clinician to determine not only the nature of the dysfunction but also the extent of the problem. (The several open-end items included provide additional flexibility.) The *ALD* also includes a unit designed to assess central language processes and a final segment for evaluating areas of functioning peripheral to symbolic language such as tactile recognition, arithmetic abilities, and the oral area (Emerick, 1971: 1)

We arranged to administer the language inventory to Mr. Tenhave at an early morning appointment when he was most alert and rested. On March 3, we met Mr. Tenhave sitting impatiently in the clinic waiting room. Ushering him into a quiet, plainly furnished office, we offered him coffee and made him comfortable at a long table. The clinician positioned himself on the patient's left side. In order to give him time to adjust to the room and the communicative situation before starting the formal testing, we engaged Mr. Tenhave in casual conversation about the weather and the visitors to his bird-feeding station. We then carefully explained the purpose of testing and provided several examples of the types of tasks to be included. Mr. Tenhave nodded that he understood and motioned eagerly toward the testing materials.

We proceeded through the ten subtests in a casual manner, pausing often, commenting about specific items, and watching carefully for signs of fatigue. At one point Mr. Tenhave objected mildly to the wording of a particular sentence, and we reinforced his criticism; if a patient can criticize the test, he will not be threatened by it. The *ALD* is carefully designed to ensure initial success by having the client begin with simple items. We agree with Toubbeh (1969) that failure, especially at the beginning of the language testing, can be devastating; indeed, it may inhibit the patient's ability to focus on all incoming stimuli (Brookshire, 1972).

> When administering a language inventory, the diagnostician should be alert for signs of auditory processing difficulty: (1) the client may miss the first part of a message due to "slow rise time"; (2) he may, as the test proceeds, experience "noise buildup"; (3) the instructions for a task, or the task itself, may overload the capacity of his input circuits; or (4) his auditory system may shut off intermittently. These processing breakdowns depend to some extent on the severity of the client's language impairment (Di Simoni, Keith, and Darley, 1983; Riensche, Wohlert, and Porch, 1983).

A portion (subtest I) of the *ALD*, containing Mr. Tenhave's responses, is included in Figure 7.6 to show the kinds of tasks employed and to illustrate his responses. We subscribe to the view of Goodglass and Kaplan (1983) that subtests are "windows" that allow us to peer through a glass dimly at the patient's underlying language competence. The total time consumed by testing, including the brief breaks and desultory conversation, was jut over seventy-four minutes. We again chatted briefly with Mr. Tenhave at the end of the formal testing; we told him that although we would need to analyze the results carefully before starting therapy, we were encouraged by his responses.

The completed *ALD* provides a protocol that outlines the severity of a patient's language disturbance and the areas (modalities) of impairment. The test does not yield a classification system nor does it attempt to place aphasics into various categories. We agree with Buck (1968: 85) that "too often our diagnostic labels blind us to the true state of affairs and prevent further investigation." It is far more useful clinically simply to identify what the patient can and cannot do with language symbols. The *ALD*, however, does provide a summary form for collating data obtained from the patient on the ten subtests. Figure 7.7 shows the completed summary form for Mr. Tenhave.

The column on the left simply lists the ten subtests. Note the five columns enumerated 1 through 5 and labeled "rating." After administering the *ALD* we rated Mr. Tenhave's performance on each subtest utilizing the following crude scale:

1.  All, or almost all, responses correct
2.  Majority of responses correct
3.  Approximately half the responses correct, half incorrect
4.  Majority of responses incorrect
5.  All, or almost all, responses incorrect

**FIGURE 7.6   Subtest I of ALD showing Mr. Tenhave's responses.**

✓ – *Correct response*
✗ – *Incorrect response*
*NR* – *No response*

1. Aural to Oral

In this subtest the examiner provides auditory stimulation and the patient responds with oral language.

A. Automatic:
   ✗1. ask patient his name "Roy"
   ✓2. ask patient to count to 10 (the examiner may provide some stimulation to get the patient started)
   ✓3. ask patient letters of the alphabet
   ✓4. ask patient days of the week

B. Imitative: the patient repeats the following words after the examiner; listen for articulation errors.
   ✗1. cat            ✓6. scissors
   ✓2. hair           ✓7. do you have a match
   ✓3. paper          ✓8. very few have freedom
   ✓4. rock           ✓9. judge not lest thee be judged
   ✓5. leaves         ✓10. six times six is thirty-six

C. Symbolic:
   1. oral opposites: have the patient supply the opposite orally.
      ✓a. thin        ✓d. fast
      ✓b. man         ✓e. living
      ✓c. strong      f. anarchy *nR*

   2. open end sentences: have the patient finish the sentence orally.
      a. you sleep on a  *"bed"*
      b. the boy picked up his bat and ball and went to play *"ball"*
      c. please get me a drink of *"milk"*
      ✗d. a bird in the hand is worth two in the _____
      e. he who hesitates is *N.R.*

   3. definitions: have the patient supply the word orally.
      a. something to read *"book"*
      b. a farm animal that gives milk *"cow"*
      c. a white cylinder of tobacco *"don't smoke"*
      d. something that registers the passage of time *"watch"*
      e. a black drink brewed from ground beans *N.R.*

   4. disparities: have the patient attempt to point out what is wrong with the following sentences.
      ✓a. They filled the car with catsup.
      ✓b. He spread his bread with butter and nails.
      ✓c. She wrote a letter with paper and peanut butter.
      ✓d. A penny saved is a penny burned.
      ✓e. No man is an Ireland. *smiled*

**FIGURE 7.7   ALD summary form for Roy Tenhave.**

ALD SUMMARY FORM

Lon L. Emerick, Ph.D.
Northern Michigan University

| Transmission | Rating | | | | | Comments |
|---|---|---|---|---|---|---|
| | 1 | 2 | 3 | 4 | 5 | |
| I. Aural-Oral | | x | | | | limited by short auditory memory span |
| II. Aural-Visual | x | | | | | |
| III. Aural-Gesture | x | | | | | |
| IV. Aural-Graphic | | | | x | | used writing brace; spells phonetically |
| V. Gesture-Visual | x | | | | | |
| VI. Visual-Gesture | x | | | | | |
| VII. Visual-Oral | | | x | | | used association |
| VIII. Visual-Graphic | | | x | | | |

IX. Central Language
    Comprehension                      Rating: 1.5
    1. Matching                        1 Peabody = 95%
    2. Sorting                         2
    3. Manding                         1

X. Related Factors                     Rating:
    1. Tactile                         5
    2. Arithmetic                      1
    3. Oral Exam                       1 normal

Observations: 1. Errors increase as length of material
                 increases.
              2. Mispronunciations are correctable by ear.
              3. Self-correction is evident.
              4. Visual field cut seems to have improved.

Roy Tenhave      71-493      March 3, 1970        E.
  Patient        Number         Date           Examiner

Thus, we have a summary profile of the patient's language abilities as manifested by his responses to the ten specific subtests.

It is also important to examine *how* the patient made his errors. Did he seem to perseverate? At what level of complexity did his responses break down? Did he give synonyms or associations for words when asked to name pictures or objects? Mr. Tenhave, for example, when asked to name a picture of a dollar bill, said, "Put it . . . pocket . . . wallet . . ." Obviously, his "error" is far better than a response of "soup" or "don't know." Was the patient attempting to correct his errors (Marshall and Tompkins, 1981)? Are his responses significantly delayed? How did he respond to various cueing techniques? What strategies does he use to attempt to retrieve words—using gestures, writing, semantic, or phonetic cues (Holland, 1982)?

We summarized the test findings, together with our impressions and prognosis, in a detailed report:

*Client*: Roy Tenhave

*Test Findings.* The Appraisal for Language Disturbance was administered and revealed the following information on each of the ten subtests:

I. *Aural-Oral* (client listens, responds with oral language). The client replied swiftly and accurately on tasks calling for automatic and imitative responses. His responses to symbolic items (oral opposites, open-end sentences, definitions) appear to be limited by reduced availability of less frequently used words. Auditory comprehension is good within the limits imposed by a reduced verbal retention span. Recognizes disparities easily.

II. *Aural-Visual* (client listens and points). Auditory recognition for objects, pictures, and simple written words is intact. Mr. Tenhave's responses were rapid and positive.

III. *Aural-Gesture* (client listens and makes appropriate gesture). The patient can follow commands (shake hand, cough) with the appropriate gesture, point to body parts when named, and demonstrate complex gestures associated with writing, using a toothbrush, and throwing a ball.

IV. *Aura.-Graphic* (client listens and writes). Mr. Tenhave was reluctant initially to attempt writing with his left hand: a Zaner-Bloser writing frame was offered, and he used it to complete the tasks.[7] Automatic items (his name, age) were accomplished easily. However, his attempts to write a series of dictated letters and numbers were limited by his reduced auditory memory span; he could retain three but not four or more digits or letters. No rotation of letters or confusion between them was noted. He missed over 50 percent of the total items included in this subtest. Several short words ("bird," "lamp") were written correctly, but in general his spelling tends to be done phonetically (e.g., "blu" for "blue," "nos" for "nose").

V. *Gesture-Visual* (clinician makes a gesture, client must select appropriate object, picture, or written word associated with the gesture). He responded accurately to each test item: he watched the clinician's gestures and selected the appropriate object, picture, and printed word from a series arrayed before him.

VI. *Visual-Gesture* (examiner shows an object, picture, or written word to the patient, and the patient makes a gesture typically associated with it). All items were done swiftly and correctly.

[7] The Zaner-Bloser Company, 612 North Park Street, Columbus, Ohio.

VII. *Visual-Oral* (client is presented a visual stimulus and is requested to read or name orally). Mr. Tenhave missed almost half of the items on this subtest. His oral vocabulary is reduced, and he frequently responded with words that were associated with the stimulus (e.g., "ring" for "bell," "eat" for "spoon," "Ford" for "car"). His reading rate is very slow; he labored over the test sentences and paragraph, pausing often to reread portions. His comprehension for reading material was good, but again, it was limited by a reduced verbal retention span. No dysarthria or apraxia was noted. He tends to mispronounce or simplify longer words; however, when he is instructed to listen carefully and is given an auditory model, he corrects his errors readily.

VIII. *Visual-Graphic* (client is presented a visual stimulus and responds by copying or writing). Mr. Tenhave had considerable difficulty with this subtest, missing more than half the items. He was able to copy letters, numbers, and written words accurately. However, he was able to identify in writing only two of the ten objects and pictures presented. When shown a drawing depicting several features, he simply enumerated three items and, after a long pause, put down the marking pen in obvious disgust. (Note: At this point the testing was stopped and the examiner and client relaxed over coffee; a respite should have been given before beginning this subtest. His concentration was so intense that it was difficult to discern when he was getting fatigued. This will have to be taken into account in therapy with him.)

IX. *Central Language Comprehension* (in this subtest, the client is given various tasks—matching, sorting, object assembly, recognition vocabulary—which more directly assess the status of the client's central sorting and integrative functioning). Matching (objects to silhouettes, pictures to pictures, objects to pictures), object assembly, and manding presented no difficulty to Mr. Tenhave. He scored at the 95th percentile on the Peabody Picture Vocabulary Test (Dunn, 1965). His errors involved sorting: he arranged the circle and squares according to color initially (note: Check to see if he has a type of color blindness—he seemed to confuse green and blue. It is rather peculiar, though, for a skilled ornithologist to be color-blind) and when the request was made to recategorize them, he was unable to do so.

X. *Related Factors* (in this subtest, areas of functioning peripheral to symbolic language are examined—tactile recognition, arithmetic ability, and motor speech behavior). Tactile recognition in the right hand is totally absent; he made two errors with his left hand. Simple arithmetic problems presented no difficulty for Mr. Tenhave; he requested several repetitions of the short story problem, however, before he could successfully complete it. This reflected his reduced verbal retention span. Oral examination revealed normal functioning.[8]

*Prognosis.* Excellent prospects for recovery. The patient's auditory recognition is intact, and his comprehension is good; both are essential to a favorable response to therapy. Another favorable sign is Mr. Tenhave's ability to detect his errors and, when provided with an auditory model, correct them. A determined attitude augurs well for his continued efforts during treatment.

The language inventory permits the clinician to identify islands of ability the client retains. In many instances, however, the clinician will want to do additional, more extensive testing in particular areas:

---

[8] Before starting therapy, Mr. Tenhave was given an audiometric evaluation; his hearing was within normal limits (see studies by Street, 1957; Miller, 1960; Needham and Black, 1970).

1. *Nonverbal intelligence.* We find *Raven's Progressive Coloured Matrices* (1960) useful to assess nonlanguage skills.
2. *Speech fluency.* Evaluation of length of utterance, rate, grammaticalness, and divergent speech tasks (Chapey, Rigrodsky, and Morrison, 1976; Chapey, 1981) assist in distinguishing fluent from nonfluent aphasia. A client's response when asked to name as many foods as he can or to list all the possible uses of an object reveals much about his verbal fluency.
3. *Reading ability.* We employ the *Reading Comprehension Battery* (LaPointe and Horner, 1979) to make an in-depth assessment of a client's reading ability.
4. *Auditory competence.* The integrity of the auditory modality is crucial prognostically: Can the client detect, localize, retain, discriminate, and sequence items she hears? We find both the *Revised Token Test* (McNeil and Prescott, 1978) and the *Auditory Comprehension Test for Sentences* (Shewan, 1980) very useful for probing a client's auditory processing abilities.

## PROGNOSIS

Selecting patients for treatment who have the best chance of recovery from aphasia is an unsettling task. Rather than abandon anyone, one's impulse is to attempt to work with every aphasic even though prospects for improvement in cases of severe language impairment are dim (Sarno, Silverman, and Sands, 1970). When there is little real progress, the patient's labors are like those of Sisyphus.

How, then, can the clinician identify aphasic clients with the best potential? A list of interrelated factors that we have found helpful for making a prognosis is presented below; however, we trust the reader's forecasting will be guided by three important maxims: (1) Do not make a final prognosis on the basis of a single evaluation session—a period of trial therapy is always highly informative; (2) do not make a prognosis solely on the basis of a single measure of behavior—for example, the client's performance on a language inventory; and (3) be sure you understand the value of predictors—they can be potent self-fulfilling prophecies.

1. *Initial severity.* The more severe the patient's language impairment is at the time of assessment, the poorer the prognosis. Three aspects of language functioning are important in predicting recovery:
   —*Auditory recognition.* Patients who make errors (even a few errors—two or three out of ten items—are significant) when identifying pictures or common objects named by the examiner have an unfavorable prognosis; an impairment at this level is apparently irreversible.
   —*Comprehension.* Patients who have marked difficulty in comprehending verbal messages make poor candidates for treatment. In fact, a reliable index of the severity of language impairment in aphasia is the degree of disturbance in comprehension.
   —*Speech fluency.* Patients who speak more fluently seem to make better recoveries. But the presence of jargon, especially when it is coupled with lack of self-monitoring, euphoria, or denial, is a poor clinical sign.
2. *Time elapsed since onset.* The longer the time elapsed since onset of aphasia

and the beginning of treatment, the poorer the prognosis. Habits of dependence, withdrawal, and possible secondary gains accruing from a nonverbal role tend to defeat therapeutic intervention.

3. *Primary stage of recovery.* The more untoward events (infantilizing, isolation, withdrawal, exposure to negative attitudes) that occur during the first few months after the brain injury, the poorer the patient's motivation will be to undertake treatment.

4. *Age.* Generally, the younger the patient the better are the prospects for recovery. Aphasics in or near retirement often lack the energy and motivation to persist in a treatment program. In addition, older patients may have more widespread cerebral damage due to arteriosclerosis.

5. *Presence of other health problems.* In our clinical experience, aphasic patients presenting health problems in addition to the brain injury (such as diabetes, systemic vascular disease, or kidney disease) often do poorly in therapy.

6. *Family response.* Patients whose families provide supportive understanding and appropriate stimulation and permit the individual to regain his role within the family unit have a more favorable prognosis.

7. *Extent of the lesion.* The more extensive the brain injury, the poorer the prospects for recovery.

8. *Location of the lesion.* Damage occurring posterior to the fissure of Rolando, especially at the junction of the parietal temporal lobe, tends to result in more persistent aphasia.

9. *Etiology.* Depending on the location and extent of the lesion, patients who have suffered traumatic brain injury tend to make better recoveries than do individuals who have had thrombotic or other vascular episodes.

10. *Premorbid personality.* The more outgoing, flexible individual generally responds better to treatment than does an inhibited, introverted person.

11. *Intelligence and education.* The more intelligent, better educated patients make better candidates for therapy. Although this is generally true, a few of our most highly educated clients were so vividly aware of the discrepancy between their premorbid abilities and their present condition, they simply withdrew in futility.

12. *Self-monitoring.* Patients who are aware of their errors and attempt to correct them have a more favorable prognosis than those who do not.

The student will want to consult the following references for further information regarding prognosis in aphasia: Smith (1971), Keenan and Brassell (1974), Kertesz and McCabe (1977), Basso, Capitani, and Vignolo (1979), Porch et al. (1980), and Marshall and Philips (1983).

HIGHLIGHT   *Motor Speech Disorders*

All the diverse structures and systems that combine to produce speech are planned and regulated by the nervous system. Any damage or disease involving this regulatory system will disrupt the normally swift movements of the speech mechanism. The disruption is reflected in distortion of the speech signal, primarily in the utterance of speech sounds.

Basically, there are two types of motor speech disorders: *dysarthria* and *apraxia.* These two disorders may coexist with aphasia or occur separately:

When paralysis, weakness, or incoordination resulting from neuro-pathology disturbs the motor control centers, all facets of speech pro-duction—respiration, laryngeal control, resonation, articulation, and prosody—may malfunction. The resultant disorder is called *dysarthria*, or more properly, *dysarthrias*, as the term includes a group of motor speech impairments that stem from disturbance of the muscular control of the speech apparatus. The patterns of dysfunction are unique to the particular neurological disorder, the impairment may be isolated (as in Bell's palsy) or multiple (as in Parkinson's disease).

*Apraxia* is the disruption of the capacity to program voluntarily the production and sequencing of speech sounds; although the individual does not show muscular paralysis, her articulation is garbled and she seems to have forgotten how to execute speech-related movements. In fact, the more volition involved in the execution of a particular act, the worse the client's performance seems to be.

## Evaluation

Because any or all aspects of speech may be involved, the clinician must make a comprehensive inventory of the mechanical and aerodynamic features of a client's speech performance. This inventory includes careful listening (each type of dysarthria has unique perceptual characteristics), direct inspec-tion of the individual's oral structures, and observation of his respiration, laryngeal control, resonance, articulation, and prosody. Due to space limita-tions, it is not possible to present an entire testing battery for motor speech disorders (see the references at the end of this Highlight);* however, to illus-trate the assessment procedure, we include a portion of a checklist prepared by a team of graduate clinicians:

> *Oral Peripheral Examination* (see Chapter 3)
>     Facial muscles:   Symmetry _____   Paralysis _____   Weakness _____
>     Lips:  Symmetry _____        Paralysis _____
>     Tongue:  Symmetry _____    Fasciculations _____
>     Mandible
>     Velopharyngeal function
>     Nonspeech movements:
>         Stick out tongue _____          Smile _____
>         Show teeth _____                Click teeth _____
>         Pucker lips _____               Clear throat _____
>         Diadochokinesis _____
>     Description of movements:  Muscle tone _____      Speed _____
>                 Range of movement _____    Speed _____   Precision _____
> *Respiratory Functioning*
>     Duration of exhalation _____           Ability to blow _____
>     Other _____

*Clinician-researchers are developing instrumentation to interpret and quantify speech deviations arising from neuropathology. Kinematic measures of respiration and physiological analysis of lip and jaw movements may offer a better way of determining how much impairment is present in the motor speech subsystems (Putnam and Hixon, 1984; Hunker and Abbs, 1984).

*Laryngeal Control*

  Duration of vowel \_\_\_\_          Steadiness \_\_\_\_

          Counting \_\_\_\_

  Loudness \_\_\_\_

  Pitch \_\_\_\_

  S/Z ratio \_\_\_\_

*Resonance*

  Hypernasality \_\_\_\_

*Articulation*

  Types of errors \_\_\_\_          Response to stimulation \_\_\_\_

  Consistency of errors \_\_\_\_

*Prosody*

  Rate \_\_\_\_     Continuity \_\_\_\_     Pause \_\_\_\_     Disfluency \_\_\_\_

  Effort \_\_\_\_          Stress/intonation \_\_\_\_

## Differential Diagnosis of Dysarthria and Apraxia

|  | DYSARTHRIA | APRAXIA |
| --- | --- | --- |
| Definition | Distinct patterns of speech due to weakness, slowness and incoordination of speech muscles. Oral movements are disrupted and reflect different types of neuropathology | Articulation errors, in the absence of muscle slowness, weakness, incoordination, due to disruption of cortical programming for the *voluntary* production of speech sounds |
| Oral peripheral examination | Obvious defectiveness: slow, weak, and incoordinated. *Vegetative* functions (sucking, chewing), disturbed as well as speech movements | No obvious dysfunction except when requested to execute *voluntary* movements. Vegetative functions performed adequately |
| Articulation | Simplification<br>a. distortions<br>b. substitutions<br>Errors consistent<br>More complex units (clusters of consonants) are more difficult<br>More errors in final position<br>Errors consistent with neurological record<br>Severity related to extent of neuromuscular involvement | Complication<br>a. transpositions, reversals<br>b. perseverative and anticipatory errors<br>c. fewer distortions, more substitutions, intrusive additions<br>Errors increase proportionate to word weight (grammatical class, difficulty of initial consonant, position in sentence and word length)<br>Fewer errors in spontaneous performance<br>Inconsistency is key sign |
| Repeated utterance | Same performance | Makes repeated attempt and may achieve correct performance. Appears to grope or struggle for correct production |

### Differential Diagnosis of Dysarthria and Apraxia (cont.)

|  | DYSARTHRIA | APRAXIA |
|---|---|---|
| Rate | Deterioration of performance with increased rate<br>Slow rate of speech | Performance improves at faster rate<br>Disturbances of prosody: stuttering-like struggle reactions; slow, labored speech during voluntary attempts |
| Response to stimulation | May alter performance slightly to match auditory-visual model. Best response to demonstration of specific articulatory gestures | Best performance if sees and hears model. Does better if provided one stimulation and given several chances to match the model |

### Additional Information

For more information regarding motor speech disorders, consult the work of Darley, Aronson, and Brown (1975) and others (Johns, 1978; Yorkston and Beukelman, 1980; Dabul, 1983; Berry, 1983; Enderby, 1983; Wertz, LaPointe, and Rosenbek, 1984).

## BIBLIOGRAPHY

ADAMS, R., and M. VICTOR (1977). *Principles of Neurology.* New York: McGraw-Hill.

ALBERT, M. L., et al. (1981). *Clinical Aspects of Dysphasia.* New York: Springer-Verlag.

AMERICAN HEART ASSOCIATION (1965). *Aphasia and the Family.* New York: American Heart Association.

BASSO, L., E. CAPITANI, and L. VIGNOLO (1979). "Influence of Rehabilitation on Language Skill in Aphasic Patients." *Archives of Neurology,* 36: 190–196.

BAYLES, K., and D. BOONE (1982). "The Potential of Language Tasks for Identifying Senile Dementia." *Journal of Speech and Hearing Disorders,* 47: 210–217.

BENSON, D. F. (1979). *Aphasia, Alexia and Agraphia.* New York: Churchill Livingstone.

BERG, L., et al. (1982). "Mild Senile Dementia of Alzheimer Type: Research Diagnostic Criteria, Recruitment, and Description of a Study Population." *Journal of Neurology, Neurosurgery and Psychiatry,* 11: 962–968.

BERRY, W., ed. (1983). *Clinical Dysarthria.* San Diego, Calif.: College-Hill Press.

BLISS, L., A. GUILFORD, and R. TIKOFSKY (1976). "Performance of Adult Aphasics on a Sentence Evaluation and Revision Task." *Journal of Speech and Hearing Research,* 19: 551–560.

BOONE, D. (1961). *An Adult Has Aphasia.* Danville, Ill.: Interstate Printers and Publishers.

BROIDA, H. (1979). *Coping with Stroke.* San Diego, Calif.: College-Hill Press.

BROOKSHIRE, R. (1972). "Effects of Task Difficulty on Naming Performances of Aphasic Subjects." *Journal of Speech and Hearing Research,* 15: 551–558.

—— (1983). "Subject Description and Generality of Results in Experiments with Aphasic Adults." *Journal of Speech and Hearing Disorders,* 48: 342–346.

BUCHANAN, A. (1957). *Functional Neuro-Anatomy.* Philadelphia: Lea & Febiger.

BUCK, M. (1968). *Dysphasia.* Englewood Cliffs, N.J.: Prentice-Hall, Inc.

BUROS, O., ed. (1978). *The Eighth Mental Measurements Yearbook.* Vol. 2. Highland Park, N.J.: Gryphon Press.

CHAPEY, R. (1981). *Language Intervention Strategies in Adult Aphasia.* Baltimore: Williams & Wilkins.

CHAPEY, R., S. RIGRODSKY, and E. MORRISON (1976). "Divergent Semantic Behavior in Aphasia." *Journal of Speech and Hearing Research,* 19: 644–677.

CHUSID, J., and J. McDONALD (1967). *Correlative Neuroanatomy.* Los Altos, Calif.: Lange Medical Publications.

COUSINS, N. (1983). *The Healing Heart.* New York: W. W. Norton & Co.

DABUL, B. (1983). *Apraxia Battery for Adults.* Tigard, Oreg.: C. C. Publications.

DARLEY, F. (1979). *Evaluation of Appraisal Techniques in Speech and Language Pathology.* Reading, Mass.: Addison-Wesley.

────── (1982). *Aphasia.* Philadelphia: Saunders.

DARLEY, F., A. ARONSON, and J. BROWN (1975). *Motor Speech Disorders.* Philadelphia: Saunders.

DAVIS, G. (1983). *A Survey of Adult Aphasia.* Englewood Cliffs, N.J.: Prentice-Hall, Inc.

DERMAN, S., and A. MANASTER (9167). "Family Counseling with Relatives of Aphasic Patients." *Journal of American Speech and Hearing Association,* 8: 175–177.

DI SIMONI, F., R. KEITH, and F. DARLEY (1983). "Tuning In and Fading Out: Performance of Aphasic Patients on Ordered PICA Subtests." *Journal of Communication Disorders,* 16: 31–40.

DUFF, R., and A. HOLLINGSHEAD (1968). *Sickness and Society.* New York: Harper & Row.

DUNN, L. (1965). *Expanded Manual for the Peabody Picture Vocabulary Test.* Circle Pines, Minn.: American Guidance Service.

EISENHOWER, D. (1965). *Waging Peace.* New York: Doubleday.

EISENSON, J. (1954). *Examining for Aphasia.* New York: Psychological Corp.

────── (1984). *Aphasia in Adults.* Englewood Cliffs, N.J.: Prentice-Hall, Inc.

EMERICK, L. (1971). *Appraisal of Language Disturbance.* Marquette: Northern Michigan University Press.

EMERICK, L., and J. COYNE (1972). *Screening Test of Aphasia.* Danville, Ill.: Interstate Printers and Publishers.

ENDERBY, P. (1983). *Frenchay Dysarthria Assessment.* San Diego, Calif.: College-Hill Press.

EVANS, R., and L. NORTHWOOD (1983). "Social Support Needs in Adjustment to Stroke." *Archives of Physical Medicine and Rehabilitation,* 64: 61–64.

FARRELL, B. (1969). *Pat and Roald.* New York: Random House.

GOODGLASS, H., and E. KAPLAN (1983). *The Assessment of Aphasia and Related Disorders.* Philadelphia: Lea & Febiger.

GRANGER, C., and G. ALBRECHT (1979). "Outcome of Comprehensive Medical Rehabilitation: Measurement by PULSES Profile and Barthel Index." *Archives of Physical Medicine and Rehabilitation,* 60: 145–154.

GRIFFITH, V. (1970). *A Stroke in the Family.* New York: Delacorte.

GRINKER, R., and A. SAHS (1966). *Neurology.* Springfield, Ill.: Chas. C. Thomas.

HARVEY, R., and H. JELLINEK (1983). "Patient Profiles: Utilization in Functional Performance Assessment." *Archives of Physical Medicine and Rehabilitation,* 64: 268–271.

HAYNES, W., and B. GREENBERG (1976). *Understanding Aphasia.* Danville, Ill.: Interstate Printers and Publishers.

HELMICK, J, T. WATAMORI, and J. PALMER (1976). "Spouses' Understanding of the Communication Disabilities of Aphasic Patients." *Journal of Speech and Hearing Disorders,* 41: 238–243.

HODGINS, E. (1964). *Episode: Report on the Accident in My Skull.* New York: Atheneum.

HOLLAND, A. (1977). "Comment on 'Spouses' Understanding of the Communication Disabilities of Aphasic Patients." *Journal of Speech and Hearing Disorders,* 42: 307–308.

────── (1980). *Communicative Abilities in Daily Living.* Baltimore: University Park Press.

────── (1982). "Observing Functional Communication of Aphasic Adults." *Journal of Speech and Hearing Disorders,* 47: 50–56.

HOLMES, T., and R. RAHE (1967). "The Social Readjustment Rating Scale." *Journal of Psychosomatic Research,* 11: 213–218.

HOROWITZ, B. (1962). "An Open Letter to the Family of an Adult Patient with Aphasia." *Rehabilitation Literature,* 23: 141–144.

HUNKER, C., and J. ABBS (1984). "Physiological Analysis of Parkinson Tremors in the Orofacial System," in *The Dysarthrias: Physiology-Acoustics-Perception-Management*, ed. M. McNeil, J. Rosenbek, and A. Aronson. San Diego, Calif.: College-Hill Press.

JENKINS, J., et al. (1975) *Aphasia in Adults*. 2nd ed. New York: Harper & Row.

JOHNS, D., ed. (1978). *Clinical Management of Neurogenic Communicative Disorders*. Boston: Little, Brown.

KEENAN, J., and E. BRASSELL (1975). "A Study of Factors Related to Prognosis for Individual Aphasic Patients." *Journal of Speech and Hearing Disorders*, 39: 257-269.

KERTESZ, A. (1979). *Aphasia and Associated Disorders: Taxonomy, Localization and Recovery*. New York: Grune & Stratton.

—— (1980). *Western Aphasia Battery*. London, Ont.: University of Western Ontario.

KERTESZ, A. and P. McCABE (1977). "Recovery Patterns and Prognosis in Aphasia." *Brain*, 100: 1-18.

KINSELLA, G., and F. DUFFY (1978). "The Spouse of the Aphasic Patient," in *The Management of Aphasia*, ed. Y. LeBrun and R. Hoops. Amsterdam: Swets and Zeitlinger.

KNOX, D. (1971). *Portrait of Aphasia*. Detroit: Wayne State University Press.

LaPOINTE, L., and J. HORNER (1979). *Reading Comprehension Battery for Aphasia*. Tigard, Oreg.: C. C. Publications.

LEUTENEGGER, R. (1975). *Patient Care and Rehabilitation of Communication-Impaired Adults*. Springfield, Ill.: Chas. C. Thomas.

LONGERICH, M. (1955). *Helping the Aphasic to Recover His Speech*. Los Angeles: College of Medical Evangelists.

LURIA, A. (1972). *The Man with a Shattered World*. New York: Basic Books.

MARSHALL, R., and D. PHILIPS (1983). "Prognosis for Improved Verbal Communication in Aphasic Stroke Patients." *Archives of Physical Medicine and Rehabilitation*, 64: 597-600.

MARSHALL, R. and C. TOMPKINS (1981). "Identifying Behavior Associated with Verbal Self-Corrections of Aphasic Clients." *Journal of Speech and Hearing Disorders*, 46: 168-173.

McBRIDE, C. (1969). *Silent Victory*. Chicago: Nelson-Hall.

McCORMICK, G., and P. WILLIAMS (1976). "The Midwestern Pennsylvania Stroke Club: Conclusions Following the First Year's Operation of a Family Centered Program," in *Clinical Aphasiology*, ed. R. Brookshire. Minneapolis: BRK Publishers.

McNEIL, M., and T. PRESCOTT (1978). *Revised Token Test*. Baltimore: University Park Press.

MILLER, M. (1960). "Audiological Evaluation of Aphasic Patients." *Journal of Speech and Hearing Disorders*, 25: 333-339.

MOSS, C. (1972). *Recovery with Aphasia*. Urbana: University of Illinois Press.

MÜLLER, D., C. CODE, and J. MUGFORD (1983). "Predicting Psychosocial Adjustment to Aphasia." *British Journal of Disorders of Communication*, 18: 23-29.

NATION, J., and D. ARAM (1977). *Diagnosis of Speech and Language Disorders*. St. Louis: C. V. Mosby.

NEEDHAM, E., and J. BLACK (1970). "The Relative Ability of Aphasic Persons to Judge the Duration and Intensity of Pure Tones." *Journal of Speech and Hearing Research*, 13: 725-730.

NETTER, F. (1958). *The Nervous System*. New York: Ciba.

ORGASS, B., and K. POECK (1969). "Assessment of Aphasia by Psychometric Methods." *Cortex*, 5: 317-330.

PAGE, I., et al. (1961). *Strokes: How They Occur and What Can Be Done About Them*. New York: Dutton.

PETERSON, J., and A. OLSEN (1964). *Language Problems After a Stroke*. Minneapolis: American Rehabilitation Foundation.

PORCH, B. (1967). *Porch Index of Communicative Ability*. Palo Alto, Calif.: Consulting Psychologists Press.

PORCH, B., et al. (1980). "Statistical Prediction of Change in Aphasia." *Journal of Speech and Hearing Research*, 23: 313-321.

PORTER, J., and B. DABUL (1977). "The Application of Transactional Analysis to Therapy with Wives of Adult Aphasic Patients." *Journal of the American Speech and Hearing Association*, 19: 244-248.

POWELL, G., S. BAILEY, and E. CLARK (1980). "A Very Short Form of the Minnesota Aphasia Test." *British Journal of Social and Clinical Psychology*, 19: 189-194.

POWELL, L., and K. COURTICE (1983). *Alzheimer's Disease.* Reading, Mass.: Addison-Wesley.

PUTNAM, A., and T. HIXON (1984). "Respiratory Kinematics in Speakers with Motor Neuron Disease," in *The Dysarthrias: Physiology-Acoustics-Perception-Management,* ed. M. McNeil, J. Rosenbek, and A. Aronson. San Diego, Calif.: College-Hill Press.

RAVEN, J. (1960). *Guide To Standard Progressive Matrices.* London: H. K. Lewis.

RIENSCHE, L., A. WOHLERT, and B. PORCH (1983). "Aphasic Comprehension and Preference of Rate-Altered Speech." *British Journal of Disorders of Communication,* 18: 39–48.

ROBINSON, R., and D. BENSON (1981). "Depression in Aphasic Patients: Frequency, Severity, and Clinical-Pathological Correlation." *Brain and Language,* 14: 282–291.

ROLLIN, W. (1984). "Family Therapy and the Aphasic Adult," in *Adult Aphasia,* ed. J. Eisenson. Englewood Cliffs, N.J.: Prentice-Hall, Inc.

SARNO, J., and M. SARNO (1973). "The Functional Life Scale." *Archives of Physical Medicine and Rehabilitation,* 54: 214–220.

SARNO, M. T. (1969). *Functional Communication Profile.* New York: Institute of Rehabilitation Medicine.

—— (1981). *Acquired Aphasia.* New York: Academic Press.

SARNO, M. T., M. SILVERMAN, and E. SANDS (1970). "Speech Therapy and Language Recovery in Severe Aphasia." *Journal of Speech and Hearing Disorders,* 13: 607–623.

SCHUELL, H. (1965). *The Minnesota Test for Differential Diagnosis of Aphasia.* Minneapolis: University of Minnesota Press.

SCHUELL, H., J. JENKINS, and E. JIMENEZ-PABON (1964). *Aphasia in Adults.* New York: Harper & Row.

SHEEHY, G. (1976). *Predictable Crises of Adult Life.* New York: Dutton.

SHEWAN, C. (1980). *Auditory Comprehension Test for Sentences.* Chicago: Biolinguistics Clinical Institutes, 1980.

SIEGEL, G. (1975). "The High Cost of Accountability." *Journal of the American Speech and Hearing Association,* 17: 796–798.

SKLAR, M. (1966). *Sklar Aphasia Scale.* Los Angeles: Western Psychological Services.

SMITH, A. (1971). "Objective Indices of Severity of Chronic Aphasia in Stroke Patients." *Journal of Speech and Hearing Disorders,* 36: 167–207.

SOLOMON, P., et al. (1961). *Sensory Deprivation.* Cambridge, Mass.: Harvard University Press.

SPELLACY, F., and O. SPREEN (1969). "A Short Form of the Token Test." *Cortex,* 5: 390–397.

SPREEN, O., and A. BENTON (1977). *Neurosensory Center Comprehensive Examination for Aphasia.* Victoria, B.C.: University of Victoria.

STEINBECK, J. (1961). *Travels with Charley.* New York: Viking.

STREET, B. (1957). "Hearing Loss in Aphasia." *Journal of Speech and Hearing Disorders,* 22: 60–67.

TAYLOR, M. (1963). *Functional Communication Profile.* New York: New York University Medical Center.

—— (1958). *Understanding Aphasia.* New York: Institute of Physical Medicine and Rehabilitation.

TIKOFSKY, R. (1984). "Assessment of Aphasic Disorders," in *Adult Aphasia,* ed. J. Eisenson. Englewood Cliffs, N.J.: Prentice-Hall, Inc.

TOUBBEH, J. (1969). "Clinical Observations on Adult Aphasia." *Journal of Communication Disorders,* 2: 57–68.

TWAMLEY, R., and L. EMERICK (1970). "The Nurses' Role in Aphasia." *Today's Speech,* 18: 30–33.

ULTAOWSKA, H., et al. (1976). "The Assessment of Communicative Competence in Aphasia," in *Clinical Aphasiology,* ed. R. Brookshire. Minneapolis: BRK Publishers.

VICK, N. (1976). *Grinker's Neurology.* 7th ed. Springfield, Ill.: Chas. C. Thomas.

WEPMAN, J. (1972). "Aphasia Therapy: A New Look." *Journal of Speech and Hearing Disorders,* 37: 203–214.

WEPMAN, J., and L. JONES (1961). *Studies in Aphasia: An Approach to Testing.* Chicago, Ill.: Education/Industry Service.

WERTZ, R. (1978). "Neuropathologies of Speech and Language: An Introduction to Patient Management," in *Clinical Management of Neurogenic Communicative Disorders,* ed. D. Johns. Boston: Little, Brown.

WERTZ, R., L. LaPOINTE, and J. ROSENBEK (1984). *Apraxia of Speech in Adults.* New York: Grune & Stratton.

WHITEHOUSE, E. (1968). *There's Always More.* Valley Forge, Pa.: Judson Press.

WHURR, R. (1983). *Whurr Aphasia Screening Test.* London: M. Phil.

WISCONSIN DIVISION OF HEALTH (1966). *Communication Status Chart.* Madison, Wisc.: Division of Health.

WULF, H. (1973). *Aphasia, My World Alone.* Detroit: Wayne State University Press.

YORKSTON, K., and D. BEUKELMAN (1980). "An Analysis of Connected Speech Samples of Aphasic and Normal Speakers." *Journal of Speech and Hearing Disorders,* 45: 27–36.

ZUBEK, J. (1969). *Sensory Deprivation: Fifteen Years of Research.* New York: Appleton-Century-Crofts.

# CHAPTER EIGHT
# VOICE DISORDERS

## INTRODUCTION

There were major changes in the assessment and treatment of voice disorders in the early part of this century. The speech pathologist became involved in processes of diagnosis and remediation that were previously the province of physicians and singing teachers (Stemple, 1984). Recently, there has been increased research in the area of normal and disordered vocal physiology. Research, assessment, and treatment are being changed further by the technological advances in microcomputers and electronics. Thus, today we possess insights into the vocal mechanism that we did not have even a decade ago. New instruments are available for diagnosis and treatment that help to objectify behaviors that previously were unobservable and fleeting. It is an exciting time for those clinicians who deal with voice disorders.

The proliferation of new instrumentation and research, however, should not obscure the fact that we have developed some very effective clinical procedures over the years that do not require machinery. Most authorities continue to believe that it is the listening skill and judgment of the well-trained clinician that are the most important tools in a voice evaluation. Voice diagnosis combines the subjective and the objective as in all clinical work, and the clinician must have and be able to employ the mental set of both the scientist and the wine taster. In this chapter we will touch on both subjective and objective aspects of vocal assessment.

Many adults and some children are referred to the speech pathologist by their physician for voice disorders resulting from medical difficulties or surgical intervention. The clinician more frequently comes in contact with children as the result of screening large numbers of youngsters in school settings or by teacher/parent referral. Prevalence figures for voice disorders among school-aged children vary considerably. Silverman and Zimmer (1975) report that 23.4 percent of the primary-grade children they evaluated possessed chronically hoarse voices, whereas Wilson and Rice (1977) postulate that 1 percent of the school-aged population needs voice therapy. Other studies range between 4 and 6 percent. From our experience it would appear that substantially less than 1 percent of school-aged children are presently receiving voice therapy (Deal, McClain, and Sudderth, 1976). The practicing speech clinician, for a variety of reasons, is not identifying the number of voice cases that the experts predict are in existence.

## DEFINITION OF VOICE

The imprecision of labels, which is the bane of voice study, begins with the term *voice* itself. Some definitions restrict the term to the generation of sound at the level of the larynx; others include the influence of the vocal tract on the generated tone; and still others broaden the definition to include ultimately aspects of tonal generation, resonation, articulation, and prosody. For the purposes of this chapter, voice is defined as the end product of respiratory power, laryngeal valving and sound generation, vocal tract resonation, and alteration of the tone. It is further categorized into pitch, quality, and loudness characteristics.

The imprecise definitions and the nebulous aspects of voice are related to several factors:

1.  The voice is a product of muscle functions that are not readily observed and are difficult to control directly. Whereas in articulation an individual can be told to elevate the tongue tip, and the success of this action can be observed and measured, the voice clinician cannot request the client to bring his arytenoid cartilages together. There is a mystique that surrounds the unobservable, and much of voice rehabilitation has been "mystical."

2.  The voice is indirectly influenced by several body systems, including the respiratory, phonatory, resonatory, endocrine, and neural. With so many systems functioning, it is often difficult to determine just which potential etiological factor is responsible for any given symptom.

3.  There are contradictory points of view on the relative influence of the physical and psychic factors of voice production. The voice is said to be a bellwether of both physiological and psychological states and is subject to insidious and hard to detect influences.

4.  There is no clear concept of just what normal voice is, as the influences of culture, age, sex, role, and specific activity alter the expected vocal output. Under certain circumstances, nearly any voice variation could be termed "normal."

5.  The various parameters of voice are subject to continuous and flowing change at the whim of the speaker. Whereas it would be considered aberrant for a speaker to alter abruptly his syntactical system or articulatory pattern, each

of us continuously changes the pitch, loudness, and quality of the voice in keeping with the meaning of the spoken signal. Such instantaneous changes make voice characteristics difficult to define precisely.

6.  The listener's perceptions of vocal characteristics are mediated through other aspects of the speech signal. For example, Sherman (1954) pointed out that the perception of nasality is partly dependent on articulatory patterns.

7.  In the literature concerning voice there has been a tendency to confuse perceptual and physical characteristics. To state that the "natural pitch" of the adult male is approximately 125 Hz (hertz) encourages confusion and imprecision.

8.  We have no clear idea of the compensatory capabilities of the vocal tract in voice production. It is not known, for example, if the resonators can and do mask phonatory differences in some individuals, or, on the other hand, if an increased exhalatory effort results in a compensating function of the vocal folds.

9.  The study of voice has been divided between the "scientists" and the "practitioners." The voice scientists and experimental phoneticians have provided the discipline with much of the hard data on which to assess clinical behavior, but there have been precious few who have been willing to make clinical suggestions from the laboratory findings. Similarly, the flow of information has not been reciprocal; clinicians have been remiss in collecting clinical data that can hold up under the critical eyes of the researchers. This situation is currently changing with the emphasis on single-case experimentation and the advent of the "clinician-researcher" (Silverman, 1977; Ventry and Schiavetti, 1980).

With this set of factors in mind, then, there is little wonder that some clinicians are poorly prepared to deal with the disordered voice. Worthley (1969) found in a survey of more than 400 public school speech clinicians that they rate their training in voice disorders poorer than in any other area.

## PARAMETERS OF VOICE AND VOCAL DISTURBANCE

A framework to conceptualize voice and voice disturbance is shown in Figure 8.1. The auditory characteristics of pitch, loudness, and quality constitute one dimension of the paradigm. They are perceptual attributes of the voice and relate generally to the fundamental frequency, amplitude, and complexity of the signal.

Pitch that is too high, too low, too invariant, or inappropriately variant for the speaker or the cirsumstances constitutes a voice disorder. The loudness of the speaking voice is usually judged according to the speaking circumstance, the aberant ranging from the total lack of voice (aphonia) to the inappropriately loud. For our purposes the term *quality* refers to the perceived pleasantness, or appeal, of the voice. This perception is linked to both the phonatory and resonatory characteristics of the speaker.

The physical systems that most directly influence vocal production are the respiratory, phonatory, and resonatory-articulatory. Although these systems have

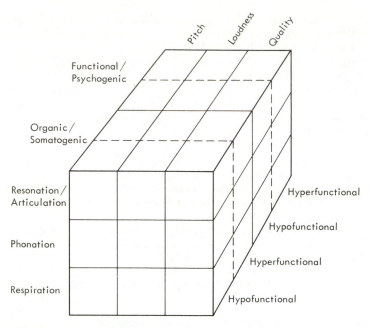

**FIGURE 8.1**    An organizational schema of voice disorders.

the most direct impact on the voice signal, they are not the only systems that influence the voice. Luchsinger and Arnold (1965) discuss the effect of the endocrine system on voice production.

The respiratory system provides the motive force for voice production, and ultimately the resultant airstream becomes the vibrator that embodies all of the characteristics that the ear eventually senses. That the airstream is important to vocal production is not really the issue at this point, but there is some question as to the influence of the respiratory mechanism on the various vocal characteristics. It appears that the respiratory mechanism must be capable of the following:

1.  Provide an adequate amount of air so that the speaker can sustain speech with ease to allow for natural phrasing and prosodic factors.
2.  Provide adequate breath support so that the vibratory pattern can be established without undue laryngeal valving tension.
3.  Provide adequate control of the flow of air so that the mechanism can, when necessary, either initiate or arrest the speech signal.
4.  Provide an airstream that is not so indebted to active muscle contraction that it encourages unnecessary muscle tension in the respiratory and phonatory mechanisms.
5.  Provide an airstream that is instantly available on demand and able to be sustained somewhat constantly for a sufficient length of time.

The physiology of the respiratory mechanism has been poorly understood. Early writings spoke incorrectly of "breathing from the diaphragm" and stressed the "proper" inward movement of the abdomen during inhalation. Some clinicians still concentrate on the respiratory function when the disorder is clearly phonatory. If a tire loses air because of a leak in the air valve, one would not attempt to fix the leak by altering the pressure within the tire; rather, one would attack the problem at the site of the breakdown.

A protracted review of the physiology of phonation is not within the scope of this text; however, some elements of laryngeal function are crucial in diagnostic evaluation. In order to be an efficient sound source, the larynx must perform a valving action on the flow of air that establishes alternate, regular pressure changes within the body of air. In order to do this the vocal folds must

1. Be capable of a wide range of valving actions, from completely open and unrestricted through closed and totally restricted.
2. Be able to valve completely along their entire length.
3. Be of approximately equal size and shape so that they can move in synchrony with one another.
4. Be able to close and open during phonation with just the right amount of energy to avoid extreme tension during the closing phase.
5. Be of appropriate size (length and mass) for the age and sex of the person.
6. Be capable of natural movement that is free from superimposed and undue tension.
7. Be capable of small, subtle instantaneous adjustments that must be made continuously to alter the various vocal characteristics. These adjustments must allow for a variety of cyclic variations in the potential time of glottal opening and closing, from the long closing time of the glottal fry to the short closing time of the falsetto voice.

The glottal tone is complex and rich in higher harmonics, but it is only through the resonant and damping effects of the vocal tract that the speech sounds achieve their identity. In order for the resonating chambers of the vocal tract to be efficient, they must be flexible in size, shape, texture, and relationship with one another. The effect of the resonators on the laryngeal valve has been discussed by several writers (Curtis, 1968; Wendahl and Page, 1967), but the exact nature of this relationship has yet to be determined.

The term *functional* should imply more than the simple absence of measurable organic deviation; it should also imply that the diagnostician has found some active agent of etiology and that the agent is nonorganic. We agree with Powers (1971) that the term *functional* has, unfortunately, come to mean diagnosis by default. Voice disorders offer an interesting testing ground for the traditional organic-functional dichotomy. This separation does not stand up on almost any basis. Murphy (1964) points out the continuous nature of vocal disorder etiologies.

Figure 8.1 identifies functional-psychogenic and organic-somatogenic as clinically meaningful categories. The term *functional* refers to those disorders where the learned, psychic, or maladaptive behavior has resulted in faulty vocal production but not in physical alteration. If physical change has resulted from the functional cause, however, the proper designation is psychogenic. Similarly, if the original factor was physical or organic, then the term *organic* is justified; but if the physical difference results in behavioral change—that is, emotional response or faulty compensatory adjustments—the term *somatogenic* is appropriate (Murphy, 1964).

The terms *hyper-* and *hypofunctioning* refer, respectively, to an excess or insufficiency of laryngeal tension and, as such, could apply to a wide variety of organic or functional disorders.

The term *voice disorders,* then, refers to abnormal pitch, loudness, or vocal quality according to sex, age, status, temporary physiological state, purpose of the speaker, and elements of the speaking circumstance. Vocal disorders may be primarily organic or functional and may be affected by any of the primary systems.

## DIAGNOSTIC FORMAT

This chapter will not cover the anatomy and physiology of the mechanisms of vocal production. This information is offered in many sources and should be studied carefully before undertaking voice diagnosis (Moore, 1971; Zemlin, 1981; Kaplan, 1971; Dickson and Maue-Dickson, 1982; Palmer, 1984; Kahane and Folkins, 1984; Daniloff, Schuckers, and Feth, 1980). We also cannot provide an elaborate description of each voice disorder type; this information is available to the student in several sources (Luchsinger and Arnold, 1965; Greene, 1980; Boone, 1983; Aronson, 1980; Stemple, 1984).

Our major focus will be on the actual planning, preparation, and execution of voice diagnoses. Diagnosis is intended to define the parameters of the problem, determine the etiology, and outline a logical course of action.

## THE PRESENTING COMPLAINT

The diagnostic process begins with a careful scrutiny of the original statement of the problem as provided by the referral source. Four perspectives guide our evaluation of this information: who, what, why, and when.

*Who makes the referral?*   It is important to know who presents the original complaint about the client's voice. We have found that the "best" source from a motivational standpoint is the client, but anyone who might have a significant impact on the client may be a satisfactory referral source.

If the client and those around her do not consider the voice to be a problem, then, in reality, there is none. With voice disorders, however, such thinking may be dangerous because some minimal changes in voice quality may reflect anatomic changes, and there is a circular pattern of cause and effect in voice disorders that is best treated early. An amazing number of people do not consider voice characteristics to be in the realm of speech disorders. The implication is that the characteristics that determine a person's voice are genetically determined and cannot be changed by training or practice. Several investigations have studied the classroom teacher's efficacy in referral of children with voice disorders (Diehl and Stinnett, 1959; James and Cooper, 1966).

*What problem is reported?*   The description of the problem in the presenting complaint is important not only in helping us to understand the difficulty better but also because it allows us to see the problem through the eyes and ears of another. When the statement comes from the person with whom we will be working, we listen not only to the actual words spoken but also to the way in which they are presented. One of the best sources of information about the impact of the problem on the individual is the way in which it is described. Invariably, when interviewing the client we find it valuable to probe the following five areas:

1. "Describe your voice." Listen for the terms used, the factors that appear to alter the voice, other sources of variance in vocal characteristics, and subtle signs of concern.

2. "How do others react to your speaking voice?" Generally we attempt to judge this answer against reality as best we can. Very often the individual will respond that no one ever mentions the voice, and the diagnostician must take care not to reinforce such reactions while at the same time not to strip the client of all defenses. It is quite possible that there has been little environmental reaction and that the client is being honest in the reply, but we are concerned with the client's perception of others' reactions. Remember that you may be the first person to ask the client such questions, and plenty of time should be allowed for responses.

3. "How severe do you consider this problem to be?" Generally, we give the client some sort of subjective rating scale on which to judge. This is very useful baseline information and is directly related to the next question.

4. "How much does this problem bother you?" We have found that the degree of concern and the judgment of severity are not always directly related, but in any case we must know just how much this individual wishes to change the voice. The clinician must be careful in such discussions because the client may respond that no problem exists and change is not necessary. Although this is important diagnostic information, it is also important to the therapy process; and the diagnostician must be able to recover the initiative and put the client back on the track.

5. "What caused the problem?" The clinician should be interested in any hypotheses the client entertains regarding the disorder. The client's opinion may be correct, or if serious misconceptions are present, these could be areas of future counseling and discussion.

Murphy (1964) presents a series of twenty questions to clarify the individual's self-concept regarding the speaking voice. Such lists often provide useful information for the diagnostician.

*Why was the referral made?*   The reason for referral to the voice clinician may vary from something as simple as an impending trip ("I just have to sound better than this by the first of August") to fears of serious medical problems. In evaluating the reasons for referral, it is important to keep in mind that contacting a speech clinician is often seen as psychologically safer than going to a medical doctor or a psychologist. This points up the importance of secondary referrals.

*When was the referral made?* Three things are of major concern here. First, it is important to know when, in the sequence of development of the problem, the referral was made. Is this a problem of long standing that has only recently become serious, or is it a relatively new phenomenon that has been detected early? Second, what is this person's age and maturational level? Whereas certain vocal changes are to be expected before puberty (Curry, 1949) and would thus be considered normal, a similar vocal quality at a later maturity level may be abnormal. Third, does this problem appear in cycles? Does the client suffer from this vocal quality only during hay fever season? The time of year of the referral may provide some important diagnostic information.

## REFERRAL BY THE SPEECH PATHOLOGIST

In most cases of phonatory voice disorders, some type of referral for medical or psychological evaluation will be necessary. Voice disorders may be caused by life-threatening situations such as carcinoma of the larynx or something as simple as vocal misuse. Structural changes such as ulcers, polyps, or nodules may be detected through laryngeal examination. Symptoms such as hoarseness or harshness of the voice should prompt the clinician to make referral, particularly if the hoarseness lasts more than ten days. It is widely accepted that ideally the speech pathologist and the laryngologist should cultivate a close working relationship when dealing with voice cases (Boone, 1983; Aronson, 1980). Each professional can provide significant information to the other, and voice treatment that attempts to alter a parameter such as pitch should not begin without a laryngological examination. A vocal hygiene program, however, can begin with many clients before a laryngoscopic examination. Thus, waiting for medical examination in cases of vocal abuse should not be used as a reason to postpone enrollment in treatment.

During an examination by a specialist, indirect laryngoscopy will be accomplished via a mirror or fiberoptiscope. In cases of infants and young children, who may be difficult to perform indirect procedures on, there is the possibility of the laryngologist using direct laryngoscopy. Radiographic techniques may also be used to supplement the laryngologist's examination of the vocal mechanim (Aronson, 1980).

The speech pathologist will be interested in the findings of the laryngeal examinations for several reasons. First, the examination can document any physical alteration to the vocal mechanism—nodules, polyps—that may account for differences in voice quality. Second, there is a possibility that surgical intervention is the treatment of choice for a particular patient and that voice therapy may not be indicated at the present time. Third, the speech pathologist will want to have the extent of any vocal fold pathology documented if voice therapy is indicated so that alterations in the client's vocal quality over time as the result of treatment might be correlated with concomitant organic changes in the future laryngological examinations. Finally, the absence of organic deviations on the laryngoscopic examination may suggest more functional or psychogenic bases for the client's disorder. In this case, other referrals may be in order.

In communicating with the laryngologist, several sources have recommended the use of forms containing drawings of the vocal apparatus on which the physician can make notes indicating the size and location of abnormalities (Boone, 1983; Weinberg, 1983; Stone, Hurlbutt, and Coulthard, 1978). This could become part of the client's record and be used for comparisons over time with other examinations.

A general medical evaluation or a specific neurological examination may be indicated in certain cases. When dysfunction of the peripheral or central nervous system appears to be a possible contributing factor to the voice disorder, referral is indicated.

## HISTORICAL INFORMATION

There are many excellent sources for guidance in taking an adequate case history with an emphasis on voice disorders, and many of these provide forms for the clinician's use (Wilson, 1979; Moncur and Brackett, 1974; Greene, 1980; Aronson, 1980; Boone, 1983). Our purpose is to identify those specific aspects within each of the historical subcategories that have particular relevance to voice diagnosis.

*Family data.* Information regarding parents' occupation, number of siblings, history of family adjustment, other voice problems within the family, and general health pattern of the family tells us a great deal about the client's social and physical milieu. Generally, the following characteristics may be considered potentially remarkable and should be explored further: (1) too much or too little structure and organization in the home; (2) premium placed on verbal competition; (3) interparental friction; (4) unusual sibling competition; (5) history of voice disorders; (6) poor parental adjustment; (7) history of extended recurrent health problems; and (8) general level of concern for physical and health problems.

*Onset of the problem.* In many instances the beginning of the voice problem will have great diagnostic significance. It is important to investigate not only the nature of the onset but the circumstances surrounding it. Physical or psychological trauma may have equally instant effects on voice production. In some cases, extended questioning may be necessary because it is common for clients to repress uncomfortable incidents of the past. Aronson (1980) indicates that a sudden onset within hours suggests the high probability of a conversion vocal disorder or a neurological cerebral vascular accident (CVA) origin, whereas many other types of vocal disturbance develop gradually (mass and approximation lesions, degenerative disease, and so on).

Although the abrupt onset of a vocal disorder is traumatic and startling, most voice disorders are of insidious origin. Many people cannot pinpoint the exact date of the onset and tend to indicate when people first noticed or remarked about their voices. Because a gradual onset is not necessarily specific to organic or functional etiologies, the examiner must look to other data for final answers. Probably more important than the rate of development is information on coincident factors such as the client's general health and emotional state.

*Course of development.*    A careful description of the developmental stages of the voice disturbance may provide helpful diagnostic information. The course of the development of the voice disorder may be found to parallel a chronic medical problem, accumulating vocational stress, certain periods of physical maturation, changes in family relationships, or developing financial crises. We want to know how the problem has changed since its onset and any circumstances surrounding variability of the voice disturbance. For instance, were there changes in the voice disorder during its development that might be correlated with changes in personal habits (smoking, use of alcohol), work conditions (excessive noise, stress), or medical conditions (sinus, allergy). The clinician will want to keep in mind that once a voice disorder has firmly been established only a minimal amount of tension or misuse or abuse will be necessary to perpetuate the problem.

*Description of daily vocal performance and problem variability.*    Questions on the course of development seek an historical perspective, but we also need information on factors the client reports to influence the voice. For instance, we might ask the client to describe his or her daily routine and relate it to talking. Does the problem become worse through the day? Does it become better as the day progresses? Boone (1983) suggests having the patient identify any situations that seem to be consistently related to good and poor vocal performance. It is especially important in cases of childhood vocal pathology to obtain an accurate picture of the youngster's typical use of voice and instances of misuse or abuse (Wilson, 1979; Boone, 1983).

*Social adjustment.*    Assessment of the personality characteristics of the individual may assist the diagnostician in interpreting other information. Formal personality testing is not within the jurisdiction of the speech pathologist, but each clinician is expected to be perceptive and sensitive to clues about the client's basic adjustment to life. The notion that the voice is closely related to the individual's self-concept and reveals inner conflict has been carefully examined by several researchers. Moses (1954) and Rousey and Moriarty (1965) present interesting views of the interaction of the personality and voice production. Classification of voice characteristics with specific personality types has not provided overwhelming evidence, but the personality and the voice interact in a complex fashion and this results in many symptomatic characteristics.

*Vocation.*    We are interested in the vocation of our voice client for two reasons. First, we must determine if the occupation demands a great deal of talking and if that talking is under adverse conditions. Not all teachers develop "teacher's nodules," however, and the vocation must be judged in relation to the person. Several writers have postulated that there is a personality type that develops vocal nodules (Jackson, 1941; Withers, 1961). We have found many of these people to be tense, energetic, high strung, and verbally aggressive. Place this type of person in an occupational setting that demands a great deal of speaking under tension, and a bit of poor judgment in choosing adaptive procedures, and the chances of finding an individual with vocal nodules could be greatly enhanced.

A second factor in our evaluation of vocation is to assess the possibility of changing aspects in the client's job routine or behavior at work if the vocation has a deleterious effect on the voice disorder:

> We worked with a college professor who taught several large lecture classes to groups of more than 150 students. His vocal abuse and misuse during these presentations had resulted in small nodules for which voice therapy was recommended. In an effort to be both audible, dynamic, and authoritative, he had been speaking loudly, with a lower pitch and excessive tension. We explored the possibility of his using a lavalier microphone in the large lecture rooms, and this effectively eliminated a significantly abusive situation that was vocationally related.

*Health.* Realizing that the voice is influenced by many physiological systems, the clinician should require a complete medical history and examination in many instances. A history of the general health and physical development of the client should be obtained, along with information about specific illnesses, surgeries, and medications. The clinician should also obtain data concerning general energy level and such health-related habits as smoking, drinking, and drug use. Luchsinger and Arnold (1965) present a particularly comprehensive discussion of vocal disorders of organic etiology. Referral of a client to a physician may uncover a medical problem of which vocal quality is a symptom:

> Sherry was identified in the speech and hearing screening program. Her voice was described as breathy, low in pitch and volume, expressionless, and varying in degrees of nasality. The case history revealed the following information: low metabolic rate, rapid fatigue, and body temperatures generally below normal. Subsequent medical referral indicated specific muscle weakness and a medical diagnosis of myasthenia gravis. It should be noted that the speech clinician's alertness to the accumulation of medical danger signs in addition to the speech characteristics resulted in a proper referral and subsequent identification of the problem.

## THE EVALUATION PROCESS: PITCH, LOUDNESS, QUALITY

The first step in voice analysis is simply listening to the client in an objective and yet analytical manner. Obviously, this listening process is largely judgmental; therefore it may be helpful to use a checklist such as Table 8.1. Many voice profiles are available for use in making assessments of all vocal parameters. The profiles typically include scales that rate a number of aspects of voice in terms of severity of any deviation. The Buffalo Voice Profile (Wilson, 1979) rates laryngeal tone, laryngeal tension, vocal abuse, loudness, pitch, vocal inflection, pitch breaks, diplo-

**TABLE 8.1    Checklist of Vocal Characteristics**

PITCH

| 1 | 2 | 3 | 4 | 5 | 6 | 7 |

| DESCRIPTION | SEVERITY | | | | | | |
|---|---|---|---|---|---|---|---|
| — Too high | 1 | 2 | 3 | 4 | 5 | 6 | 7 |
| — Too low | 1 | 2 | 3 | 4 | 5 | 6 | 7 |
| — Invariant | 1 | 2 | 3 | 4 | 5 | 6 | 7 |
| — Pitch breaks | 1 | 2 | 3 | 4 | 5 | 6 | 7 |
| — Diplophonia | 1 | 2 | 3 | 4 | 5 | 6 | 7 |
| — Repetitive pattern | 1 | 2 | 3 | 4 | 5 | 6 | 7 |

LOUDNESS

| 1 | 2 | 3 | 4 | 5 | 6 | 7 |

| DESCRIPTION | SEVERITY | | | | | | |
|---|---|---|---|---|---|---|---|
| — Excessive | 1 | 2 | 3 | 4 | 5 | 6 | 7 |
| — Inadequate | 1 | 2 | 3 | 4 | 5 | 6 | 7 |
| — Uncontrolled variation | 1 | 2 | 3 | 4 | 5 | 6 | 7 |
| — Repetitive pattern | 1 | 2 | 3 | 4 | 5 | 6 | 7 |
| — Invariant | 1 | 2 | 3 | 4 | 5 | 6 | 7 |
| — Tremulous | 1 | 2 | 3 | 4 | 5 | 6 | 7 |

QUALITY

| 1 | 2 | 3 | 4 | 5 | 6 | 7 |

| DESCRIPTION | SEVERITY | | | | | | |
|---|---|---|---|---|---|---|---|
| — Hoarseness | 1 | 2 | 3 | 4 | 5 | 6 | 7 |
| — Harshness | 1 | 2 | 3 | 4 | 5 | 6 | 7 |
| — Breathiness | 1 | 2 | 3 | 4 | 5 | 6 | 7 |
| — Hypernasal | 1 | 2 | 3 | 4 | 5 | 6 | 7 |
| — Hyponasal | 1 | 2 | 3 | 4 | 5 | 6 | 7 |
| — Other (describe) | 1 | 2 | 3 | 4 | 5 | 6 | 7 |

JUDGMENT OF VOCAL TENSION

— Aphonia/whisper
— Breathy phonation
— Normal
— Hypertension
— Hypertension/intermittent phonation

OVERALL JUDGMENT OF VOICE

| 1 | 2 | 3 | 4 | 5 | 6 | 7 |

Note: 1 = normal; 7 = severely disordered

phonia, resonance, nasal emission, rate, and overall voice efficiency. The voice profiles designed by Wilson and his colleagues (Wilson, 1972; Wilson and Rice, 1977) have received wide acceptance and can be used reliably (Starr and Wilson, 1976). Boone (1983) also offers a children's voice rating scale. Wilson (1979) recommends obtaining samples of the client in conversation, reading, counting, and sustained vowel productions.

Ratings on these scales should be a helpful starting point in voice evaluation, and the clinician who notes disturbance in any parameter of vocal production can move on to more specific analysis techniques that illuminate further the affected aspect of voice. We recommend tape recording the client's sample on a high quality audio recorder to document the condition of the voice for later comparison.

### Respiration

Our concern for the respiratory process involves both the vegetative processes and breathing for speech. There are six areas of concern for the diagnostician.

*Air volume.* The maximum amount of air that can be exhaled following maximal inhalation is called vital capacity (Wood, 1971). The relationship of vital capacity to speech production is somewhat a matter of conjecture at this point. Vital capacity is apparently related to several factors, such as body size, physical condition, and sex (Gray and Wise, 1959; Van Riper and Irwin, 1958). There is little or no research to vindicate those who have worked to increase the vital capacity of their voice clients. On the other hand, it is logical to assume that an individual with an extremely small amount of air available would find it difficult to sustain phonation and might resort to increased laryngeal tension and forcing to maintain normal or near-normal phrasing. It is probably not so much the volume of air as it is the individual's ability to control the airflow (Hardy, 1961).

There appears to be no satisfactory substitute for the spirometer to measure vital capacity. Clinically, however, we have found that a vital capacity insufficient for normal speech purposes was so obvious from normal observation that further formal testing was not necessary. Vital capacity measurements may be of particular concern in cases of emphysema, later stages of Parkinson's disease, and children with cerebral palsy. Related to lung volume are indications of the client's tidal volume, inspiratory reserve volume, and expiratory reserve volume, which some authorities recommend measuring clinically (Boone, 1983).

*Respiratory type.* The methods of respiration have been classically designated as clavicular, thoracic, and abdominal. The terms refer to the area of greatest excursion during inhalation. There appears to be general agreement that respiratory type has little influence on vocal characteristics except in the case of extreme upper chest or clavicular breathing, which tends to encourage great laryngeal tension and insufficient intake of air volume. Observation appears to be the most satisfactory method of determining the type of respiratory process.

*Respiratory rate ratio.* Vegetative respiratory rate varies considerably, depending on the age and activity level of the individual. A rate of thirty to forty respirations per minute is not uncommon in the very young infant, but beyond one and one-half to two years of age the rate should have stabilized in the low twenties. With some clients an extremely high respiratory rate appears to interfere with contextual speech development, just as most people find it difficult to carry on a conversation while jogging. The continual interruption of the speech for respiratory purposes makes flowing speech difficult.

While observing the respiratory rate, it may be helpful to make note of the rhythm of respiration as well. Inconsistency in the rhythm of breathing may indicate neuromuscular problems and is quite typical in some cerebral palsied individuals.

Respiratory patterns are altered significantly during speech. The inhalatory phase is shorter in duration and generally the volume of air intake is greater; the exhalation phase is more controlled and gradual, with pulses of air being released in each syllable. Whereas the ratio of inhalation to exhalation time is approximately equal in normal respiration, during speech it may vary around a ratio of 1 to 7. Too frequent inhalation patterns may alter the flow of speech and so may inhalations that take too long to accomplish.

It is by no means an easy task to measure the temporal aspects of respiration without the aid of graphic representation. In those cases where there is some serious question regarding the respiratory ratio, it may be necessary to video- and audiotape the person and make careful evaluation.

*Duration and flow.* The maximum duration of sustained exhalation reveals the respiratory mechanism's ability to regulate exhalatory factors (rib recoil, muscle relaxation, lung tissue pressure, and gravity) so as to provide a continuous flow of air without interruption. Boone (1983) recommends a pneumotachometer to measure airflow rate. Normative data on children, adults, and voice disorder types are available for use in comparison. Patients with certain changes in vocal fold mass (polyps or nodules) may exhibit greater airflow rates because of an inability to adduct the vocal folds completely.

Several investigations have examined the maximum duration of voiced and voiceless exhalations (Ptacek and Sander, 1963; Bless and Saxman, 1970; Tait, Michel, and Carpenter, 1980). More recently, Eckel and Boone (1981) and Boone (1983) have advocated the use of the $s/z$ ratio in voice screening and diagnosis. The $s/z$ ratio is computed when the client prolongs the $/s/$ phoneme as long as possible and then the $/z/$ for three trials each. The ratio of $/s/$ to $/z/$ is typically near 1.0 in clients with normal laryngeal function. Eckel and Boone (1981) demonstrated that individuals exhibiting a variety of vocal fold pathologies revealed $s/z$ ratios of more than 1.4, whereas the normal voice and "functionally" voice disordered clients with no pathology scored near 1.0. Thus, the duration of $/s/$ and $/z/$ should be almost equal in patients having no glottal margin pathologies, and the duration of the $/z/$ tends to be shorter as the vocal fold pathology increases, due to the escape of air.

Boone (1983) demonstrated that progress in treatment and reduction in the size of vocal fold abnormalities can be documented with the $s/z$ ratio. This measure appears to have clinical utility; however, further investigation is needed to document clearly its efficacy with children and individuals with a variety of vocal fold pathologies.

*Associated tension.* Exhalation for speech purposes involves more than just the controlled relaxation of the inhalatory musculature. There is also a series of pulselike and sustained contractions of the thoracic and abdominal muscles. In some instances this process could result in tension that has an overflow effect on the laryngeal musculature and may result in faulty phonatory behavior. In examination this would be most evident upon sustained utterance. Once the person gets below her resting lung volume, additional muscle tension of both the respiratory and phonatory structures may be present in order to maintain sufficient subglottic pressure. What we are looking for is an inordinate amount of additional tension that can sometimes be visually observed or felt by placing the fingers lightly on the individual's neck beside the thyroid cartilage.

*Associated sounds.* In the healthy structure the vegetative respiratory process is fairly silent. Unwanted noise upon inhalation or exhalation may be a critical sign of a wide variety of problems ranging from laryngeal polyps and enlarged adenoidal tissue to laryngeal webs, adductor paralysis, or various types of neoplasms. Inspiratory stridor should be medically investigated immediately.

### Auditory Skills

Routine testing for auditory acuity is suggested for all voice cases. We sometimes go beyond simple acuity measures to evaluate the individual's discrimination ability. We want to get an idea of the client's abilities in discrimination of pitch, loudness, and quality differences, both interpersonally and intrapersonally.

## EVALUATION OF VOCAL PRODUCTION

It is generally advisable to evaluate each of the vocal characteristics of pitch, loudness, and quality, no matter which dimension is the primary contributor to the vocal disorder. As in evaluating other parameters of communication (fluency, articulation, language), the clinician must realize that the type of sample obtained will influence performance. It is preferable for certain types of cases to make the sample an "ecologically valid" one. For instance, in the case of a child with vocal nodules who is suspected of being a vocal abuser, it would be ideal to observe the youngster in a play situation with others and, if possible, in the school or home environment (Wilson, 1979). Most often, a variety of sampling activities is used in the evaluation ranging from conversation, coughing and counting to the production of isolated vowel sounds and singing (Weinberg, 1983; Wilson, 1979; Boone, 1983). The point here is that the clinician should be aware that a broad sampling of vocal performance is needed in order to make correct judgments on any parameter of voice.

The following discussion parcels the evaluation process into the three primary categories of pitch, loudness, and quality. Remember, though, that we generally try to evaluate as many aspects of vocal production at one time as possible.

### Loudness

Inappropriate loudness is seen in patients exhibiting some dysarthrias, vocal fold paralyses, vocal abuse, and occasionally disorders of psychological origin. Although some of the following measurement techniques are somewhat subjective, they may be helpful in analyzing loudness:

1. Determine the normal conversational loudness level of the individual under a variety of speaking situations. The clinician's judgment is the best means for evaluating loudness. Because loudness changes in its appropriateness with the communication situation, even objective measurements with instruments need to be interpreted by the clinician. First, open the conversation with your client seated a few feet away and gradually move back until you are ten to fifteen feet away. In order to determine the ability to adapt the voice to the speaking circumstance, you may wish to provide a background noise such as a radio or tape-recorded conversation. Generally, we are listening to the loudness level at this point, but we also observe such factors as undue tension, pitch, quality change, and inability to alter vocal performance with the circumstance.

2. The ability to project the voice can be evaluated by bringing the client to a large lecture room or an auditorium.

3. The ability to vary loudness with changes in meaning can be evaluated by using vocal variety drills such as those in the drillbooks of Fairbanks (1960) or Hanley and Thurman (1970). We generally ask the client to read "with feeling" sentences such as the following:
    Get out of here, get out of here!
    I don't know, I said I don't know!
    I need more money, Dad, I'm broke!
    Where did she go, I can't find her?
    Will you cut that out!

4. The ability to produce isolated vowel sounds is examined under a variety of conditions. First, the examiner must generally determine if the client can produce front and back and high, mid, and low vowels at various loudness levels. We listen for steadiness of tone, improved volume with changes in the resonant characteristics of the vowel, and the ability to project without concomitant changes in other variables such as quality of pitch. We also determine the ability to produce a steady, unwavering tone at various loudness levels.

5. A sound level meter could provide an objective measurement of a client's loudness level (Boone, 1983). Another objective measure that could be used is the Vocal Loudness Indicator, a feedback instrument with eight blinking lights showing loudness increments.[1] Also, Voice Lite[2] provides visual feedback to a client as the voice reaches a preset intensity level.

[1] Linguisystems, Inc., Moline, Ill.
[2] Behavioral Controls, Inc., 1506 West Pierce Street, Milwaukee, Wis.

## Pitch

Pitch is a perceptual phenomenon that correlates directly with the valving rate of the vocal folds. Obviously, the pitch level of most voices varies continuously and flowingly, and for this reason it is sometimes difficult to measure it precisely. As the clinician attempts to formulate a diagnostic format to evaluate pitch characteristics, several factors must be considered. First, there is probably a most efficient pitch range for each speaking voice. Second, each voice has a range of pitch variation. Third, there is a habitual pitch level during the contextual speech, and this may or may not coincide with the most efficient pitch level for a particular individual. Fourth, several factors have a direct influence on the pitch level of a given voice.

*Optimal pitch.*   The concept of optimal performance is attractive. The term implies efficiency (we always strive for an optimum performance in everything from our car to our golf swing). As voice clinicians, we are concerned not only with the acoustic end product and its appropriateness but also with the vocal mechanism's operating efficiency. Performance at nonoptimal levels implies greater constriction and strain of the vocal mechanism, with greater potential for abuse. The notion of determining optimal pitch in an evaluation is not without controversy (Weinberg, 1983; Thurman, 1958). Some advocate abandoning the search for this phenomenon in clients altogether; others, however, still recommend its determination (Boone, 1983). It should be emphasized that optimal pitch is not a single note, but is a range of notes where the vocal mechanism appears to function best with the least muscular tension.

The determination of optimal pitch is by no means precise. Several methods have been described in the literature. Generally, when pitch level is of paramount concern, it is best to use a combination of measures. It has been noted in both children and adults that there is significant variability in basal pitch levels both within and between days, implying multiple samples might be appropriate before arriving at optimal pitch (Cooper and Yanagihara, 1971; Austin and Leeper, 1975). The procedures for determining optimal pitch described by Fairbanks (1960), Murphy (1964), and Boone (1983) are most frequently used by speech clinicians. They include the following:

1.  The procedure described by Fairbanks is widely used. Essentially, it requires the client to determine the total pitch range, including falsetto, in full musical steps. For the adult male the optimal pitch is one-fourth of the total range up from the lowest level, and for the adult female it is considered to be two notes lower than one-fourth of the way up from the lowest note.
2.  Murphy describes the following procedures: (a) the loud-sigh technique: take a deep breath and intone "ah" on expiration; (b) the swollen tone technique: stop up the ears, sing "ah" or hum "m" up and down the scale until the pitch level at which the tone swells or is loudest is identified.
3.  Boone adds two techniques to the above: (a) it is suggested that the client yawn and sigh with the phonation of the sigh expected to be at or near the optimal level; (b) the patient is asked to say "uh-huh" in an affirmative voice,

and this utterance, made automatically, may approximate the optimal pitch level.

4. Boone (1983: 94) advocates the use of the Visi-Pitch (1980) in determining a client's optimal pitch level. This instrument can provide frequency as well as intensity data on a vocal sample. Boone says

> . . . optimal pitch is usually the frequency that is slightly louder and clearer in quality; both relative changes in intensity and in quality can be determined by the scope tracings (greater vertical excursion indicates greater intensity, and improved sharpness of tracing line indicates better periodicity or improved quality).

*Pitch range.*    The pitch range is determined in relation to the tests for optimal pitch level. Information about the client's pitch range tells us something about the flexibility and control of the respiratory and laryngeal structures. Some clients will have great difficulty humming up and down the musical scale, and consequently the clinician may have to demonstrate or sing along with them. It may be helpful to have the person produce the highest and lowest tones possible by using a pitch pipe or piano. The examiner can then calculate the total range. We also are looking for pitch breaks while talking and moving up and down the scale.

*Habitual pitch.*    The pitch level around which a person's voice varies in contextual speech is termed the habitual pitch level. Obviously this level will vary with the circumstance, but our main concern is the chronic use of a pitch level too high or too low for the individual's vocal mechanism. Once again this process is probably best done through instrumental analysis of the vocal signal; however, it is possible to train the ear to listen to the client's running speech and identify the fundamental pitch level. Probably the best method of doing this is to tape-record the client and concentrate on the pitch level while listening. Make every attempt to disregard content. The client should be totally unaware of the fact that you are recording for the purposes of evaluating pitch level, because this may affect the performance.

Boone (1983) suggests taking a tape-recorded sample and stopping the recorder a number of times on the playback and determining the pitch level by matching it with a pitch pipe. The process then results in a modal pitch level, which is the level most frequently occurring in the sample, and this is usually interpreted as the habitual pitch. Boone (1983) also recommends the Visi-Pitch for determination of habitual pitch, as well as other instruments such as Tonar II (Fletcher, 1972), and Tunemaster III (1974).

### Pitch Variations

Mass, effective valving length, and tension of the vocal folds are among the physical variables that influence pitch level. In an evaluation, however, we are interested in observing the changes in pitch during both intentional and unintentional activities. For example, we can listen to the client's vocal productions as he sings, follows inflectional changes, matches the pitch produced by the examiner, and attempts to maintain a steady pitch level for ten seconds. This will provide further data on the client's pitch range and will give the clinician an indication of the person's auditory discrimination abilities. Imitative responses are often useful prognostically. On the unintentional side, we should listen specifically for pitch changes during alterations in loudness and quality of vocal production. Also, there might be pitch changes during physical exertion, postural changes, or alterations of head position.

### Quality

The most difficult vocal characteristic to evaluate is quality. Involving both phonatory and resonatory characteristics, quality is that component which gives primary distinction to a given speaker's voice when pitch and loudness are excluded from judgment. Quality variations are essentially limitless but become of concern to the speech clinician when they take on an unpleasant and distracting character or are the precursors of physical abnormality. The variables of pitch and loudness can be scaled according to both physical and perceptual attributes, but the quality variable is still dependent on an array of subjective terms. For a discussion of the various terms used to describe vocal qualities, the reader is directed to the writings of Moore (1971), Murphy (1964), and Perkins (1971). The diagnostician must give the quality a label and describe it, determine the impact of various variables, and identify associated characteristics of the individual's vocal production.

*Description.* Most authorities maintain that despite the sophisticated instrumentation available today, the best assessment of vocal quality can be made through critical listening by an experienced clinician (Aronson, 1980; Boone, 1983; Weinberg, 1983). Because quality disorders may be either phonatory or resonatory, one of your first tasks is to make this differential determination. Following this judgment, it is useful to label the quality for purposes of communication with other professionals as well as to conceptualize the problem. There is some agreement on the meaning of hoarseness, harshness, breathiness, hypernasality, and denasality (Moore, 1971; Fairbanks, 1960), so we can feel fairly confident in using them.

Another method of rating quality without having to assign a single descriptor such as hoarse is to use a voice profile such as that recommended by Wilson (1972). The voice profile allows a clinician to rate the laryngeal valving on a scale from $-4$ to $+3$, where the former represents totally open vocal folds and the latter suggests a closed glottis. A voice having both breathiness and tension might be characterized as a $+2-2$. Whatever method the clinician uses, the description of the voice quality should be made as the client performs on a variety of tasks such as those used in evaluating pitch and loudness.

Vocal quality can also be investigated using instrumentation. The sound spectrograph can measure periodicity, changes in amplitude (shimmer), and changes in frequency (jitter) (Boone, 1983). The Visi-Pitch can also depict some aspects of quality in demonstrating aperiodicity and glottal attack differences associated with hoarseness (Boone, 1983).

*Associated characteristics.* Additional characteristics of quality may be investigated. The nature of the glottal attack in contextual speech should be determined. This is sometimes a rather difficult attribute to identify, so we generally have the person produce a series of words, vowels, and syllables. We also listen for the method of phonatory termination.

Another variable to investigate is the degree of laryngeal constriction, or tension, in phonation. Many vocal quality disorders are directly related to laryngeal hyperfunction. We depend primarily on four measures to determine the degree of vocal tension: observation, primarily for visible signs of strain; auditory cues that indicate a greater than normal degree of laryngeal valving; placing the hand lightly on the neck while the individual is speaking; and the client's self-report on the degree and locus of tension without the speaking mechanism.

### Prognosis

Prognosis has several aspects. First, there is the question of spontaneous remission of the presenting symptoms. Will this individual display an improvement in vocal quality without intervening voice therapy? Second, how much improvement can be expected following the prescribed clinical program? That is, to what degree is the voice therapy as projected going to be effective? Third, how permanent are the gains shown in therapy going to be? Is the vocal quality such that continuous therapy will be necessary to maintain optimal voice performance? Finally, would some other clinical procedure be of greater benefit to the client?

A variety of factors have potential prognostic value in voice cases. Some of the variables are directly observable and subject to quantification; others are much more subjective. The factors appear to fall into three broad categories: characteristics of the disorder, the person, and the environment.

1. Duration of the problem. Generally, disorders of long standing have greater resistance to clinical treatment.
2. Etiological factors. Two factors are relevant here. First, is the cause of the problem identifiable? Second, is the cause of the problem alterable? And, if so, is the type of habilitating service required available?
3. Degree of secondary psychological components. Generally, the greater the degree of psychological disturbance, the poorer the prognosis.
4. Variability and general flexibility of the voice. Generally, the more the client is able to alter his vocal behavior, the better the prognosis.
5. Auditory and imitative skills. The better the client is at hearing differences in quality, pitch, and loudness, coupled with the ability to imitate these differences, the more favorable the prognosis.
6. Impact or degree of disability. The greater the impact of the voice difference on the individual, the better the chances for cooperation. Generally, too, if the family of the client is supportive, the outlook is more favorable.

7. Structural integrity of the vocal mechanism. Clearly, the more the speech mechanism is disrupted anatomically or neurologically, the worse the prognosis will be.

## DIAGNOSIS OF THE LARYNGECTOMEE

We provide a separate section on assessment of clients who have undergone a laryngectomy because this group of people requires slightly different diagnostic considerations. Laryngeal surgery is primarily undertaken to preserve the life of the patient; however, the surgeon is continuously conscious of the need to provide as great a chance for continued vocal function as is possible. Surgery may include excision of the total larynx, half of the larynx, one vocal fold and part of the other, removal of the anterior section of the thyroid cartilage and both vocal folds, or various other combinations. There are also some recent surgical procedures that attempt to reconstruct a serviceable larynx and preserve voice. It is important that the speech clinician know exactly what procedures were undertaken, as the relearning process will vary relative to the amount and type of tissues remaining.

The exact nature of the diagnostic evaluation will vary, depending on when the client is seen. The preoperative evaluation will be markedly different from that of an individual who has been struggling to learn esophageal speech for some time. There are, however, three primary goals of the diagnostic process with the laryngectomee: to provide information, support, and release; to determine the speech potential; and to provide therapy direction.

*Providing information, support, and release.* A preoperative visit by the speech pathologist may be the first contact with the client, who has to be emotionally and physically capable of dealing with the issues of this meeting. Most speech clinicians depend on the referral of the physician for this initial contact. The clinican must remember, in the preoperative visit, that the client is facing a trauma unparalleled in her lifetime. Fears of death, loss of communication, loss of job, and social and marital adjustments plague her. The first confrontation is no social chat and may well demand all of the professional proficiency the clinician can muster. Occasionally, the clinician might find that the client is not capable of dealing rationally with the topic immediately before surgery and, in these cases, it may be preferable to postpone detailed discussion until after the client has recovered from the surgery.

One of the major goals of the first meeting is to provide some information about the operation and the implications for speech. After consultation with the physician, every attempt should be made to present a clear discussion of the anatomical changes. Charts and diagrams are often helpful. We generally use a demonstration tape of excellent esophageal speech, or have an exemplary esophageal speaker accompany us on this first visit (Boone, 1983). We stress that esophageal speech is a major goal, but not the only one. Several options are discussed such as the electrolarynx and written communication. Any of a number of nonvocal communication devices may be appropriately considered by the clinician in certain circumstances (Silverman, 1980). Although further information is sometimes provided in this first discussion, generally it is best to deal with related problems after surgery or as they arise. Many times even the discussion of the anticipated communication problem has little impact until after the patient has experienced muteness.

Providing adequate information to the family can have far-reaching clinical implications. The spouse and immediate family must understand the anatomy of the operation. Often, clinicians stress what the laryngectomee is unable to do, and although this information is important, it is also important to stress to the family what the patient will be able to do. We generally attempt to have a frank discussion with the spouse about the typical reactions of the family. If a pattern can be identified before it develops, it may be easier to control. The tendency to dominate the silent mate or parent must be controlled, as must the inclinations to infantilize, overindulge, and pity. Often we have to warn the family not to shout at the patient. Some families readily admit to a feeling of repulsion caused by the client's physical changes; such feelings are easily conveyed to the client because of his heightened sensitivity about the operation. The silent mate is sometimes excluded from conversation and decision making in the family.

The clinician must be sensitive to the fact that the spouse will have significant concerns. The fear of death, reduced income, new responsibilities, social changes, and alterations in the marital relationship may be topics for discussion. One of the primary purposes of the clinician's first visit with the laryngectomee and the family is to let them know that their feelings are understood. It is expected that the clinician will be warm, sincere, and insightful, but we resist the temptation to dictate any specific attitude beyond this because each patient will require a somewhat different approach. Some need to be dealt with gently, others straightforwardly and frankly. Find the level and type of interaction your client responds to best and use it.

*Determine the potential for speech.*    A thorough case history is helpful with laryngectomized patients, but three facets are particularly crucial. It is important to know the extent of the surgery, the degree of involvement of related structures such as the tongue or pharynx, general health of the client, and medical prognosis. The second critical area is the individual's vocation and interests. We find it most helpful to plan our clinical work about the client's preferred activities. It is also important to know if the person will be able to continue in a vocation and hobbies that involve communication. A third variable related to the client's potential for learning esophageal speech is attitude and motivation. Some clients are depressed, discouraged, and unmotivated, whereas others evidence a high level of interest in recovering their communication abilities. This is a subjective judgment on the clinician's part, but it is one of those intangible variables that certainly relates to the potential of the client to speak again.

It may also be necessary to examine the client's oral anatomy. Generally, we evaluate the tongue, lip, and jaw mobility. Some information about the previous articulation, speech, and language patterns of the client is helpful, but this is not always available.

If the client has already begun to learn esophageal speech, some measure of the current performance level is necessary. Most authorities would agree that a clinician with critical listening ability is the most effective means for evaluating esophageal productions. It is perhaps best to judge the overall effectiveness of the client's speech and then focus on more specific parameters. According to Martin (1979), an average male esophageal speaker will have a fundamental frequency of about 65 Hz, which is about half that of a normal speaking male. The intensity of the esophageal speech signal will be slightly less than normal with a smaller range of loudness.

The clinician should take note of the ease with which the client can inject air into the esophagus and the latency between injection and phonation. Martin (1979) indicates that any searching behavior prior to injection of air should be noted because this contributes to latency and interrupts communicative flow. The air volume in the esophagus is far less than in the lungs, so the client must inject air more often during esophageal speech as compared to inhaling during normal speech. Difficulties with injection of air or this searching behavior prior to inflation makes the speech interrupted and less smooth. After air has been injected into the esophagus, the clinician should record the duration of esophageal vowel phonation on one air charge.

Esophageal speakers exhibit some problems unique to their disorder. All distracting mannerisms should be diagnosed early because they are more easily eradicated before a great deal of practice occurs. When a client injects air too rapidly into the esophagus a "klunking" sound can occur. Some clients exhibit multiple "klunks" when they attempt more than one inflation before phonation. Another distracting behavior is stoma noise (stoma blast), which is caused by the client forcing exhalations through the stoma at the time he is phonating esophageally. Sometimes the stoma noise masks the esophageal speech to the point of affecting intelligibility. A final mannerism is facial grimacing during injection of air into the esophagus. The clinician should note these types of behavior in esophageal speakers and attack them early on in the treatment program.

The clinician can also rate the client's esophageal speech production on one of many scales available for this purpose (Wepman et al., 1953; Robe et al., 1956; Barton and Hejna, 1963; Shipp, 1967). An example of a seven-point scale is that of Wepman et al. (1953):

1. Automatic esophageal speech
2. Esophageal sound produced at will with continuity of word grouping
3. Esophageal sound produced at will; single-word speech
4. Voluntary sound production most of the time; vowel sounds

5. Voluntary sound production part of the time; no speech
6. Involuntary esophageal sound production; no speech
7. No esophageal sound production; no speech

In forming a prognostic statement, the clinician might consider variables thought to be critically related to learning esophageal speech by Berlin (1963):

1. Ability to phonate reliably on demand. If the client can inflate the esophagus and phonate 100 percent of the time on demand for twenty trials, there is a more favorable prognosis for esophageal speech learning.
2. Maintaining short latency between injection of air and phonation. If the client is timed with a stopwatch from beginning of inflation to phonation over ten trials, a latency of 0.2 to 0.6 second is associated with a better prognosis.
3. Adequate duration of phonation. Berlin noted that clients who could sustain phonation longer than 1.8 seconds had a better prognosis.
4. Sustaining phonation while articulating. This has to do with coordination of articulation with esophageal phonation and perhaps is most successful when the client injects air while articulating plosive sounds. At any rate, if this coordination is good, the person has a better prognosis. A variety of speech tasks that vary in phonemes and number of syllables will be helpful. Careful analysis should be made of the client's method of air intake and associated mannerisms. It is generally easier to prevent poor speaking habits than to correct them.

An assessment of the client's hearing acuity may prove helpful. Because a high percentage of laryngectomees are males above the age of fifty-five, it is common to find a degree of hearing loss. A moderate to severe hearing loss may make the learning process more difficult but not impossible.

Thus, at the end of the evaluation sessions, we should have obtained pertinent case history data as well as provided information to the client and the spouse about the anatomical changes and potential communication methods. We should also have a good idea about the patient's current method of communication and potential for treatment.

## RESONANCE DISORDERS

Resonance problems are most frequently seen in clients who have had clefts of the soft and hard palate. It is also possible that resonation will be affected by certain neurologically based disorders (cerebral palsy, spastic and flaccid dysarthria, myasthenia gravis) or postsurgical differences following an adenoidectomy. Our discussion will focus mainly on the cleft palate population as resonance difficulties in this group are most common. This emphasis is not meant to minimize the importance of judging resonatory function in all clients, however.

In diagnosis of resonance problems associated with cleft palate, the speech clinician is typically a member of a team. The "cleft palate team" is a well-accepted clinical entity, and in many communities represents the ultimate in interdisciplinary cooperation among speech pathologists, audiologists, psychologists, surgeons, otolaryngologists, prosthodontists, orthodontists, pedodontists, and education personnel (Wells, 1971; Bzoch, 1979). The speech clinician is expected to inform the team members about the child's speech, predict the effects of contemplated rehabilitative procedures, and serve as the primary agent for change in the client's speech development. The dramatic growth in the development of surgical and other rehabilitative procedures for the cleft palate child during the past three decades has been encouraging.

The routine case history data may need to be augmented for the cleft palate client. Knowledge of the type of cleft, as well as a description of the surgical, prosthedontic, orthodontic, and other rehabilitative procedures performed would be helpful. Some statement of the child's current medical status and plans for the future will also help direct the evaluative process. If the clinician is not a formal member of a cleft palate team, copies of reports from other professionals who have dealt with the client should be obtained.

*Critical listening.*    Although the initial interaction between clinician and child should be free and relatively unstructured, the clinician has a most demanding task. Once the patient is interacting and conversing in a spontaneous manner, the clinician must apply critical listening ability to assess the child's total communication effectiveness.

The first task involves systematically shifting perceptual sets from one aspect of the child's speech to another. The clinician should listen for the degree of nasality and the type. Although trained judges are able to identify nasality fairly adequately, the clinician may wish to tape-record the child and listen to several playbacks, or play the tape backward to isolate the nasality from articulation (Sherman, 1954; Spriestersbach, 1955). After noting the degree of nasality or denasality, preferably on some scaling device, the clinician should listen to the general articulatory pattern without recording actual errors. Is there an obvious preponderance of a particular type of error (glottal stops, pharyngeal fricatives)? Does the articulation appear to alter with differing communication situations, rates, or stress patterns? Next, listen to the language of the child and check for appropriate word choice, sentence complexity, and structure. The rate and rhythm of the child's speech should be noted. Are there any other vocal quality differences? Finally, are there any particular mannerisms that attract your attention? Is there a facial grimace, a constriction of the nares, or any other behavior that detracts from the child's total effectiveness.

*Articulation testing.*    Standard articulation testing may be satisfactory for cleft palate children, but there are several special considerations. Certainly, all of the functional, perceptual, and sensory factors that affect the normal child could be active, but in cleft palate children there are added possibilities. Most important are the degree of velopharyngeal closure and the resultant airflow and intraoral pressure. The deviant geography of the oral cavity may contribute to this problem, which is also complicated by the fact that the oral structure may well have undergone several architectural changes within the first few years of life. The diagnostician must keep in mind that this child has been trying to produce standard sounds with a nonstandard structure and, under these conditions, unique compensatory adjustments may have been made. The child may have increased the airflow in order to build up adequate oral pressure or minimized it to lessen nasal escape. It is entirely possible that the habits developed before the final surgical adjustments may persist, even though the child can now make the correct articulatory movements. Articulation errors may also be related to an existing or prior hearing loss.

Articulation testing, in addition to providing an inventory of the client's sound productions, can indicate the adequacy of velopharyngeal closure (Boone, 1983). Certain sounds have a higher probability for error than others. Research has shown that affricates, fricatives, and plosives are more often associated with nasality or nasal emission than are other phonemes (Moore and Sommers, 1974). The speech pathologist should obtain a thorough sample of these sounds in articulation testing. Because articulation involves dynamic and overlapping movements, the clinician should be certain to get samples of the client producing isolated sounds, syllables, words, and connected speech. In certain cases of assimilation nasality, it is necessary to evaluate specific phonetic contexts containing nasal and non-nasal sounds to determine if the client can make the rapid velopharyngeal alterations. Many authorities have reported that two characteristic articulatory substitutions found in cleft palate children are the glottal stop and pharyngeal fricative; the clinician should be especially aware of these.

When listening to the speech of the child, the clinician should note weak consonants with a light articulatory contact and inadequate plosive pressure. Any other specific anatomical adjustments the child is making in order to produce sounds should be observed; for instance, some children exhibit nasal emission of air when producing continuant phonemes.

Several formal test instruments have been traditionally associated with cleft palate articulatory assessment. Bzoch (1971) has devised an Error Pattern Articulation Test. Also, part of the Templin-Darley (1969) Tests of Articulation, called the Iowa Pressure Test, focuses on forty-three responses that assess pressure consonants in a number of contexts. Several authors recommend the use of phrases or reading passages containing no nasal consonants or a preponderance of fricatives and plosives to measure hypernasal and hyponasal resonance qualities (Boone, 1983; Vandemark, 1964).

*Nasal resonance.*   Resonatory voice disorders are generally described as variations of two types: hyper- and hyponasality. Hypernasality is generally the result of inadequate velopharyngeal closure, which in turn may be related to functional factors, such as tension, fatigue, or learning, or organic factors, such as neurological disorders or cleft palate. Listener evaluation of the nasality of a speaking voice is the best way for the clinician to judge this parameter.

*The oral peripheral examination.*   There are several reasons to perform an oral peripheral examination with clients manifesting resonation disorders. First, it is an initial step to determine the general relationships of the structures in the vocal tract. For instance, the clinician can get a gross picture of palatal shape and length and movement of the velum in relation to the pharyngeal walls. It is important for the clinician to realize that it is not possible to actually view the site of velopharyngeal closure because it is above the lower portion of the velum. It is possible, however, to make a general judgment regarding the mobility of the velum during various vowel productions (Boone, 1983). A second goal of the examination is to determine any oral cavity deviations that may interfere with speech and to discover any fistulas present in the hard or soft palates. If the speech pathologist has any concerns regarding structure or function, the physician should be consulted. General information on conducting an oral peripheral examination is provided in Chapter 3.

*The velopharyngeal mechanism.*   As indicated previously, the articulation test is an indirect measure of the client's velopharyngeal adequacy (Boone, 1983; Wilson, 1979). Fox and Johns (1970) describe a technique for measuring static closure whereby the child is required to maintain intraoral pressure by puffing up the cheeks. If this is accomplished, the child is then asked to protrude the tongue and then puff up the cheeks (to prevent lingual valving). The examiner holds the child's nostrils while this is done to aid in impounding pressure. If no air escapes when the nostrils are released, it is assumed that velopharyngeal closure is adequate.

Boone (1983) summarizes a variety of evaluation measures that have been used in assessing velopharyngeal adequacy. There are aerodynamic measures, which provide information on airflow in the oral and nasal cavities (Mason and Warren, 1980). There are pressure measures involving use of the U-tube manometer or Hunter Oral Manometer.[3] Also, acoustic measures, such as the sound spectrograph and Tonar II (Fletcher, 1972), analyze nasal resonance in connected speech. Radiographic instruments, such as lateral x-ray and multiview cinefluorography, can provide visual evidence of velopharyngeal function during articulation in a variety of speech tasks (Skolnick, Glaser, and McWilliams, 1980; Skolnick et al., 1975). Finally, there are visual probe instruments, such as the oral endoscope and oral panendoscope, some of which use fiberoptic techniques to view the velopharyngeal port from either above or below. The clinician may or may not have access to some of the instruments described above but should know that they are available. In this age of high technology it can be expected that access to such equipment in universities, medical centers, and clinics will become easier and more widespread.

*Auditory acuity and language ability.*   The high incidence of auditory acuity problems among cleft palate children has been well documented (Loeb, 1964; Sataloff and Fraser, 1952). For this reason it is absolutely essential that every cleft

[3]Hunter Manufacturing Co., Iowa City, Iowa.

palate child have a hearing examination. These examinations should include both air and bone conduction testing and should be a part of every speech diagnosis.

Several researchers have documented the existence of a language deficit among cleft palate children (Nation, 1970; Smith and McWilliams, 1968; Morris, 1962). The clinician should examine the child's traditional language abilities and pay particular attention to his expressive skills. The procedures discussed in Chapter 4 should be sufficient for this evaluation.

The speech clinician will wish to see the cleft palate child as soon as possible. During this early contact the parents can be informed regarding the need for normal speech and language stimulation, what to expect from their child regarding speech production, and the need for frequent audiometric testing. Some speech clinicians use established language stimulation programs as a preventive measure with these children.

## CONCLUDING REMARKS

The evaluation of voice disorders is a challenge to the speech pathologist. It requires the ability to deal with older adults as well as young children. The clinician must often work closely with medical personnel and other allied health workers, which necessitates knowing procedures and terminologies that are peripheral to speech-language pathology. The clinician must also remain abreast of current technological developments in electronics, surgery, and medical technology. Finally, the clinician must keep interpersonal clinical skills finely honed so that psychological aspects of vocal disorders can be detected and dealt with through treatment or referral. Beginning students are encouraged to read widely about voice disorders, seek out clients with vocal problems, and gain as much clinical experience as they can in this interesting area.

HIGHLIGHT  *Voice Image and Vocal Type*

Voice is an area that most beginning clinicians tend to associate with organic components. There is an emphasis on anatomy, physiology, instrumentation, and acoustics, with sometimes the subtle psychological aspects of vocal performance being overlooked. In an evaluation, the clinician should be aware that there is a significant relationship between the client's psychological state and her voice. Cooper (1973: 36) talks about the importance of a person's vocal image, which he defines as

> . . . the sound or voice that the individual either likes or dislikes, either identifies with or disinclines to identify with. Unfortunately, many voice patients have a desire or need to seek voices that assuage their ego rather than meet with their vocal abilities. The vocal image creates counterfeit voices which most individuals find attractive or appealing. Using a counterfeit voice creates vocal misuse and abuse.

According to Cooper, the vocal image concept is fostered by our culture, peer group, and the media. A person can gravitate toward a particular vocal image or attempt to avoid a type of vocal performance. The vocal image can be associated with pitch, quality, intensity, or breath support. Thus, any parameter of the voice can be affected by a person's psychological perception of what his voice should be.

Superimposed on our vocal image are various "voice types" that are used consciously or without awareness during the course of a day. Cooper indicates that one type of voice is the "put-on voice," which may be used temporarily in certain situations for effect. Another voice type reported by Cooper is the "intimate or confidental voice." This voice type is one that exudes confidence and intimacy. Other vocal types listed by Cooper are the "telephone voice," the "sexy (bedroom) voice," and the "authoritarian voice." There may be other voice types that Cooper does not report; however, the basic concept is the most important point. The voice is intimately tied to the personality, and the diagnostician must take this into account when dealing with clients. Some questions during the interview can probe the client's perceptions of what a good voice should be. It is important to know if the client has a particular vocal image she is striving to attain or escape, especially if the voice is not optimal for the person's mechanism.

## BIBLIOGRAPHY

ARONSON, A. (1980). *Clinical Voice Disorders.* New York: Thieme-Stratton.

AUSTIN, M., and H. LEEPER (1975). "Basal Pitch and Frequency Level Variation in Male and Female Children: A Preliminary Investigation." *Journal of Communication Disorders,* 8: 307–315.

BARTON, J., and R. HEJNA (1963). "Factors Associated with Success or Nonsuccess in Acquisition of Esophageal Speech." *Journal of the Speech and Hearing Association of Virginia,* 4: 19–20.

BERLIN, C. (1963). "Clinical Measurement of Esophageal Speech. I. Methodology and Curves of Skill Acquisition." *Journal of Speech and Hearing Disorders,* 28: 42–51.

BLESS, D., and J. SAXMAN (1970). "Maximum Phonation Time, Flow Rate, and Volume Change During Phonation: Normative Information on Third Grade Children." Paper presented to the American Speech and Hearing Association.

BOONE, D. (1983). *The Voice and Voice Therapy.* Englewood Cliffs, N.J.: Prentice-Hall, Inc.

BZOCH, K. (1971). "Measurement of Parameters of Cleft Palate Speech," in *Cleft Lip and Palate: Surgical, Dental and Speech Aspects,* ed. W. Grabb, S. Rosenstein, and K. Bzock. Boston: Little, Brown.

—— (1979). *Communicative Disorders Related to Cleft Lip and Palate.* Boston: Little, Brown.

COOPER, M. (1973). *Modern Techniques of Vocal Rehabilitation.* Springfield, Ill.: Chas. C. Thomas.

COOPER, M., and N. Yanagihara (1971). "A Study of the Basal Pitch Level Variations Found in the Normal Speaking Voices of Males and Females." *Journal of Communication Disorders,* 3: 261–266.

CURRY, E. (1949). "Hoarseness and Voice Change in Male Adolescents." *Journal of Speech and Hearing Disorders,* 14: 23–24.

CURTIS, J. (1968). "Acoustics of Speech Production and Nasalization," in *Cleft Palate and Communication,* ed. D. Spreistersbach and D. Sherman. New York: Academic Press.

DANILOFF, R., G. SCHUCKERS, and L. FETH (1980). *The Physiology of Speech and Hearing: An Introduction.* Englewood Cliffs, N.J.: Prentice-Hall, Inc.

DEAL, R., B. McCLAIN, and J. SUDDERTH (1976). "Identification, Evaluation, Therapy and

Follow-Up for Children with Vocal Nodules in a Public School Setting." *Journal of Speech and Hearing Disorders,* 41: 390–397.

DICKSON, D., and W. MAUE-DICKSON (1982). *Anatomical and Physiological Bases of Speech.* Boston: Little, Brown.

DIEHL, C., and C. STINNETT (1959). "Efficiency of Teacher Referrals in a School Speech Testing Program." *Journal of Speech and Hearing Disorders,* 24: 34–36.

ECKEL, F., and D. BOONE (1981). "The S/Z Ratio as an Indicator of Laryngeal Pathology." *Journal of Speech and Hearing Disorders,* 46: 147–150.

FAIRBANKS, G. (1960). *Voice and Articulation Drillbook.* 2nd ed. New York: Harper & Row.

FLETCHER, S. (1972). "Contingencies for Bioelectronic Modification of Nasality." *Journal of Speech and Hearing Disorders,* 37: 329–346.

FOX, D., and D. JOHNS (1970). "Predicting Velopharyngeal Closure with a Modified Tongue-Anchor Technique." *Journal of Speech and Hearing Disorders,* 35: 248–251.

GRAY, G., and C. WISE (1959). *The Bases of Speech.* 3rd ed. New York: Harper & Row.

GREENE, M. (1980). *The Voice and Its Disorders.* Philadelphia: Lippincott.

HANLEY, T., and W. THURMAN (1970). *Developing Vocal Skills.* New York: Holt, Rinehart, & Winston.

HARDY, J. (1961). "Intraoral Breath Pressure in Cerebral Palsy." *Journal of Speech and Hearing Disorders,* 26: 309–319.

JACKSON, C. (1941). "Vocal Nodules." *American Laryngological Association,* 63: 185.

JAMES, H., and E. COOPER (1966). "Accuracy of Teacher Referral of Speech-Handicapped Children." *Exceptional Child,* 30: 29–33.

KAHANE, J., and J. FOLKINS (1984). *Atlas of Speech and Hearing Anatomy.* Columbus, Ohio: Chas. E. Merrill.

KAPLAN, H. (1971). *Anatomy and Physiology of Speech.* New York: McGraw-Hill.

LOEB, W. (1964). "Speech, Hearing and Cleft Palate." *Archives of Otolaryngology,* 74: 4–14.

LUCHSINGER, R., and G. ARNOLD (1965). *Voice-Speech-Language.* Belmont, Calif.: Wadsworth.

MARTIN, D. (1979). "Evaluating Esophageal Speech Development and Proficiency," in *Laryngectomee Rehabilitation,* ed. R. Keith and F. Darley. Houston, Tex.: College-Hill Press.

MASON, R., and D. WARREN (1980). "Adenoid Involution and Developing Hypernasality in Cleft Palate." *Journal of Speech and Hearing Disorders,* 45: 469–480.

MONCUR, J., and I. BRACKETT (1974). *Modifying Vocal Behavior.* New York: Harper & Row.

MOORE, G. (1971). *Organic Voice Disorders.* Englewood Cliffs, N.J.: Prentice-Hall, Inc.

MOORE, W., and R. SOMMERS (1974). "Phonetic Contexts: Their Effects on Perceived Nasality in Cleft Palate Speakers." *Cleft Palate Journal,* 11: 72–83.

MORRIS, H. (1962). "Communication Skills of Children with Cleft Lips and Palates." *Journal of Speech and Hearing Research,* 5: 79–90.

MOSES, P. (1954). *The Voice of Neurosis.* New York: Grune & Stratton.

MURPHY, A. (1964). *Functional Voice Disorders.* Englewood Cliffs, N.J.: Prentice-Hall, Inc.

NATION, J. (1970). "Vocabulary Comprehension and Usage in Preschool Cleft Palate and Normal Children." *Cleft Palate Journal,* 7: 639–644.

PALMER, J. (1984). *Anatomy for Speech and Hearing.* New York: Harper & Row.

PERKINS, W. (1971). "Vocal Function: Assessment and Therapy," in *Handbook of Speech Pathology and Audiology,* ed. L. Travis. New York: Appleton-Century-Crofts.

POWERS, M. (1971). "Functional Disorders of Articulation-Symptomatology and Etiology," in *Handbook of Speech Pathology and Audiology,* ed. L. Travis. New York: Appleton-Century-Crofts.

PTACEK, P., and E. SANDER (1963). "Breathiness and Phonation Length." *Journal of Speech and Hearing Disorders,* 28: 267–272.

ROBE, E., et al. (1956). "A Study of the Role of Certain Factors in the Development of Speech After Laryngectomy. 1. Type of Operation." *Laryngoscope,* 66: 173–186.

ROUSEY, C., and A. MORIARTY (1965). *Diagnostic Implications of Speech Sounds.* Springfield, Ill.: Chas. C. Thomas.

SATALOFF, J., and M. FRASER (1952). "Hearing Loss in Children With Cleft Palates." *Archives of Otolaryngology,* 55: 61–64.

SHERMAN, D. (1954). "The Merits of Backward Playing of Connected Speech in the Scaling of Voice Quality Disorders." *Journal of Speech and Hearing Disorders,* 19: 312–321.

SHIPP, T. (1967). "Frequency, Duration and Perceptual Measures in Relation to Judgments of Alaryngeal Speech Acceptability." *Journal of Speech and Hearing Research,* 10: 417–427.

SILVERMAN, E., and C. ZIMMER (1975). "Incidence of Chronic Hoarseness Among School-Age Children." *Journal of Speech and Hearing Disorders,* 40: 211–215.

SILVERMAN, F. (1977). *Research Design in Speech Pathology and Audiology.* Englewood Cliffs, N.J.: Prentice-Hall, Inc.

—— (1980). *Communication for the Speechless.* Englewood Cliffs, N.J.: Prentice-Hall, Inc.

SKOLNICK, M., E. GLASER, and B. McWILLIAMS (1980). "The Use and Limitations of the Barium Pharyngogram in the Detection of Velopharyngeal Insufficiency." *Radiology,* 135: 301–304.

SKOLNICK, M., R. SHPRINTZEN, G. McCALL, and S. ROKOFF (1975). "Patterns of Velopharyngeal Closure in Subjects with Repaired Cleft Palates and Normal Speech: A Multiview Video-fluoroscopic Analysis." *Cleft Palate Journal,* 12: 369–376.

SMITH, R., and B. McWILLIAMS (1968). "Psycholinguistic Abilities of Children with Clefts." *Cleft Palate Journal,* 5: 238–249.

SPRIESTERSBACH, D. (1955). "Assessing Nasal Quality in Cleft Palate Speech of Children." *Journal of Speech and Hearing Disorders,* 20: 266–270.

STARR, C., and F. WILSON (1976). "Reliability Considerations of a Voice Profiling System." *Human Communication,* 1: 47–56.

STEMPLE, J. (1984). *Clinical Voice Pathology: Theory and Management,* Columbus, Ohio: Chas. E. Merrill.

STONE, E., N. HURLBUTT, and S. COULTHARD (1978). "Role and Laryngological Consultation in the Intervention of Dysphonia." *Language, Speech and Hearing Services in Schools,* 9: 35–42.

TAIT, N., J. MICHEL, and M. CARPENTER (1980). "Maximum Duration of Sustained /s/ and /z/ in Children." *Journal of Speech and Hearing Disorders,* 45: 239–246.

TEMPLIN, M., and F. DARLEY (1969). *The Templin-Darley Tests of Articulation.* 2nd ed. Iowa City: University of Iowa Bureau of Educational Research and Service.

THURMAN, W. (1958). "Frequency-Intensity Relationships and Optimum Pitch Levels." *Journal of Speech and Hearing Research,* 1: 117–123.

TUNEMASTER III (1974). Berkshire Instruments, Inc., 170 Chestnut Street, Ridgewood, N.J. 07450.

VAN RIPER, C., and J. IRWIN (1958). *Voice and Articulation.* Englewood Cliffs, N.J.: Prentice-Hall, Inc.

VANDEMARK, D. (1964). "Misarticulations and Listener Judgments of the Speech of Individuals with Cleft Palates." *Cleft Palate Journal,* 1: 232–245.

VENTRY, I., and N. SCHIAVETTI (1980). *Evaluating Research in Speech Pathology and Audiology.* Reading, Mass.: Addison-Welsey.

VISI-PITCH (1980). Kay Elemetrics Corp., Pine Brook, N.J.

WEINBERG, B. (1983). "Phonatory Based Voice Disorders," in *Diagnosis in Speech-Language Pathology,* ed. I. Meitus and B. Weinberg. Baltimore: University Park Press.

WELLS, C. (1971). *Cleft Palate and Its Associated Speech Disorders.* New York: McGraw-Hill.

WENDAHL, R., and L. PAGE (1967). "Glottal Wave Periods in CVC Environments." *Journal of the Acoustical Society of America,* 42: 1208.

WEPMAN, J., et al. (1953). "The Objective Measurement of Progressive Esophageal Speech Development." *Journal of Speech and Hearing Disorders,* 18: 247–251.

WILSON, D. (1979). *Voice Problems in Children.* Baltimore: Williams & Wilkins.

WILSON, F. (1972). "The Voice Disordered Child: A Descriptive Approach." *Language, Speech and Hearing Services in Schools,* 4: 14–22.

WILSON, F., and M. RICE (1977). *A Programmed Approach to Voice Therapy.* Austin, Tex.: Learning Concepts, Inc.

WITHERS, B. (1961). "Vocal Nodules." *Eye, Ear, Nose and Throat Monthly,* 40: 35–38.

WOOD, K. (1971). "Terminology and Nomenclature," in *Handbook of Speech Pathology and Audiology,* ed. L. Travis. New York: Appleton-Century-Crofts.

WORTHLEY, W. (1969). "The Report of a Survey for the Speech Clinician." Unpublished.

ZEMLIN, W. (1981). *Speech and Hearing Science.* Englewood Cliffs, N.J.: Prentice-Hall, Inc.

# CHAPTER NINE
# THE DIAGNOSTIC REPORT

Only one very important phase of the evaluation remains to be considered: the preparation of the diagnostic report. Put the clinical situation, the interview, testing methods, results, and impressions in writing *as soon as possible*. Never trust a memory. Commit it to paper while the facial characteristics and voice inflections can still be remembered. Make the report "alive" so that others can experience what occurred in time and place just by reading about it. The raw data are of limited value to the clinician or other workers until they are assembled in a clear, precise, and orderly fashion.

A diagnostic report is a written record that summarizes the relevant information we have obtained—and *how* we have obtained it—in our professional interaction with a client. It serves the following functions: (1) It acts as a guide for further services to the client—providing a clear statement of how the person was functioning at a given point in time, so that we can document change or lack of change; (2) it communicates our findings to other professional workers; it provides answers to a number of clinical questions, including: Does the person have a problem? How severe is the problem? Will therapy be helpful? And will referrals be necessary? and (3) it serves as a document for research purposes.

The importance of the first function should be obvious: Intelligent clinical plans evolve naturally from carefully prepared reports. The second purpose of diagnostic reports is to answer questions about clients so that other professionals can plan and provide appropriate services. In addition to transmitting necessary information, a carefully prepared examination report will tend also to establish the credibility of the clinician in the eyes of other workers. To state it another way, a written document is an extension of the diagnostician, and even minor errors in spelling or grammar may cast doubt upon her accuracy and attention to detail with respect to substantive material. Although the clinician may be highly skilled in testing and interviewing, his competence may be evaluated by his written communications. Clinical reports are the principal way we relate to other professions.

## FORMAT

There are several ways to organize a diagnostic report (Knepflar, 1976; Darley and Spriestersbach, 1978; Hutchinson, Hanson, and Mecham, 1979; Hollis and Dunn, 1979; Tallent, 1980; Peterson and Marquardt, 1981; Flower, 1984). Because reports may vary, depending on the intended reader, no single schema is appropriate for all circumstances; in many instances the format will be dictated by the agency the clinician serves.

For example, clinicians working in a medical setting record their findings in a "problem-oriented" format (Kent and Chabon, 1980). Problem Oriented Medical Records (POMR) feature a carefully defined and "documented list of problems which encompass all the significant difficulties a patient is experiencing" (Enelow and Swisher, 1972: 69). The list includes the presenting complaint as well as those problems identified by the members of the treatment team. All available information about the person is then organized under four headings (Bourchard and Shane, 1977), which form the acronym SOAP:

| SUBJECTIVE | OBJECTIVE | ASSESSMENT | PLAN |
|---|---|---|---|
| Interview and case history | Test results | Collation of subjective and objective information | Additional testing Treatment options |

Public school clinicians report their diagnostic findings in a client-focused record called an Individualized Educational Program (see Highlight).

Regardless of the format employed, a diagnostic report should be organized for easy retrieval of information (Pannbacker, 1975) and prepared in a manner that reflects high professional standards. Here are additional criteria we use to judge a diagnostic report: Is it *accurate*? Is it *complete*? Is it *efficiently* written (clearly and with an economy of words)? Was it prepared *promptly*?

We have found the following generic format (see Figure 9.1) quite effective and recommend it to the beginning clinician. It contains several major sections.

I. Routine Information

Name:                                  File no.:

Sex:                                   Date:

Address:                               Phone no.:

Birth date:                            Age at Evaluation:

Parents:                               Referred by:

Evaluated by:                          Address:

II.   Statement of the Problem
III.  Historical Information
IV.   Evaluation
V.    Clinical Impressions
VI.   Summary
VII.  Recommendations

_____

                                       Clinician

_____

                                       Supervisor

**FIGURE 9.1   Format for diagnostic report.**

### Routine Information

In this section we present basic identifying information—client's name, sex, address, date of birth, telephone number, parent's name where relevant, and of course the date of the examination; an undated report is of very little use. In addition to these routine data, we generally identify the referral source (parent, teacher, physician) and the evaluator. If the client is a school-aged child, we note the name and location of his school and the names of his teacher and the principal. The keystone of this initial section of the report is meticulous attention to *accuracy*.

### Statement of the Problem

In this section we include a succinct statement of the presenting problem. What is the complaint and who is making it? Be sure to distinguish between the client's complaint and the problem stated by the referral source. In most instances the reason for referral is stated in the client's (or her parent's) own words—always indicated by quotation marks.

### Historical Information

Before seeing a client for evaluation, many speech clinicians request that the individual fill out a brief case history form (see Figure 9.2). Although we prefer to obtain a complete history in a face-to-face interview, the information obtained in a brief questionnaire provides information useful for planning the diagnostic session.

**FIGURE 9.2  Case history form.**

---

Speech and Hearing Clinic
Northern Michigan University
Marquette, Michigan
49855

Date:_____

If the case history is for an adult, only the information indicated by asterisk (*) is required. If the history is on a child, please fill in both pages.

NAME OF PERSON COMPLETING THIS FORM          RELATIONSHIP TO CHILD

IDENTIFICATION

*Name_____*Date of birth_____*Sex_____*Age_____

*Address_____*Phone_____

Mother's name_____ Address_____ Age_____

Mother's occupation_____ Education_____

Father's name_____ Address_____ Age_____

Father's occupation_____ Education_____

List names of brothers and sisters, their ages, and if they have a history of speech, hearing, or other health problems.

_____

_____

_____

*Referred by_____*Address_____

*Name of family doctor_____*Address_____

*STATEMENT OF THE PROBLEM

Briefly describe the problem, indicating when it was first noticed and its development.

---

Note: This form is mailed to the client and returned prior to the diagnostic session.

**FIGURE 9.2  (cont.)**

*General Development*: Describe any illnesses, accidents, or problems relating to the mother or child during pregnancy, birth, or during infancy.

*Medical History*: Indicate at what ages any of the following illnesses or operations occurred. Please indicate severity.

| | Age | Severity | | Age | Severity |
|---|---|---|---|---|---|
| Whooping cough | | | Earaches | | |
| Mumps | | | Running ears | | |
| Scarlet fever | | | Chronic colds | | |
| Measles | | | Head injuries | | |
| Chicken pox | | | Venereal disease | | |
| Pneumonia | | | Asthma | | |
| Diphtheria | | | Allergies | | |
| Croup | | | Convulsions | | |
| Influenza | | | Encephalitis | | |
| Polio | | | High fevers | | |
| Headaches | | | Typhoid | | |
| Sinus | | | Tonsillitis | | |
| Meningitis | | | Tonsillectomy | | |
| Rickets | | | Adenoidectomy | | |
| Rheumatic fever | | | Mastoidectomy | | |
| Pleurisy | | | Thyroid | | |
| Tuberculosis | | | Heart trouble | | |
| Smallpox | | | Enlarged glands | | |

Have the child's ears been examined? _____ By whom? _____

**FIGURE 9.2** (cont.)

Results _____

Is he now under the care of a doctor? _____ For what reason? _____

_____

Is he presently taking any medication? _____ For what reason? _____

*Speech and Hearing History*: Briefly describe any abnormalities noticed during the development of your child's speech and hearing.

Information obtained from referral letters, the case history, and the intake interview are included in this section. Material regarding the client's development (general and speech and language), medical, educational, and familial history, and estimates of personality and behavioral adjustments are summarized. Only the most pertinent items are included in the diagnostic report. Because most of the historical information is obtained by questioning the client, a parent, or other informants, we suggest that you briefly describe the interview situation—type of rapport established, the frankness and completeness of the respondent's answers, and any other pertinent observations.

### Evaluation

The results of the various tests and examinations are delineated in this section. Before describing the assessment procedures and results, however, we include an opening statement that describes how the client approached the clinical setting and the tasks used to evaluate her communication abilities. Was she apprehensive, bored, fatigued, cooperative? The name of each test, an explanation of what it does and how it was administered, and the results obtained should be included. Should the clinician include statements about communication skills that are within normal limits at the time of the evaluation? Knepflar (1976) believes that a complete diagnostic report should mention, even if briefly, all aspects of a client's speech, hearing, and language performance so that subsequent assessments can utilize the information as baseline observations. The information is simply presented, not interpreted, in this section of the report.

### Clinical Impressions

In this section we summarize our impressions of the individual and his communication impairment. What type of speech or language problem does he have? How severe is it? What caused it? What factors seem to be perpetuating it? What impact has it had on the client and his family? How much does it interfere with his everyday functioning? What are the prospects for treatment? Although we can offer interpretations here, we must still be able to support our impressions with information obtained during the interview or testing. Speculations based on clinical experience, such as similarity between the client and other cases the diagnostician has examined, should be clearly labeled as such.

### Summary

The summary should be a concise (not more than a short paragraph) statement abstracting the salient features of the whole report. What is the communication disorder? What are the primary features of the disorder? What is the probable cause of the disorder? What is the prognosis (and general estimate of the predicted time frame) for recovery?

### Recommendations

This is perhaps the most crucial portion of the report. We must now translate our findings into appropriate suggestions or directions that will help the client solve his communication and related problems. Do we recommend further speech and language evaluations? Is a medical referral necessary? Is treatment indicated? What direction should be taken? By whom, and when? The task, then, is to crystallize all the disparate interaction we have had with the individual, collate all the data, and then provide a flexible blueprint for further action. We must attempt to answer the question: What happens now; where do we go from here? Try to make the recommendations specific and brief. Suggestions for treatment or a more lengthy plan of therapy can be outlined in a letter or follow-up report. One final warning: Do not recommend specific evaluations or remediation procedures to workers in other professions. It is improper, for example, to recommend a client for electroencephalography to a neurologist, or for dental braces to an orthodonist; the speech clinician would be chagrined if a physician referred a child and recommended the administration of the *ITPA*. Be sure that your referrals for additional assessment are based on sound evidence; it is expensive, time consuming, and stressful to the client to make recommendations for comprehensive medical or psychiatric evaluation without serious and compelling reasons:

> Early in the diagnostic session with five-year-old Mark we suspected the possibility of brain injury. Mindful of the family's limited finances, we wanted to document carefully all signs of apparent cerebral dysfunction before making a referral for a complete pediatric neurological evaluation. Observation revealed a number of serious symptoms: difficulty with motor coordination; labile emotions; rapid and slurred speech; perseveration; and blanking out spells. The necessity for referral was then obvious.

## CONFIDENTIALITY

In our view, confidentiality is basic to any helping profession. All reports and records should be kept secure so that no harm or embarrassment comes to the persons we serve. When a diagnostic report is released, we prefer to mail it to a specific person rather than send it to the agency. Before releasing *any* information about a client, however, we must secure the client's permission in writing; most speech and hearing centers have permission forms, which are completed prior to or during the diagnostic session.

Because clients and parents have a legal right (Public Law 93-380, Family Educational Rights and Privacy Act of 1974) to read any report containing information about them, we often find it is useful to send them a copy of the diagnostic findings. Before mailing the report, however, we always review our findings and recommendations with them. By going over the report with the clients or parents, we can be sure that they understand its contents.

Figure 9.3 is an example of a diagnostic report prepared according to the format just described:

**FIGURE 9.3**   Diagnostic report.

---

### DIAGNOSTIC REPORT

Name: Craig J. Frieble                     File no.: 83-178
Sex: Male                                  Date: 1/20/83
Address: Box 223, Lake Linden, Mich.       Phone no.: 245-2819
Birth date: 5/20/79                        Age: 3.7
Parents: Rebecca and Bert Frieble          Referred by: M. Mannisto
Evaluated by: L. Miller, R. Kapala                      224 South Lake Street
                                                        South Range, Mich.

*Statement of the Problem*

Craig Frieble was brought to the Northern Michigan University Speech and Hearing Clinic for a diagnostic evaluation by his parents. The child was referred to the clinic by Marilisa Mannisto, speech clinician at the Copper County Intermediate School District. Mr. and Mrs. Frieble expressed their concern about Craig: "He has difficulty saying words. He doesn't seem to use his tongue appropriately. Craig is trying to talk, but we cannot understand him."

*Historical Information*

*Family history.* Craig lives at home with his parents and younger brother Chad (age four months). Mrs. Frieble is a homemaker and Mr. Frieble works as an cabinetmaker. Mrs. Frieble indicated that there was no history of speech or hearing disorders in either her husband's or her own family. She said that Craig's maternal grandmother has asthma and that his paternal grandfather died of a heart condition. There was no other history of health problems that might relate to communication impairments.

*Speech and language development.* Mrs. Frieble reported that Craig began to babble at four months and said the word "nice" (pronounced "ice") at thirteen months.

---

**FIGURE 9.3** (cont.)

Since then the child's vocabulary has consisted of approximately ten words; all are nouns and all are difficult to understand. According to Mrs. Frieble, Craig does not use two-word utterances, nor does he use pronouns. The youngster's main mode of communication is vocalizing and gesturing. He communicates his needs by pointing or taking his parents' arm and directing them to the desired object. The mother *believes* that Craig understands just about everything that is said to him. She added that Craig spends a lot of time talking to himself and on a play phone. The child does not make toy or animal sounds during play.

*Developmental history.* Reportedly, Craig was early in regard to motor development. He rolled over at one month, sat unassisted at six months, and crawled at nine months. Mrs. Frieble stated that Craig walked at thirteen months with no previous steps or assistance. The youngster has difficulty dressing himself (managing buttons), but is able to undress appropriately. He is toilet trained and dry at night. Craig is predominantly left-handed; the parents noticed his laterality preference at an early age.

Both parents noted that Craig has considerable difficulty chewing food; he takes very small bites. Swallowing appears to be normal. Craig has difficulty getting to sleep and is often awake three or four times a night.

*Medical history.* Mrs. Frieble reported that her pregnancy with Craig was normal. The child weighed six pounds and seven ounces at birth. He had a mild case of jaundice and was released from the hospital five days after Mrs. Frieble went home. Since that time Craig has not been hospitalized. He received immunizations for the typical childhood illnesses; he has had only a mild case of chicken pox. Craig does, however, have asthma for which he must take medication; because he refuses to take pills orally, the child has to have an injection periodically. Except for the asthma, which seems to be controlled by medication, Mrs. Frieble stated that Craig's general health is good.

*Psychosocial history.* Both parents believe that Craig is a very active and temperamental child. Reportedly, however, he interacts socially (except for communication) in an appropriate manner. According to Mrs. Frieble, Craig "has a mind of his own and becomes extremely upset when attempts are made to discipline him." She believes that because Craig is the first grandchild he receives a lot of attention and added, "He is pretty spoiled!"

Mrs. Frieble revealed that both she and her husband are quite concerned about Craig's lack of speech development. "He's getting more and more frustrated," she stated, "and I feel he definitely needs therapy."

*Rapport.* The Friebles, particularly Craig's mother, seemed to be open and honest in their responses. Rapport was established easily and remained good throughout the interview.

### Evaluation

All observation and testing was conducted in the Speech and Hearing Clinic on January 20, 1983, at 1:30 p.m. The testing environment consisted of a small table, four chairs, two large cabinets, and the testing materials. Craig's father was present throughout the evaluation. Following the case history interview, Mrs. Frieble participated in the last twenty minutes of the diagnostic session.

*Client's reactions.* Craig entered the examining room without reservation; his parents left immediately. After a few moments of interaction with the examiner, however, Craig attempted to leave the room. After several unsuccessful attempts to interest the child in play activities, the examiner asked Mr. Frieble to return to the testing room; he was present during the entire evaluation.

**FIGURE 9.3** (cont.)

Throughout the session Craig displayed uncooperative behavior—getting out of his chair, running about the room, shaking his head "no" when presented a testing task. He exhibited frustration whenever he was thwarted by either the clinician or his father. Mr. Frieble noted that Craig was somewhat fatigued by the long car trip to the clinic and the lengthy audiological evaluation that directly preceded the speech and language assessment. Later in the session, however, Mr. Frieble observed that Craig is typically "headstrong" and very difficult to manage in the home.

*Auditory testing.* A complete audiological evaluation (1/20/83) revealed that Craig's hearing acuity was within normal limits.

*Oral peripheral.* No structural abnormalities or paralysis were noted during the oral examination. Craig was unable to move his tongue or lips volitionally when asked to do so; he tried to imitate the examiner's model but was unable to. After taking a drink of water, however, the child immediately licked his lips. Tongue protrusion at this time (after drinking) appeared to be normal. Other oral movements (puckering, smiling, side-to-side tongue movement) were also noted on the automatic level but he could perform none voluntarily.

*Vocal parameters.* Craig did not produce any words during the evaluation. He did, however, vocalize on a consistent basis. The pitch range of his vocalizations (typically the vowel /ʌ/) was very limited. Loudness levels did vary slightly and resonance appeared normal.

*Receptive language.* Craig's attention was only fleeting during the formal testing procedures. When he interacted with his parents informally, the child responded inconsistently to verbal directives (four correct responses of ten attempts). Craig responded primarily to directives that involved interaction with agents other than the examiner (his father, a doll, a puppet). He refused to respond when asked to point to pictures, imitate block patterns, or to show knowledge of color or spatial concepts.

*Expressive language.* The child was nonverbal throughout the evaluation. But he did express himself through a combination of undifferentiated vocalizations and gestures. Phonologically, Craig produced the vowels /ʌ/, /a/, and /o/ and the consonant /m/. He did not imitate the examiner's modeling of words, syllables, or sounds.

*Motor skills.* Craig was able to jump in place, stand on one foot (momentarily), and throw a ball overhand. His gait while running and walking appeared normal.

The child exhibited left-hand dominance. He was able to open a covered box with a latch, stack four blocks, and manipulate a pencil well. He did not copy a circle and could not cut with a pair of scissors.

*Cognition.* The child displayed appropriate interaction with all the objects in the testing room. His play with the toys present was at the symbolic level. Although his play was context-bound (the objects were present), Craig was able to use a doll as an agent (combing her hair, washing her face, giving her a drink) rather than acting upon himself. Symbolization of objects was noted also in his ability to recognize pictures of objects and in pretending to knock at the picture of a door. In one play sequence, Craig dialed a play phone, held a brief "conversation," and then placed the receiver carefully back on the hook. Means-ends sequences were also noted, although he became frustrated at the first sign of failure.

*Clinical Impressions*

Craig displayed the behavioral characteristics of developmental apraxia of speech. The support systems for oral communication (auditory, motor, cognition) are intact. His receptive language abilities are slightly below but almost age-appropriate. The most con-

FIGURE 9.3   (cont.)

vincing feature of developmental apraxia was the child's inability to perform volitional oral movements. Additionally, Craig exhibited a great deal of frustration, which is also characteristic of apraxia in children.

*Recommendations*

1. It is recommended that Craig receive speech therapy a minimum of four sessions per week.

2. It is recommended that the treatment plan include (a) use of a consistent routine or regimen of expected behavior (focusing, attending); (b) use of nonverbal tasks such as simple form boards or puzzles to provide initial success; (c) use of visual and tactile cues to implement imitation; (d) use of simple motor patterns for creating CV combinations (starting with the phonemes /m/, /b/, /p/, and /t/).

3. It is recommended that a program of parent education be implemented to train the parents to use behavior modification strategies to control Craig's negative behaviors.

(Signed) Lori Miller
            Renee Kapala

Graduate Speech Clinicians

## STYLE

An extended discussion of prose style for report writing is not possible within the scope of this text. The reader will want to consult several of the following sources for more definitive statements about common modes of report writing: Huber (1961), Jerger (1962), Moore (1969), Good (1970), Fishbein (1972), Pannbacker (1975), Knepflar (1976), Hollis and Dunn (1979), and Tallent (1980). In the interest of brevity, then, we shall simply enumerate several principles of style that we have found useful:

1. Make your presentation straightforward and objective, using a topical outline. Use simple, brief but complete sentences. It is often helpful to write for a specific reader; picture the reader in your mind—classroom teacher, physician, speech clinician—and then simply tell the story of what you observed and recommend regarding a particular client. When in doubt about a reader's level of understanding, it is better to err on the side of simplicity.

2. Use an impersonal style. Some clinicians use the first person when writing diagnostic reports, but in our view it is preferable to keep the "I" out of it; a reference to "the clinician" or "the examiner" is more in keeping with professional reports. We prefer to individualize the *client* described in the report, not the writer. Furthermore, we believe that not only does an impersonal style help to minimize the writer's verbal idiosyncracies, it also tends to encourage objectivity.

3. Edit the report carefully to make certain that spelling and use of tenses, grammar, and punctuation are accurate. Errors. even trivial ones, undermine the confidence of the reader in the diagnostician. Remember, competence is judged to a great extent by the precision of your reporting.

4. Watch your semantics. Be wary of overused or nebulous words such as "nice," "hopefully," "good," and the like. Avoid pet expressions or stereotyped ways of phrasing information. One clinician used the phrase "in terms of" thirteen times in a two-page diagnostic report. Another laced his reports with currently popular words like "input," "interface," and "scenario." Some writers use the word "feel" inappropriately in statements like "The clinician felt the client understood the diagnostic task"; we believe (not feel!) that the word should be reserved for discussing emotions or tactile sensations. Use abbreviations sparingly. Avoid superlatives unless they are clearly indicated.

5. Avoid preparing an "Aunt Fanny" report (Sunberg and Tyler, 1962)—a bland written statement that could represent anyone, or is so filled with qualifications ("perhaps," "apparently," "tends to") that it reveals nothing; nothing, that is, except a timid diagnostician.

6. Make the report "tight." Don't leave gaps or ambiguity where it is possible to read between the lines. If findings in certain areas are unremarkable, always state this explicitly. Don't leave the reader to guess whether you have investigated all possible aspects.

7. A diagnostic report is no place to display your learning or to parade a large vocabulary. Pedantic reports are misunderstood or unread.

8. Stay close to the data until you wish to draw the observations together and make some interpretations. For example, tell the reader which sounds were in error instead of simply stating that the child sounds infantile.

9. The very essence of good style is the willingness to take the time and energy to write and rewrite the report until it communicates what we did and what we found in the diagnostic session.

## THE WRITING PROCESS

Many students have difficulty writing reports. Most of them have found the task onerous, and a few are threatened and overwhelmed by the prospect of a blank sheet of paper in the typewriter. It has been our experience, however, that rather than a writing *deficiency* most of these students have a writing *bias*—they do not think they can do it. There are, of course, no quick and simple solutions; but we offer the following suggestions that have proven helpful to more than one beginning report writer.

Write on a daily basis. Each night—before retiring, for example—sit down and write a descriptive paragraph concerning something that happened to you that day. It may be easier for you to tap into your own creative power by starting with material that arouses strong feelings (see Macrorie, 1968, 1970). At first it may be halting and difficult; as in any new task, your writing "muscles" will be sore. Don't wait for an inspiration, for that magic moment when, suddenly, it will *come* to you. *Go* to it. At the end of the week, review the writing you have done; edit, revise, ask yourself what you meant by each word or phrase. The best way to learn to write, in our opinion, is to write.

Get the message out and revise it later. It is especially important in writing reports to commence work as soon as possible while the material is still fresh in your mind. A common error that some beginning writers make is to attempt to produce perfect writing in the initial draft. It doesn't matter how it looks at this point; you can always edit or have someone help you edit. When you meet barriers or mental blocks, don't linger; jump over them and go on with the rest of the report. When you come back later, you will find that your mind has filled in the blank spots.

It is helpful to have someone read and comment on the initial draft of your report. Although it is difficult to submit one's prose for dissection, ask the reader to be frank and honest in his editing. So many times, a phrase that seems clear to the writer who conceived it is vague or obscure to an objective reader. If writing continues to be a problem consult the work of Strunk and White (1959) and others (Ferguson, 1959; Kelly, Roth, and Altshuler, 1969; Jones and Faulkner, 1971; Wubben, 1971; Berke, 1972; Mayes, 1972; Leggett, Mead, and Charvat, 1974).

## FOLLOW-UP

The clinician's responsibilities do not end when the diagnostic report is finished and filed. A complete evaluation includes one final important task: a careful follow-up. It is the examiner's professional obligation to determine that the diagnostic activities and recommendations are translated into action; it is useless, perhaps even harmful, to identify and describe problems unless the individual is seen for further testing or treatment as soon as possible. When, as often is the case, the diagnostician is also the clinician, the follow-up can be handled directly and with a minimum of paperwork. In an agency such as ours, however (a university speech and hearing clinic), we regularly refer clients to other workers for further assessment or therapy. We use the following questions as guidelines in implementing a follow-up program.

1. Did the intended readers receive the report? The best of secretaries occasionally misfiles a document, so we generally call the referral source within a week after the diagnostic to determine if the report has arrived.
2. Does the reader understand the contents of the report? What questions did it raise, if any, about the client? We always log these phone calls in the client's folder.
3. What is the disposition of the client? Is he being seen for further testing? Is he on a waiting list or being seen for treatment?
4. How is the client responding to treatment? We call the local worker, usually on a monthly basis, to assess how the client is doing in therapy relative to our recommendations. Not only does this convey our interest and assistance, it also helps the diagnostic team evaluate the efficacy of its work.

HIGHLIGHT    *The Individualized Educational Program*

During the past decade, particularly since the passage of the Education for All Handicapped Children Act (Public Law 94-142, 1975), the role of the public school speech and language clinician has expanded considerably. All handicapped children between three and twenty-one years of age must be identified, a careful assessment made of their needs, and a comprehensive plan or individualized educational program (IEP) developed.

The IEP is a case-focused (child-centered) plan devised by the child's teachers, school administrators, special remedial workers, and, last but not least, parents. The plan is spelled out in response to very specific questions:

1. *What* is the problem(s)?
2. *Where* is the child at now?
3. *Who* will do *what* with the child and *how often*?
4. *When* and *how* will progress be measured?

Here is a portion of an IEP prepared for a child with a phonological disorder:

## INDIVIDUALIZED EDUCATIONAL PROGRAM

Student: David Grabowski      Birthdate: 1/7/78      Address: 224 Orchard
Parents: Gerard and Julie      District/school: Beaver Grove Schools
Grade: First                  District of residency: Marquette County
IEP conference date: 9/12/83   Projected IEP review date: 9/10/84

*Eligibility Statement*: (What decision/description requires this service?)

David has difficulty with frictional manner of articulation production resulting in several substitutional errors: th/s, th/z, s/sh, ts/ch, dz/dj.

*Current Educational Level*: (Where is child currently functioning?)

David is enrolled in a developmental first-grade classroom.

| Special Services | | |
|---|---|---|
| Goals | Objectives | Service description |
| 1. David will produce *s, z* correctly at the word and sentence level. | 1. David will discriminate target sounds from other sounds with 90% accuracy. | Speech therapy |
| 2. David will produce *sh* correctly at the word and sentence level. | 2. David will produce target sounds at the beginning, middle, and end of single words with 90% accuracy. | |
| 3. Progress reports will be sent to parents and teacher twice a year. | 3. David will correctly produce target sounds within sentences with 80% success. | |

| Dates of Services | | Time in Programs | Responsible Individuals |
|---|---|---|---|
| Start | End | Daily | |
| 9/19/83 | 6/1/84 | Within small-group 20-minute sessions 2 times a week | Speech-language clinician |

*Evaluation Plan*: (How is it planned to ascertain that goals have been reached?)

1. Goldman-Fristoe Test of Articulation
2. Pre- and posttherapy word list containing target sounds
3. Five-minute sample of spontaneous speech

*IEP Committee Members*:

| Name | Position |
|---|---|
| Ellen Mattson | Teacher |
| Roy Brown, Jr. | Principal |
| Rebecca Clark | Speech-language clinician |
| Gerard and Julie Grabowski | Parents |

## BIBLIOGRAPHY

BERKE, J. (1972). *Twenty Questions for the Writer*. New York: Harcourt, Brace, Jovanovich.

BOURCHARD, M., and H. SHANE (1977). "Use of the Problem-Oriented Medical Record in the Speech and Hearing Profession." *Journal of the American Speech and Hearing Association,* 19: 157–159.

DARLEY, F., and D. SPRIESTERSBACH (1978). *Diagnostic Methods in Speech Pathology.* 2nd ed. New York: Harper & Row.

ENELOW, A., and S. SWISHER (1972). *Interviewing and Patient Care*. New York: Oxford University Press.

FERGUSON, C. (1959). *Say It with Words.* New York: Knopf.

FISHBEIN, M. (1972). *Medical Writing.* Springfield, Ill.: Chas. C. Thomas.

FLOWER, R. (1984). *Delivery of Speech-Language Pathology and Audiology Services.* Baltimore: William and Wilkins.

GOOD, R. (1970). "The Written Language of Rehabilitation Medicine: Meaning and Usages." *Archives of Physical Medicine and Rehabilitation,* 51: 29–36.

HOLLIS, J., and P. DUNN (1979). *Psychological Report Writing.* Muncie, Ind.: Accelerated Development.

HUBER, J. (1961). *Report Writing in Psychology and Psychiatry*. New York: Harper & Row.

HUTCHINSON, B., M. HANSON, and M. MECHAM (1979). *Diagnostic Handbook of Speech Pathology.* Baltimore: Williams & Wilkins.

JERGER, J. (1962). "Scientific Writing Can Be Readable." *Journal of the American Speech and Hearing Association,* 4: 101–104.

JONES, A., and C. FAULKNER (1971). *Writing Good Prose.* New York: Scribner's.

KELLY, M., A. ROTH, and T. ALTSHULER (1969). *Writing Step by Step.* Boston: Houghton Mifflin.

KENT, L., and S. CHABON (1980). "Problem-Oriented Records in a University Speech and Hearing Clinic." *Journal of the American Speech and Hearing Association,* 22: 151–158.

KNEPFLAR, K. (1976). *Report Writing.* Danville, Ill.: Interstate Printers and Publishers.

LEGGETT, G., C. MEAD, and W. CHARVAT (1974). *Handbook for Writers.* 6th ed. Englewood Cliffs, N.J.: Prentice-Hall, Inc.

MACRORIE, K. (1968). *Writing to Be Read.* Rochelle Park, N.J.: Hayden.

—— (1970). *Uptaught.* Rochelle Park, N.J.: Hayden.

MAYES, J. (1972). *Writing and Rewriting.* New York: Macmillan.

MOORE, M. (1969). "Pathological Writing." *Journal of the American Speech and Hearing Association,* 11: 535–538.

PANNBACKER, M. (1975). "Diagnostic Report Writing." *Journal of Speech and Hearing Disorders,* 40: 367–379.

PETERSON, H., and T. MARQUARDT (1981). *Appraisal and Diagnosis of Speech and Language Disorders.* Englewood Cliffs, N.J.: Prentice-Hall, Inc.

STRUNK, W., and E. B. WHITE (1959). *The Elements of Style.* New York: Macmillan.

SUNBERG, N., and L. TYLER (1962). *Clinical Psychology.* New York: Appleton-Century-Crofts.

TALLENT, N. (1980). *Psychological Report Writing.* Englewood Cliffs, N.J.: Prentice-Hall, Inc.

WUBBEN, J. (1971). *Guided Writing.* New York: Random House.

# APPENDIX A
# LANGUAGE ASSESSMENT INTERVIEW PROTOCOL

**CHILD LANGUAGE ASSESSMENT INTERVIEW PROTOCOL**

GENERAL INFORMATION

Referral source:

Parents' statement of the problem:

History of prior assessments:

History of prior treatments:

Parents' treatment attempts:

Preschool status:

School status:

Number and relationships of people living at home:

Parental occupations:

BIOLOGICAL PREREQUISITES

*Birth and General Health*

Pregnancy:

Birth:

Present physical health:

History of illnesses:

*Auditory Status*

History of frequent colds:

History of earaches and ear infections:

Parents' estimation of hearing acuity:

*Neurological status*

Concussions:

Unconsciousness:

Seizures:

Has the child been seen by a neurologist? For what?

Does the child evidence any motor ability difficulties?

SOCIAL PREREQUISITES

Approximate time spent in social interaction on typical day:

Who are the people the child frequently interacts with?

What are the activities associated with social interactions?

Does the child exhibit any antisocial or socially inappropriate behaviors (avoiding inter-actions, consistent playing alone, and so on)?

Does the child exhibit any self-stimulating behaviors (for example, rocking or arm flapping)?

Does the child maintain eye contact?

Does the child regulate your behavior nonverbally?

Does the child use objects or repeat actions to get your attention?

Does the child vocalize in his social interactions?

Does the child joint reference with caretaker?

Describe the child's typical day in detail:

## COGNITIVE PREREQUISITES

Does the child exhibit play routines and behavior that would indicate the following attainments?

Object permanence:

Means-end:

Immediate imitation:

Functional use of objects:

Deferred imitation:

Symbolic play with surrogate object:

Symbolic play with appropriate object:

What are the child's most frequent play activities?

## LANGUAGE

Does the child exhibit phonetically consistent forms?

Parents' estimation of the number of single words used expressively (follow up on word checklist):

Parents' estimation of MLU:

Reports of presyntactic devices:

Parents' report of semantic relation types:

Parents' estimate of language comprehension:

Parents should provide anecdotal information on the following:

Phonetic inventory:

Phonological processes:

Intonation patterns:

Estimate of intelligibility:

Grammatical morpheme use:

Questions/negatives:

Embedding/conjoining:

# APPENDIX B
# CODING SHEET
# FOR EARLY MULTIWORD
# ANALYSIS

**CODING SHEET FOR EARLY MULTIWORD ANALYSIS**

| CHILD UTTERANCE | SEMANTIC RELATION | FUNCTION | INITATION | POST-STAGE I ELEMENT |
|---|---|---|---|---|
| Push car | Action + object | Regulation | CI | |
| Push it | Action + object | Regulation | CI | |
| Car going | Instrument + action | Comment | CI | -ing |
| More car | Recurrence + X | Regulation | CI | |
| Car allgone? | X + disappearance | Questioning | CI | |
| Juice up there | Entity + locative | Elicited imitation | AI | |
| Gimme juice | Action + object | Regulation | CI | |
| That truck | Nomination + X | Answering | AI | |

# APPENDIX C
# SUMMARY SHEET
# FOR EARLY MULTIWORD
# ANALYSIS

---

**SUMMARY SHEET FOR EARLY MULTIWORD ANALYSIS**

Child: _____ Age: _____ Birth date: _____

Date of sample: _____ Context of sample (include people present): _____

Length of Sample in Time:

Activities Performed During Sample:

Mean length of utterance:

Total number of child utterances:

Longest utterance in morphemes:

Number of single-word responses:

Semantic relations evident in sample:

Functions evident in sample:

Syntactic constituents used most often:

Ratio of child-initiated to adult-initiated utterances:

Post-stage I elements noted:

Semantic relations missing from sample:

Functions missing from sample:

Recommendations for further sampling/treatment:

---

# APPENDIX D
# DATA CONSOLIDATION FOR CHILD LANGUAGE EVALUATION

---

**DATA CONSOLIDATION FOR CHILD LANGUAGE EVALUATION**

IDENTIFYING INFORMATION

Name:                                          Address:

Telephone:                                     Parents:

Date of evaluation:

---

DATA OBTAINED (check and specify)

Case history _____                        Nonstandardized tasks _____

Reports from professionals _____          Cognitive scale _____

Hearing screening _____                   Comprehension test _____

Oral peripheral _____                     Imitation test _____

Behavioral observation of caretaker-           Language battery _____
  child _____

Behavioral observation of child _____     Articulation test _____

Spontaneous language sample _____         Other _____

---

ANALYSES PERFORMED (check and specify)

MLU _____                                 Vocalization analysis _____

Distributional analysis _____             Phonological analysis _____

Syntactic complexity analysis
  package _____

Phonetic inventory _____

Descriptive analysis of syntax _____

Phonological analysis _____

Early multiword analysis of semantic
  relations and functions _____

Caretaker-child interaction
  analysis _____

Sensorimotor performative
  analysis _____

Scoring of Formal Procedures _____

Gross cognitive prerequisite
  analysis _____

Other(s) _____

---

REMARKS ON THE DATA

Remarkable case history information:

Remarkable results from prior reports and tests:

Remarkable interview information:

Behavioral observation results:

Informal testing results:

Formal test results:

SYNTHESIS OF FINDINGS

   A.  *Specific Areas of Interest*
       1.  Prerequisites to communication
          a.  Biological
             1.  Hearing:

             2.  Neurological:

             3.  Medical:

             4.  Anatomical:

          b.  Cognitive
             1.  Approximate Piagetian state attainment and characteristic behaviors. List strengths and weaknesses.

   c. Social
      1. Interpersonal manner (attachment, eye contact, reciprocity, affect, and so on):

      2. Caretaker model of communication:

      3. Nonverbal functions (include protoimperative/declarative):

      4. Evidence of self-stimulation or abuse:

2. Communicative effectiveness:
   a. Nonverbal:

   b. Phonetically consistent forms (PCF):

   c. Single-word utterances (describe):

   d. Presyntactic devices (PSD):

   e. Stage I (Brown, 1973) forms and functions (describe):

   f. Stage II:

   g. Stage III:

   h. Stage IV:

   i. Stage V:

   j. Conversational pragmatics:

   k. Phonetic inventory (describe):

   l. Phonological processes (describe):

   m. Intelligibility:

B. *Areas of Strength and Concern*

Child's age: _____ MLU: _____

Primary language stage: nonverbal   single word   early multiword   syntactic

Mark areas of strength (+) and concern (−):

| | |
|---|---|
| Biological prerequisites _____ | Phonology _____ |
| Cognitive prerequisites _____ | Pragmatics _____ |
| Social prerequisites _____ | Phonetic inventory _____ |
| Delayed language _____ | Parental model/cooperation _____ |
| Deviant language _____ | |

RECOMMENDATIONS

   A.   The child has no language impairment and no referrals are needed:

   B.   Referrals:

   C.   Recommended further testing:

   D.   Prognosis for treatment and treatment suggestions:

   E.   Results of parent counseling and recommendations for further interviews:

# NAME INDEX

# SUBJECT INDEX